The Future
of the Disabled in
Liberal Society

REVISIONS
A Series of Books on Ethics

GENERAL EDITORS
Stanley Hauerwas and Alasdair MacIntyre

The Future
of the Disabled in
Liberal Society

AN ETHICAL ANALYSIS

Hans S. Reinders

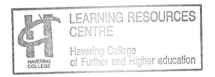

UNIVERSITY OF NOTRE DAME PRESS
Notre Dame, Indiana

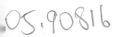

163201

Manufactured in the United States of America

Library of Congress Cataloging-in-Publication Data

Reinders, Hans S.
    The future of the disabled in liberal society : an ethical analysis / Hans S. Reinders.
        p.   cm. — (Revisions)
    Includes bibliographical references and index.
    ISBN 0-268-02856-7 (cloth : alk. paper) — ISBN 0-268-02857-5 (pbk.: alk. paper)
    1. Sociology of disability.   2. Handicapped—Social conditions.   3. Handicapped—
Government policy.   4. Eugenics—Moral and ethical aspects.   I. Title.   II. Series.
HV1568 .R45 2000
305.9'0816—dc21

                                                                    00-029891

Contents

Preface   ix

1. Introduction   1
   1.1 A Paradigmatic Shift   1
   1.2 Widening the Scope of the Debate I   4
   1.3 Widening the Scope of the Debate II   9
   1.4 The Argument   12

PART ONE

2. The 'Liberal Convention'   21
   2.1 The Context of the Debate   21
   2.2 The 'Liberal Convention'   22
   2.3 Implications of Starting with the 'Liberal Convention'   24
   2.4 Morality among Strangers   26
   2.5 Instrumentalism, Formalism, or Conventionalism?   30
   2.6 Beyond a Narrow Conception of Morality   35

3. Genetics and Prevention in Public Morality   37
   3.1 Initial Distinctions   37
   3.2 'Morally Permissible' and 'Morally Required'   39
   3.3 Preventing Conception and Preventing Birth   40
   3.4 'Impairment', 'Disability', and 'Handicap'   42
   3.5 'Disease' and 'Disability'   44
   3.6 'We' as Individuals and 'We' as a Political Community   46
   3.7 Two Questions   49

4. "The Condition, Not the Person"   51
   4.1 The Charge of Negative Evaluation   51
   4.2 The DPC Argument   53

4.3 Actual and Future People   56
4.4 Evaluating Other People's Lives   57
4.5 Disability and Identity   59
4.6 The Fallacy of Geneticization   61
4.7 What Are Clinical Geneticists Doing?   63

5. Disability, Prevention, and Discrimination   66
   5.1 Negative Side Effects?   67
   5.2 Two Types of Reasons   68
   5.3 Discrimination and Exclusion   70
   5.4 Discrimination and the Value of Life   73
   5.5 The Social Position of the Disabled   75
   5.6 The Future of Disability   78
   5.7 No World without Disabled People   81

6. Restrictions on Reproductive Choice?   84
   6.1 'Free Choice' in Human Reproduction   84
   6.2 Restriction of Reproductive Freedom?   86
   6.3 The Charge of Discriminatory Attitudes   91
   6.4 Restrictive Policies against Selective Abortion   94
   6.5 Restrictive Policies to Control Genetic Testing   96
   6.6 Degrees of Seriousness?   99
   6.7 The Weakness of the Liberal Convention   101

PART TWO

7. The Inclusion of the Mentally Disabled   105
   7.1 The Moral Standing of Disabled People   105
   7.2 Persons in the Social Sense   108
   7.3 Justice and Beneficence   109
   7.4 Recipients of Justice   113
   7.5 Public Morality as Overlapping Consensus   116
   7.6 The Parasitic Nature of Liberal Morality   118

8. Imperatives of the Self   122
   8.1 Two Claims   122
   8.2 Kenzaburo Oë: A Personal Matter   125
   8.3 An Inward Voyage   127
   8.4 Himiko's Theory   130
   8.5 Constancy and Truthfulness   132
   8.6 Accountability as Self-Narration   135

9. Responsibility for Dependent Others   139
    9.1 On Accepting Responsibility   139
    9.2 'The Ethical Demand'   142
    9.3 Social Norms and Moral Judgment   143
    9.4 'Life as a Gift'   146
    9.5 Convention and Commitment   148
    9.6 Appropriate Motivations   153

PART THREE

10. The Presumption of Suffering   159
    10.1 A Remaining Question   159
    10.2 Reasons Regarding Quality of Life   162
    10.3 Ways of Suffering   164
    10.4 Enrichment? In What Way?   166
    10.5 Identification, Not Resignation   171

11. The Transformation Experience   175
    11.1 Incoherent Views?   176
    11.2 Two Different Perspectives   177
    11.3 A Capacity for Alienation   180
    11.4 "From Devastation to Transformation"   183
    11.5 Transformation and the Power to Respond   187

12. The Meaning of Life in Liberal Society   193
    12.1 Discovered or Made?   193
    12.2 Some Conceptual Clarifications   194
    12.3 Bricoleurs Rather Than Engineers   197
    12.4 Culture as a 'Context of Choice'   198
    12.5 The Redundancy of Choice   200
    12.6 Caring for the Disabled in Liberal Society   203
    12.7 Conclusion   206

Notes   209
Bibliography   259
Index   271

Preface

In 1996 the Dutch Association of Bioethics invited me to write an essay on the ethical implications of human genetics and its possible impact on persons with mental disability, to be discussed at its annual conference that same year. The question put before me was "Should we prevent disabled lives?" It was a timely moment for a discussion of this question, given the extensive debate a few months earlier in the national media in The Netherlands on the moral issue of 'selective' abortion.

A case had been widely publicized of a couple who decided to have a pregnancy terminated because their future child would have suffered from *retinitis pigmentosa,* a genetic disease that causes severe visual impairment or complete blindness at an early age. The focus of the debate in this particular case was whether using genetic testing for reasons of preventing a disabled life implies a negative evaluation of the lives of handicapped people. This issue of negative evaluation was relatively new. The most prominent issues in the bioethical literature thus far raised questions about the rights and duties of 'primary agents' (researchers, doctors, patients, insurance companies, and employers), agents who use genetic information because they are interested in risk assessment with regard to health. Dominant themes were the issues of 'eugenics' (the question of whether people may use genetic information for reasons of enhancing certain desired features in their offspring), of 'privacy' (the question to what extent doctors must respect the private lives of their patients' families in case they diagnose a genetic disorder), of 'non-directivity' (the question of whether genetic counseling ought to be guided by particular values about responsible reproductive choices), of "the right not to know" (the question of whether people at risk of genetically affected offspring should seek information about possible future risk for their children), and of "the right to health care provisions" (the question of whether health insurance premiums may be adjusted for the carriers of genetic disorders).

Much less attention has been paid to a different kind of question, namely, how genetic testing affects our views of people whose lives may be indirectly implicated, i.e., whether genetic testing implies a negative evaluation of the lives of disabled people. Apparently, the general opinion was that there is not much to be discussed here. Who would like to be disabled anyway? One can only speculate about reasons for the absence of serious discussion of this question, but the influence of 'free choice' would be an important factor, together with popular views on the burden of living a disabled life. Whenever the disabled appear in the bioethical literature, their existence appears as part of what seems to be the problem.

Having worked for a number of years in the area of ethics and *mental* disability—which is the primary concern of the present book—I took the invitation of the Dutch Association of Bioethics to be an acknowledgment of shifting interests. As a matter of fact, for me, moving into that largely unexplored area meant moving out of the field of bioethics as it has been understood over the last thirty years. The medical paradigm that dominated the bioethical agenda not only renders the existence of disabled people intrinsically problematic, it turns to 'prevention' as the obvious solution to the problem. It is this obviousness that I wanted to question. In looking at the issue of genetics and prevention from the perspective of the mentally disabled, I seek to press a different set of questions, for example, to what extent mentally disabled are threatened by conceptions of the human good that turn their existence into a 'problem', or whether genetic testing paves the way for a form of biological perfectionism that is dangerous to people whose bodies are deemed imperfect. To raise such questions, I believe, is in itself an important contribution to public debate.

The present text has many subtexts, however, not unlike other texts on ethics, be they philosophical or theological. One subtext is the continuing debate concerning the strengths and weaknesses of liberal morality that dominates contemporary society. Another subtext, closely related to this one, is the debate about how moral argument in the public sphere relates to conceptions of the human good. Both of these subtexts determine the construction of the main argument as well as the composition of the book. The main argument is that people with mental disability and their families have reasons to be worried about their future in liberal society. The rapid proliferation of genetic testing may have discriminatory effects, I will argue, because it brings the birth of disabled children within the focus of 'reproductive choice', which makes their parents answerable to the charge of 'irresponsible behavior'.

Although liberal democracy is often and widely applauded for its stance against discrimination, its options for protecting disabled citizens against the possibly discriminatory effects of medical genetics will appear surprisingly weak. If anything, adequate moral support for disabled persons will depend on a particular kind of moral life rather than on public policies installed by liberal democracy. That is to say, the democratic state will be able to sustain adequate support for the disabled and their families to the extent that its citizens are the kind of people who are prepared to share their lives with them and who have the character and skill to do so.

Popular culture sends the message that life is more worth living the less trouble it takes. Only people who know this myth to be utterly distortive of human life will be capable of accepting lives with limited capacities as valuable and worthwhile in their own right. If true, this suggests that the extent to which disabled people may expect solidarity and support depends on a different conception of the human good *and* on the moral character necessary in order to live such a conception. To have a conception of the good is one thing. To be capable of living it is quite another. Liberal democracy can be a powerful instrument in the protection of vulnerable people, such as the mentally disabled necessarily are, but only insofar as its citizens live from moral sources other than the narrow conceptions of public morality on which it is based.

With regard to the composition of the book, it may be helpful to add a few remarks. In the first chapters the focus is largely on framing the issues within the domain of public morality as it is currently understood in liberal society. The discussion is aimed at questions regarding negative evaluations of disabled lives and their potentially discriminatory effects. But on a different level, the objective is to push the framework of liberal morality to its limits, in order to suggest that the debate needs to be expanded so as to include questions beyond the scope of the narrow conception of morality that currently dominates much of the bioethical literature. We desperately need to tap other moral sources in order to discuss the more profound issues that mentally disabled children confront us with. The strategy to expand the debate on genetics and prevention is a strategy against this narrow conception. Given the political context within which the moral debate on genetics and prevention evolves, expanding or reducing its scope will have its effects upon mechanisms of inclusion and exclusion. To think about disabled lives primarily as possible sources of meaning, rather than as the cause of deficit, is an attempt to make that scope as wide as possible in order to include disabled people as full members into our moral community.

The original essay for the Dutch Society of Bioethics has been elaborated and expanded considerably. Included in the text are a few unpublished texts and some texts that have not been published in English before. Also a couple of new chapters were added. Consequently, the present text comprises work over the last four years during which there have been many occasions to discuss parts of it with colleagues and friends both at home and abroad. Apart from the discussion in the Dutch Society of Bioethics, the original essay has received stimulating comments from my colleagues in The Netherlands, Paul van Tongeren (Catholic University of Nijmegen) and Marjan Verkerk (Erasmus University of

Rotterdam). In an early stage of the project some of the material was presented as a paper at the Kennedy Institute of Ethics at Georgetown University, on which occasion I received helpful comments from John Langan, Tom Beauchamp, and Bob Veatch. During my sabbatical year at the University of Notre Dame, I had the opportunity to converse with Alasdair MacIntyre on the implications of moral identity for one's ability to live one's moral convictions, which took shape in chapter 9. Conversations in the "ethics reading group" that same year with David Solomon, Paul Weithman, and Jim Sterba, among others, provided a great source of inspiration. I am particularly indebted to Kees van Kooten Niekerk from the University of Aarhus in Denmark, who was of great help with his comments on my use of ideas developed by the Danish philosopher Knut Eljert Løgstrup. The last chapter, on the meaning of life in liberal society, has benefited from discussions in the Institute of Ethics at my own university and the Research School of Ethics in The Netherlands. I am indebted to Rene van Woudenberg, Wessel Stoker, Henry Jansen, and Sander Griffioen for helpful comments. Jan Bransen of Utrecht University was a critical but stimulating reader who pointed out several ambiguities and mistakes. The same holds for Gijs van Oenen from Erasmus University, Rotterdam, and Brenda Almond from the University of Hull. Last but not least, I am particularly grateful to Professor MacIntyre and Professor Hauerwas for their comments on earlier versions of the manuscript.

Although critical readers and commentators are vital to any author, there is a yet more important contribution, which is that of academic friendship. It is from our friends that we receive support at times when we are only beginning to sense what it is that we want to say about our subject. For this book I have received this kind of invaluable support most of all from Reinhard Hütter from the Lutheran School of Theology at Chicago, whose patience in enduring my laborious reports of "work in progress" has been angelic; from David Solomon, University of Notre Dame, who continues to remind me that a theologian who tries to write philosophy need not try to become a philosopher; and from Stanley Hauerwas, Duke University, who in many ways has deeply influenced my thoughts about ethics and disability and who has been a constant source of encouragement in the writing of this book. I am indebted to my colleague Henry Jansen, who took the trouble of trying to improve my use of the English language. Needless to say, the remaining mistakes are entirely my own responsibility.

ONE

Introduction

> It takes considerable rhetorical agility to urge the public to support
> screening programs so as to prevent the conception of handicapped in-
> dividuals while at the same time insisting that full respect be paid to
> such developmentally disabled adults as are already among us.
>
> *Daniel Wikler*

1.1 A Paradigmatic Shift

Public debate on human genetics has been largely shaped by the question of
what this new technology has to offer with regard to genetic diseases. The apparent assumption behind this question is that to be burdened with a genetic
disease is to be burdened with a life that one would rather avoid. Accordingly
the medical uses of gene technology are perceived in the context of helping
people avoid a cause of serious suffering in their lives. This perception is emphatically expressed in the following quote from Dr. Francis S. Collins, Director
of the National Center for Human Genome Research in the United States:

> The mandate to alleviate human suffering is one of the most compelling of all
> expectations of humanity. . . . When genetics is seen to fall into that larger man-
> date, it is hard to argue with its potential goodness. In fact, given that potential,
> it can be argued that the most unethical approach of all would be to insist that
> genetic research be stopped; because if it were, those individuals, present and
> future, who suffer from the ravages of genetic diseases would be doomed to
> hopelessness.[1]

The centrality of the notion of genetic disease indicates that the ethical debate on genetics has evolved within a medical paradigm. The main issues have
been shaped by the question of what doctors can do and should be allowed to

do for their patients. Within this paradigm, the lives of people who are affected by genetic disorders cannot but appear in a negative light. Their 'quality of life' is tainted by a 'defect'. Given this medically inspired attitude, developing new methods for detecting genetic disorders is often presented as a way of enhancing the possibility of reproductive choice. Whereas people in previous times had to live with genetic disease as imposed upon them by fate, they now have the chance to prevent such an ordeal. Public response to the new technology has been driven primarily by the fact that people who are at risk of having a child affected by genetic disorder can now ask, "Is there anything we can do to prevent this?" That this question can be raised is due only to the option of genetic screening and counseling that is now available. Prevention is therefore one of the more important—if not the most important—goals for further technological development that provides people at risk with new hope.[2]

In this inquiry I will raise moral questions regarding this goal from the perspective of disabled people, particularly mentally disabled people. Since the early seventies, people within the disability community have grown very critical of the dominant medical approach. Many of them discovered that their lives changed significantly once they began to look upon themselves as human beings with their own gifts and potential. Many of them did succeed—often after a difficult struggle with the helping professions—in shedding the negative identity that comes with the image of inability and neediness. More often than not professionals adhered to the medical paradigm and its preoccupation with bodily disfunction, to the effect that the disabled person was seen primarily as someone with a problem, a 'case' to be treated. Much of this has changed because the medical paradigm has been replaced by a new paradigm in which the approach to disability has been shifted from 'defect' to 'potential'. This new approach is now firmly established as the paradigm of 'normalization'.[3] People with disabilities are approached as potential participants in social life if only given the chance to do so.[4]

Under the inspiration of this new paradigm, the strategies that have been developed for enhancing opportunities have transformed social services and caring institutions beyond recognition in many countries.[5] The question to be addressed here is what this new paradigm implies for ethical reflection on questions regarding the use of genetic information for prevention of disability. If normalization policy aims at equal respect for the disabled in society, and if legal standards are established to enhance their opportunities to participate, why is using gene technology for preventing mentally disabled lives generally accepted as a matter of course? If the assumptions of normalization policy are valid, to the effect that the disabled are to be accepted as our equals, why does our society think that preventing their existence is the rational thing to do?

In looking at the development of gene technology from the perspective of normalization, one need not deny that genetic disorders may cause specific medical problems that demand to be treated, nor need one deny that disabled lives have more than average limitations. As people from the disability community are apt to point out, however, there are many other stories to be told about disabled people besides the medical ones. Many of these people reject the suggestion that either they or their relatives are living deplorable lives that would better not have been brought into existence. Whether the cause of their disabling condition is called a genetic 'defect' or not, they do not think of their lives as such as being defective. Rather, they view their lives as valuable because of what they are capable of doing, just like anybody else. From their point of view, the goal of prevention is obviously informed by social and cultural images that enter into negative perceptions of 'disability'.

Although people in the medical world can justifiably claim the moral intention of combatting disease, it is this very claim that confirms, in a sense, that of which they are accused by the opponents of the genetics approach to disability. In conceiving disability primarily from a medical perspective, people tend to ignore its social and political dimensions. Persons with disabilities are not simply the victims of nature, but they are also often victims of a lack of opportunities in life. In ignoring the wider social and economic dimensions, the medical perspective fails to do justice to the daily experiences of disabled people and their families. The question of whether a genetic disorder causes a disability depends as much on how our society responds as it does on biological conditions.

To draw attention to this causal connection, the World Health Organization has adopted a definition of disability that focuses on the relation between individual capacities and sociocultural environment.[6] Being deaf limits one's possibilities of communication only in an environment within which no one has learned how to use sign language. If one is unable to walk due to a condition of permanent paralysis, one is still able to go anywhere by wheelchair, provided that one's environment is designed in such a way as to be accessible for persons in wheelchairs. There is no need for people in wheelchairs to be lacking in self-respect unless others treat them in a condescending way. Likewise, many people with mental disabilities are capable of learning if society would only provide them with adequate forms of education.[7] Given the relevance of these wider dimensions for understanding the daily experiences of disabled people, we should oppose, it is said, any approach that defines the lives of disabled persons primarily in terms of medical problems and makes their lives appear as dependent upon how much help the medical profession can provide.[8]

Curiously enough we find ourselves confronted by two different worlds with respect to disability. One is the world of normalization, which depicts disabled people as people not unlike ourselves, people who have been wronged by their unnecessary exile from ordinary life and who, therefore, deserve our support. The other world is the world of prevention, which depicts living with a disability as a fate that can be worse than death and offers a rationale for justifying the practices of selective abortion and infanticide in the case of severely disabled children. In this other world, the world of modern medicine, preventing such a child from being born often appears as the only rational thing to do. Within these two contrasting worlds people find themselves confronted by different questions. In the world of medicine they face the question of whether they run the risk of having a disabled child, a question that only members of the medical profession can answer. In the world of normalization they find themselves facing the task of sharing their lives with their disabled child and doing the best they can. With regard to this state of affairs, it appears as though our society is simultaneously sending two messages to the disabled and their families.[9] The first message says, "Since you're here, we're going to care for you as best we can," but the second says, "But everyone would be better off if you were not here at all."[10] While officially these messages remain separated, many people within the disability community are troubled by the relation between them.

1.2 Widening the Scope of the Debate I

As indicated, my intention in this book is to think about the ethics of the prevention of disability by following the shift from the medical to the normalization paradigm. The policies and strategies developed within this new paradigm are concerned with providing disabled people with opportunities to participate in society just like other people. In that sense 'normalization' appears to be at odds with the suggestion of defective human lives within the medical paradigm. Even though it can be argued that medical practices such as clinical genetics seek to enhance the well-being of patients, it is very well possible that they contribute to side effects for disabled people and their families in other domains of social life. This possibility is grounded in the fact that these practices reflect and probably reinforce particular beliefs and attitudes towards handicap and disability in society. The International League of Societies for Persons with Mental Handicaps (ILSPMH) has expressed this concern as follows:

> Language as 'defect', 'abnormality' and 'congenital malformation' is sometimes used to describe fetuses in which a disability has been detected. This frames disability in the context of individual pathology, rather than in a social context. With renewed ideological acceptance of the medical model and the emerging genetic model of disability, there is a danger that efforts and resources that should

be directed to removing handicapping barriers in society could be diverted into genetic research.[11]

Inasmuch as the genetics approach to disability reflects the notion of defective lives that can be prevented from coming into existence, the League claims, it can influence people's perceptions of priorities in public policy. Hence the question of how the proliferation of genetic testing will affect disabled people with respect to, for example, their access to social services, education, health care, and the labor market. Raising this issue requires that we widen the scope of the ethical debate on genetics and ask how it may affect our views on social and political issues regarding disabled people outside the medical domain.

It has been reported, in this connection, that philosophical publications on the topic of disabilities or handicaps in the 1970s and 80s showed that over 75 percent were concerned with the issues of euthanasia and so called 'non-treatment decisions'.[12] The prevailing philosophical concern in those days seemed to be whether or not it is permissible to kill or let die a genetically affected fetus or neonate. Occasionally one encountered allusions as to the possibility that in the long run the genetics approach to disability may undermine the social position of disabled persons in our society.[13] But only recently has a wider scope to the debate on human genetics begun to emerge in which different moral concerns are expressed.[14] As has been noticed more than once, however, scientists do not appear to be very keen on including wider issues of public policy in the debate on genetic research. For example, the editors of *Nature*, the leading British journal of science, reflecting on the recent report on the cloning of sheep, argued that

> the growing power of molecular genetics confronts us with future prospects of being able to change the nature of our species is a fact that seldom appears to be addressed in depth. Scientific knowledge may not yet permit detailed understanding, but the possiblities are clear enough. This gives rise to issues that in the end will have to be related to people within the social and ethical environments in which they live.[15]

This recognition that science interacts with and operates within a cultural context that mediates the social and moral implications of its results is exactly what causes worries of the kind that are expressed by the ILSPMH. No doubt, the intentions of many people involved in genetic research are to serve patients as best they can, but that does not diminish the importance of questioning the social and political impact of their practices.

One explanation for the lack of serious attention to possible side effects in the long run may be the fact that in matters of extrapolations about possible future dangers we have little or no empirical evidence to go on. At least this is how Lee Silver, professor in molecular biology at Princeton University, explains this fact in *Remaking Eden:*

> As the technologies of reproduction and genetics have become ever more powerful over the last decade, most practicing scientists and physicians have been loathe to speculate about where it may all lead. One reason for reluctance is the fear of getting it wrong. It really is impossible to predict with certainty which future technological advances will proceed on time and which will encounter unexpected roadblocks.[16]

Reluctance because of the fear of 'getting it wrong' may be one explanation but there is more. Particularly in the earlier days, the phrase 'wild speculation' often was used against the suggestion that the emerging technologies generated reasons for moral concern about their social and cultural effects in the long run. According to Silver, scientists prefer to abstain from discussing such wider issues because of their reluctance to become involved in 'politics'.[17] Publicly authorized procedures of control are seen as interfering with the scientific process. The attitude characteristically resulting from such interference is one of frustration. Scientists seem to believe that all too often their work is hindered by a zeal for public control that is more often than not inspired by ignorance.

An instructive example of this attitude can be found in a recent collection of essays by leading scholars in the field of molecular biology and genetics called *Genetics and Society.* In the opening essay of this collection Dr. Robert Pritchard, professor of genetics at the University of Leicester, claims that the responsibility for developments in human genetics should be in the hands of those who are directly involved: "Obviously knowledge can be exploited in undesirable ways, and its application may have unexpected and deleterious side-effects. Yet, on any scale of rational values, the record surely shows that the balance has been overwhelmingly positive, and that there is an immeasurably greater problem—that of ignorance" (*Genetics and Society,* 3).[18] The greatest difficulty, according to Pritchard, is not the exploitation of knowledge in undesirable ways but the creation of barriers to the expansion of knowledge by the ignorant.[19] Medical doctors and their patients should be credited for knowing how to use scientific knowledge in a socially responsible way. People learn to control the risks and to behave responsibly when they know that they will be held personally accountable. In the field of human genetics and its medical uses, this means that the control of risks should be the responsibility of doctors and their patients. Interference generated by public concern is in Pritchard's view anything but helpful: "All my experience suggests that, if people are given responsibility and equipped with the knowledge to enable them to make informed decisions, most will behave responsibly. They will certainly behave as responsibly as those who think it their job to determine what others should think and do because they are too frail and too selfish to do so for themselves" (*Genetics and Society,* 11). Pritchard clearly favors individual freedom and responsibility as the overriding moral concern in thinking about the use of gene technology in a medical context. If one accepts that decisions are best left to those who are directly involved, the central moral issue becomes that of making sure that they are given the freedom to do so. This requires the public space of a permissive and participatory society.[20]

Given the emphasis on individual freedom and responsibility, extensive debate on the direction in which our society should go is of little use or purpose because this question is decided by the choices made by individuals. Public responsibility regarding this question extends no further than the task to safeguard 'free choice'. In this sense Pritchard's view reflects a deep-seated democratic impulse, namely the tendency to believe not only that people are entitled to make decisions regarding their own lives, but also that only they know what is best for them and that they will behave responsibly in making these decisions.[21]

As we will see, however, the argument for individual freedom in the area of human genetics and reproduction creates an awkward problem for public policy. If there are serious reasons to think that the new technology will have deleterious side effects on the lives of disabled people and their families, then it is a question of public responsibility how to control these effects. In that case we can no longer afford to ignore a potential conflict between opposing moral interests, which implies that the scope of the debate must be widened as to include questions about the cultural, social, and political effects of gene technology beyond the domain of medicine.

In her own contribution to *Genetics and Society,* Baroness Mary Warnock rejects this suggestion by taking a position that is comparable to Pritchard's. She contends that individual treatment of genetic disease should not be linked to issues regarding the common good:

> We need not raise questions about the future of society as a whole. For the life of an individual (and thus, of course, in the long run, and indirectly, the life of society at large) would be infinitely better if that individual did not suffer from that disease. . . . in the case of individual gene therapy, there is simply no need to raise this kind of problem. We have to think how best to alleviate individual human suffering. (*Genetics and Society,* 112)

The problem with this claim is that, obviously, the Baroness takes a position on the very question that she wants to lay at rest. Whether our society should give priority to the alleviation of individual suffering over its socio-cultural and economic side effects is itself a question about what is best for society as a whole. If there are reasons to think that this medical focus on alleviating individual suffering may have deleterious effects for certain people in the long run outside the domain of medicine, as I will suggest,[21] then our society cannot afford to ignore questions as to where it should go with regard to controlling the use of the new technology. But at the same time, to justify public control in this area will be difficult without questioning the decisions that individual providers and their clients make. More specifically, to justify the protection of some people against the side effects of other people's choices will be problematic with respect to the freedom to make these choices.

Against this suggestion it may be argued, however, that there is no need for ethical reflection on the use of genetics from the perspective of disabled people because the two worlds that were spoken of in the previous section exist alongside one another without causing any conflict. The world of clinical genetics is driven by a concern for 'future people', whereas, in contrast, concerns about the normalization of disabled lives in contemporary society are about 'actual people'. While the latter are already members of our society, the former are people who do not yet exist and who—if preventive strategies work as they should—never will exist. Couples who are at risk of having a genetically affected child worry about the future of such a child as well as about their own lives with that child. In the event that they decide not to have that child, they are not in any way judging the lives of disabled people. Neither are they in any way implying that society has no responsibility to provide disabled people with equal opportunities. Given the distinction between 'actual' and 'future people', so the objection concludes, there is no conflict between the moral concerns about disability expressed within the medical paradigm, on the one hand, and the normalization paradigm, on the other, because the lives of existing people with disabilities are not at all implicated in strategies of prevention.

In my view this objection is mistaken for a number of reasons. Extensive argument is required to show why this is so, but at this introductory stage only a few remarks can be offered to indicate how the argument might run. Decisions to use prenatal diagnosis and selective abortion for reasons of prevention can be morally justified, of course, by arguing that in making such decisions people are simply exercising their individual liberties to make decisions regarding their own offspring. This justification ignores the question of the grounds on which these decisions are made. In pursuing this question, one will inevitably find that at some point or other images of disabled lives play a crucial role. In any given case, the only reasonable answer to the question of why a disabled child should not be born is by reference to what one thinks about the lives of people actually living with the same disorder. Obviously one can say that, regardless of what the reason for their decision may be, people are entitled to their own judgment on these matters. One can even go so far as to say that in exercising this right people are not required to give any reason for their decisions at all. Granted all that, it is nonetheless true that *if* someone were to give a reason intended to justify the decision, this could not be done independently from an evaluative judgment on the prospect of sharing one's life with a disabled child. One may certainly refrain from making this judgment explicit, but the evaluation as such must be implicit in one's reasoning. This suggests that the lives of existing people with disabilities are at least indirectly implicated in strategies of prevention, because without such evaluations these strategies could not make sense.

1.3 Widening the Scope of the Debate II

There is yet another sense in which widening the scope of the debate on ethics and the prevention of disability will prove to be unavoidable. This has not so much to do with moral concerns regarding other people besides the providers and users of genetic services. Instead it has to do with bringing a particular kind of moral conviction and belief to the debate. Let me quote once more from the document on genetics by the ILSPMH:

> Modern scientific practices such as selection by prevention cannot help but be informed by paradigms about disability and the human ideal. Certain commonly held assumptions put people with disabilities at risk in relation to genetic and reproductive technology. These include such questionable assumptions as: people with disabilities suffer because of their disability; human value is judged according to intellectual or physical qualities of the individual; the human race can and should be improved; and we need only consider genetic factors to comprehend human difference. If the application of genetic research is driven by these sorts of spurious assumptions, the lives and rights of people with disabilities may be at risk. (*Just Technology?*, 7)

As appears from this claim, the scientific practices in question are guided by a set of assumptions that exceed the realm of scientific knowledge, for example, assumptions regarding the relation between disability and suffering as well as the different value attached to specific human qualities. In philosophical terms these assumptions can be characterized as assumptions concerning the good life for human beings. Moral questions about genetics and its uses in medicine are not only about dealing with deplorable health conditions arising from natural accidents. Neither are they only about combating human suffering, nor about the right to decide for oneself in critical situations. Lurking behind these questions is a more profound moral issue, namely, the question of what it means to live a human life with physical or mental limitations, or both.[23] All of us hold certain views about what makes our lives worthwhile and it is on the grounds of these views that we come to evaluate the meaning of disability. Since such views are part of our general perspective on the nature and value of human life, it will be unavoidable to discuss the presuppostions underlying genetic research in terms of these general perspectives.

Obviously, given the success of modern medicine in prolonging our lives we cannot evade the question of what it means to live our lives with limited physical and/or mental capabilities.[24] The nature of our bodily existence and the changes affecting it over time is such that all of us will be confronted, in one way or another, with such limitations. Without an answer to the question of what it means to live a human life with limited capabilities, it would be difficult to make sense of the genetics approach toward disability in the first place. However, extensive discussions of this question are virtually absent from the bioethical literature, including the literature that deals with human genetics. Generally speaking, there is a strong tendency in this literature to discuss moral issues regarding the prevention of disability in terms of individual rights and responsibilities. The reason for this tendency can only be surmised, but there are at least two possible explanations at hand.[25]

One is that bioethics in general since its revival in the 1950s has taken on the role of an emancipatory movement with a strong commitment to patient autonomy against the growing impact of medical decisionmaking.[26] Consequently, the emphasis has mainly been on the interaction between doctors and their patients within the institutionalized forms of medicine that modern society has come to know in the last decades.[27] This main interest in discussing the rights and duties of the providers and users of health-care services explains the limited interests in deeper philosophical issues. To put it somewhat crudely, if the aim is to create a moral space for patients within which they have the right to make their own decisions, then there is little patience for questioning both the reasons on which their decisions are based and the social and cultural contexts that generate these reasons.[28] As a result, there has been a remarkable shift in the ethics of health care professionals in the direction of respecting their patients' rights to make decisions according to their own conceptions of the good.[29]

The second explanation is that ethics in general has been strongly preoccupied in recent decades with the fact of 'moral diversity'. People in our society, it is commonly accepted, disagree with one another when it comes to their general perspectives on life, so that little progress can be made in ethical debate unless the scope of that debate can be limited to issues of public morality. Given moral diversity, the suggestion of grounding ethical reflection on the convictions and beliefs of particular people is a bad idea because it favors one particular moral perspective over other perspectives. Hence the philosophical project of laying out the rules and principles of a moral discourse that is genuinely 'public' in the sense of arguing on the basis of moral considerations that can be shared by all participants. This project has generated a 'minimalist' approach to ethics and to ethical theorizing that is known under various names, such as 'the exclusion of ideals', 'the method of avoidance', and 'the priority of the right'. These designations point to a particular characteristic of the minimalist approach, which is to avoid any appeal to substantial convictions and beliefs regarding the good life for human beings. If moral discourse in our society is to be guided by reason rather than force, then the scope of convictions and beliefs with which it operates should be as narrow as possible.

This objection to widening the scope of moral debate as to include considerations regarding the good life reflects an important distinction in contemporary moral philosophy between two conceptions of morality. There are different ways of identifying these two conceptions depending on the particular aspect that one wants to discuss. One way is to speak of a 'narrow' as distinct from a 'wide' conception of morality.[30] This distinction focuses on morality's object. According to a narrow conception, the object of morality is secure social cooperation among individuals who are not sufficiently well disposed toward one another to make cooperation between them a matter of course.[31] On this view, the major task for thinking about morality is to specify moral rules and principles that will guide social cooperation and conflict in ways that are justifiable in the eyes of all who are concerned. These rules are social rules, and the conception of morality that they specify is concerned with social morality. A wide conception of morality, in contrast, is concerned with the question of the good life for human beings. Morality, on this view, necessarily proceeds on the basis of general philosophical or religious perspectives on the nature and meaning of human life because the structure of our moral lives is thoroughly teleological. In being directed towards the good, the object of morality in the wide sense is the perfection of human beings *qua* human beings.[32]

If ethical reflection is committed to a narrow conception of morality, as has been the case for most of contemporary bioethics, any plea for widening its scope will be met with suspicion.[33] In order to widen its scope, in the sense described here, one must proceed from a particular philosophical or religious perspective on fundamental questions regarding the good, which creates problems for the possibility of public justification. In connection with our topic—the ethics of the prevention of disability—questions on what it means to live one's life with a disability are better avoided, on the minimalist view, because such questions cannot be addressed without appeal to particular moral convictions and beliefs. The fact that there is little to be found on these questions in the bioethical literature that starts with the problem of moral diversity should not come as a surprise, therefore.

Given this narrow conception of morality, my suggestion to reflect on the prevention of disability from the perspective of the mentally disabled and their families must appear as questionable. The reason is that these people have their own set of values based upon their particular convictions and beliefs about living a disabled life. Whatever these convictions and beliefs may be, they will certainly not be acceptable to all the participants in the debate. Even when it is conceded that we certainly should take seriously the experience of disabled people in our society, it does not follow that we should adopt the convictions and beliefs of these particular people as a normative framework for the debate, because it represents only one way of understanding these experiences. On the contrary, the argument may go, the fact of moral diversity requires that we try to disengage ourselves from any particular perspective in order to conduct our discussion as a genuinely public debate.

It is important to see the political implication of the issue between both conceptions of morality: narrowing or widening the scope of the ethical debate has direct implications for excluding or including particular moral concerns of particular people. No doubt, the more pragmatic route with respect to actual policy decisions—given the fact of pluralism—is to avoid potentially divisive questions as much as possible. However, to exclude such questions from the agenda is to exclude the people whose moral interests are implicated in those questions. In that sense, widening or narrowing the scope of the debate is inevitably a political act. To discuss the issues of genetics and the prevention of disability only in terms of the interaction between 'providers' and their 'clients', as suggested by Professor Pritchard and Baroness Warnock, is to exclude the perspective of disabled people whose lives are indirectly implicated in this discussion. Having said this, let me respond to the objections against widening the scope of the debate by laying out the general argument of this inquiry.

1.4 The Argument

The issue of how the use of genetics for reasons of prevention may affect the lives of disabled people—which is the issue of side effects—is an intricate one: not only because it brings two worlds in opposition that are usually regarded as existing separately without any apparent conflict between them,[34] but also because in raising this issue we stumble on implicit assumptions that invoke deeper philosophical questions about suffering, about normality and abnormality, as well as about human perfection and the meaning of life. On top of this comes the fact, noted above, that moral discourse in our society tends to refrain from raising such questions insofar as it intends to be public discourse. Furthermore, since the issue of side effects concerns responsibility for disabled people in society outside the domain of medicine, it inevitably leads towards questions about public policy. Consequently, in bringing this issue to the attention of society, we should be prepared to discuss it in terms of public discourse. If I am right that in discussing it we cannot avoid the deeper philosophical questions, then our discussion will include a debate on convictions and beliefs that presumably exceed what can be publicly justified.

To deal with this intricacy, we need some sort of account of public discourse in our society in order to see where its moral resources can take us in the reflection on the prevention of disability. Like any other debate, the debate on genetics does not proceed in a moral vacuum but uses the moral resources that are available to respond to the issue at stake. With regard to our society the moral sources of public debate are predominantly regarded as 'liberal', but it is not at all clear what that notion entails. The problem appears to be that the concept of liberal morality belongs to so called 'essentially contestable concepts', which are characterized by the fact that there is no fixed order of priority with regard to the necessary and sufficient conditions for their correct application.[35] So, in order to identify the moral convictions and beliefs that can be appealed to in a public debate on the ethics of prevention, we have to specify some of the core elements characterizing the use of 'liberal' that is pertinent to this inquiry. I suggest that the following account covers a wide variety of interpretations, even though many interpreters will insist on a more nuanced account with regard to certain aspects or details.

Public debate in liberal society evolves on the basis of convictions and beliefs centering upon the values of freedom and equality for individuals. Various liberal interpretations of public morality notwithstanding—'egalitarian', 'libertarian', 'communitarian', 'republican'—the crucial importance assigned to the values of freedom and equality is what qualifies them as liberal. Public morality in the liberal view does not provide people with a conception of the good life, religious or otherwise, by the light of which they conduct their personal lives, but confines itself to specifying the conditions that enable individuals to acquire such a conception and live according to its precepts.[36]

Obviously, the practical implications of these liberal values have to be specified with regard to any given practical problem, but as such these values generate the core elements of public moral discourse in liberal society. Given the inevitability of social conflict, the values of freedom and equality—on virtually any interpretation—will support a distinction between the 'private' and the 'public'. These two spheres of social life separate between on the one hand, what can be left to individuals to decide for themselves with regard to their own lives, and on the other, what must be a matter of public concern because it affects the lives of some or all of them. On this account of liberal morality, other values of public morality such as, for example, self-determination, equity, or justice have no independent standing but are ultimately justified on the basis of (some interpretation of) freedom and equality. Consequently, public justification in liberal society proceeds on the basis of the recognition that individuals are free to live their own lives as they prefer, provided that they allow other people equal freedom to do the same, and provided that they accept and receive a fair share in the burdens and benefits of the social cooperation. Within this normative framework moral discourse in liberal society seeks to resolve any issue that invokes the question of public responsibility. Surely there are more demanding moral values such as, for example, the values of benevolence and generosity that are conducive to a civilized and flourishing society, but they are not necessary for the possibility of public justification. Even if people are not sufficiently well disposed to be concerned with the well-being of others, they may still be expected to accept—as all reasonable persons should—that these others are treated with equal concern and respect. This account of liberal morality represents by and large the narrow conception of social morality that informs much of the debate on health care-issues as they are understood in the literature of contemporary bioethics.[37]

If we approach the issue of possible side effects of genetic testing for reasons of prevention within this normative framework, we will find that it presents itself as an issue about genetic discrimination. On any interpretation, discrimination has to do with treating people unequally without regard for their capacities as moral agents. People are discriminated against when they are treated for what they are—female, black, Jew—rather than for what they do. To raise the issue of side effects of genetic testing from the perspective of the disabled is to raise the issue of whether it may result in unequal treatment of these people for reasons of their being disabled. Two questions arise. Can the position of disabled people in society be affected in such a way that public policy may be called upon to protect them on the grounds of equal concern and respect? If so, what kind of protection can be implemented that is justifiable from a liberal point of view in the sense explained?

To answer the first question, a number of empirical assumptions must be made with regard to future developments. The strongest possible argument for the claim that discriminatory side effects may undermine the position of disabled people in society proceeds from the following speculations. Assuming that disabled people will always be among us, that the proliferation of genetic testing will strengthen the perception that the prevention of disability is a matter of responsible reproductive behavior, and that society is therefore entitled to hold people personally responsible for having a disabled child, it is not unlikely that political support for the provision of their special needs will erode. If this development takes place, their access to social services, welfare, education, and the labor market will be in danger, or so I will argue. At any rate, it will be much more in danger than when the general conviction is that disabled people should enjoy these social goods because of the special needs that they have without any fault of their own. Assuming that this is a plausible case for genetic discrimination and that it represents a serious threat to disabled people in the long run, the question arises as to what can be done about it.

With regard to this second question various possibilities arise. Negatively defined, none of them is based on attempts to secure access to social goods for the disabled in the long run *independently* from the developments in the field of genetics and reproductive medicine. The reason is that any such attempt would be question begging since the developments in this field are assumed to cause eroding public support for the disabled in the first place. The alternative that suggests itself is, positively defined, a policy of restricting 'reproductive choice' in one way or another. Some uses of individual freedom may have consequences for other people that require intervention by the state. Should it be unfair toward parents of disabled children to be held responsible for having these children; will the state in that case be justified in restricting access to, and distribution of procedures for genetic testing if that is arguably part of the cause? The answer to this question must be that, given its commitment to equal opportunity, the liberal democratic state seems to be justified in proceeding in this direction as a matter of principle, but from a pragmatic point of view it has no feasible instruments to implement a restrictive policy. It may either try to restrict the range of genetic disorders that people can legally prevent—for example by ruling out certain disabling conditions as justifiable grounds for 'selective abortion'—or it may try to restrict what people can legally find out about the conditions of their future offspring, for example by ruling out certain disorders from genetic testing and screening. More closely considered, however, none of these policies will pass the test of public justification because in any case the restriction of reproductive choice presupposes a substantial view about what specific genetic disorders imply for the quality and meaning of the lives that people with these conditions are capable of leading.

This disappointing—and embarrassing—result from the liberal point of view becomes even more poignant when we see that ultimately it is the liberal justification of public morality itself that is responsible for the failure to include disabled people on the basis of equality. In this respect the feature that characterizes people with *mental* disabilities is particularly relevant, because of the problem it creates for the moral standing of these people in liberal theory. Put generally, people with mental disabilities are lacking to a greater or lesser extent the powers of reasons and free will. Since these are the powers that bring substance to the core values of the liberal view on public morality, mentally disabled people never acquire full moral standing in this view. This is because its moral community is constituted by 'persons' and these, in turn, are constituted by the powers of reasons and free will. This conception of the person is particularly problematic with respect to the inclusion of severely mentally disabled citizens, since on the liberal view only persons in the sense of rational moral agents can be the recipients of equal concern and respect.

These problems notwithstanding, however, liberal morality is to be recommended for holding itself accountable for the inclusion of the mentally disabled, as we will have ample opportunity to see.[38] That is to say, liberal morality—or should I rather say its philosophical proponents?—is at least not insensitive to the problem of excluding particular groups of human beings from an equal moral standing. Being proud of its own record of respect for the dignity of human beings, the exclusion of 'defective' human beings cannot but offend the humanism of its moral consciousness, even though it has insufficient resources to accommodate this problem.

How is one to proceed from here, now that the convictions and beliefs entailed in the liberal conception of morality have been taken to the limits of what they are capable of justifying as a matter of public concern? The answer to this question may be stated in terms of 'the parasitic nature' of liberal morality. With this I mean that liberal morality must fail to make good its promises unless it is supported by convictions and beliefs that exceed the limits of its narrow conception of morality.[39] Put positively, liberal morality is capable of accepting moral responsibility for such dependent others as the mentally disabled because there are people in our society who practice convictions and beliefs wider and deeper than what the narrow framework of that morality is capable of justifying. In other words, with regard to the inclusion of 'nonpersons' and the moral consideration their interests receive, public morality feeds upon implicit convictions and beliefs 'borrowed' from nonliberal practices of moral responsibility.

The response to objections against widening the scope of moral debate in either of the two senses described in this chapter is, then, that the inclusion of dependent people and the special provision our society makes for them would be incomprehensible and unjustifiable should we try to account for them strictly in terms of the 'narrow' view of liberal morality. Our society proves to have moral sources to sustain both the practices of caring for dependent others and the institutions within which these practices take shape beyond what narrow conceptions of its public morality can recognize.

The last stage of the argument is to provide a positive account of some aspects of a wider conception of our moral lives that can help to fill out the gap that public morality in the liberal view leaves behind. Characteristic of this conception is that it includes ideals of human perfection that are grounded in views about what human beings 'really' are. Among these ideals is the acceptance of moral responsibility for dependent people regardless the fact that we have no relation of reciprocity with them. It is not that we owe them equal treatment and respect because and insofar as they owe us the same. What we owe them cannot be justified by specifying the individual capacities of moral agency that they share with us. In other words, moral responsibility for dependent others must have a different basis than a conception of the person in the liberal sense.

To suggest what this alternative basis may be, I turn to an account of the moral life according to which the other person is 'given' to us in the sense that, prior to the rules and principles of social morality, the presence of the other in our lives constitutes our responsibility. Moral responsibility arises neither from contractual relationships nor from the cooperative exchange between independent individuals. Instead it arises from the nature of the moral self that discovers itself within a network of social relationships. Our moral lives are social lives and our moral selves develop within the social relationships that we find ourselves to be part of. To accept responsibility for other people, we must regard our own lives in terms of those relationships. That is to say, only when we regard our own lives as received from others that have accepted responsibility for us, will we be able to assist and support those who have nothing to offer in terms of reciprocating our actions. Even if it is often suggested that it is 'rational' to act on the principle *do ut des,* the constitution of human life is such that this principle is more appropriately reversed: we can give because—and to the extent that—we have been and continuously are given.

The argument is that if human beings are necessarily part of one another's world, they cannot claim sovereignty over their own lives on the basis of which moral obligations arise as the result of a mutual and voluntary exchange of claims and counterclaims. The demand that we care for the other person's life is rooted in the fact of our indebtedness for all the things we have received: intelligence, meanings, speech, love, and much more. But even when this is acknowledged as true, it does not follow that we are also motivated to respond accordingly. It is not cognition but motivation that matters. Human agents need their moral resources to be nourished by the experience of love, sympathy, and friendship. Mutuality in moral relationships is therefore different from that in contractual relationships, because the latter is conditioned by expected benefits, whereas the former is not. The benefits bestowed by love and friendship are consequential rather than conditional, which explains why human life that is constituted by these relationships is appropriately experienced as a gift.

A society that accepts responsibility for dependent others such as the mentally disabled will do so because there are sufficient people who accept something like the above account as true. Without this supposition, I will argue, we cannot make sense of the effort our society puts into the practices of caring, and in revising institutions and programs according to the normalization paradigm, regardless of the fact that its effort regards people who *cannot* bear responsibility for others as others do for them. Among the moral resources it must have available, therefore, are the convictions and beliefs of those who are engaged themselves in caring for dependent others. Ultimately the question of why our society accepts responsibility for its mentally disabled members depends on the question of whether there are sufficient people who have the character and the skills necessary to engage themselves in sharing their lives with them. For the liberal justification of public morality this creates the awkward problem that its failure to include disabled people as recipients of justice and equality is made good by people whose moral convictions and beliefs it prefers to ignore as part of what sustains the public domain. Whether or not the proliferation of genetic testing in society will undermine their support does not so much depend on what public policy can do to avert the threats of genetic discrimination, but on what sort of people we—the ones who find handicapped people to be part of our communities—are capable of being.

Part One

TWO

The 'Liberal Convention'

It is unclear to me why the agreement not to talk about fundamental disagreements in public is any less loaded and controversial an assumption than the idea of a "veil of ignorance" which asks us to feign ignorance about our conception of the good.

Seyla Benhabib

If the basic liberal goal is to ensure that individuals are not imposed upon as they go about forming moral convictions and moral commitments—and this, after all, is the *point* of liberal anxiety about the state—then the moral ideal here is indeed 'the privatization of the good'. And this brings me back to my bedrock objection: Having privatized the good, are we still able to render critical judgments on the global way of life in which these putatively 'self-governing' individuals nonetheless participate?

Ronald Beiner

2.1 The Context of the Debate

The task of determining the moral context that provides the background of the present inquiry leads us toward a characterization of liberal morality that dominates much of the contemporary bioethical literature. The tendency to abstain from questions about the good life for human beings leads contemporary bioethics to regard the issue of genetics and the prevention of disability as an issue about reproductive freedom. As a consequence this issue presents liberal bioethical thinking with an awkward dilemma that it cannot adequately address within its own narrow framework.[1] But before I develop the argument for this claim in the coming chapters, we will first consider a principled defense of the narrow approach to bioethics. It is provided by H. T. Engelhardt's *The*

Foundations of Bioethics, in which the author sets out to explain the internal logic of contemporary moral minimalism in the area of health care. It is Engelhardt's contention that bioethics has to refrain from any substantial view regarding the human good and should limit itself to the principles of a purely procedural morality. I have chosen to discuss Engelhardt's view because I consider it to be one of the most rigorous defenses of this position that have been offered in recent years.[2]

2.2 The 'Liberal Convention'

The key feature of morality in liberal society is commonly taken to be its diversity. People disagree widely and deeply about fundamental questions of right and wrong, good and evil. And they disagree widely and deeply about the sources from which valid judgments on these matters can be inferred. But diversity cannot extend across the board, it is often said, because it would then be impossible to appeal to a substantial *public* morality by means of which people can cooperate despite their disagreements. Accordingly, the context of moral debate in liberal society is provided by the convictions and beliefs that enable its members to maintain their particular society. I will refer to these convictions and beliefs as the 'liberal convention'.[3] The liberal convention encompasses the views to which many people in our society subscribe in the public debate on genetics and the prevention of disability.[4] The following account offers the most important of these views.

First and foremost, the liberal convention includes the paramount moral value of 'free choice'. This means that people have a right to decide matters concerning their private lives. The paramountcy of individual freedom reflects the idea that human beings are capable of choosing the kind of life they prefer and of acting upon their preference. Consequently, 'free choice' implies a further belief regarding the legitimacy of public responsibility and control. When people have the right to act upon their own preference, it then follows that society has no right to interfere. Sir Isaiah Berlin famously coined the term 'negative freedom' to characterize this idea.[5] It implies the notion of a moral space within which, other things being equal, the individual is at liberty to act in accordance with his or her own desires. But, of course, things may not be equal. There can be situations that eventually justify society's interference with 'free choice'. Not only are there catastrophic situations brought about by natural disasters, of course, there are also many other situations in ordinary social life where the use of freedom by some, means lesser freedom for others. Negative freedom is therefore extended to a right to equal freedom. Individuals are free to act according to their own preferences as long as they do not violate the equal freedom of others to do so as well. In this respect the belief in 'free choice', as expressed by the liberal convention, is strongly attuned to the preferences and ideals of individual agents. In the moral ontology of liberalism the individual precedes society.

Closely connected with this is the view that the liberal convention holds regarding 'the value of life'. Once it is accepted that people have a right to choose for themselves the kind of life they prefer, the value of their lives cannot be measured by standards derived from some external authority. That is to say, it cannot be right that the value of my life is assessed on grounds other than those that are accepted by me. This view implies the belief that the value of life in liberal society ought to be decided on grounds accepted by the person whose life it is. A valuable life is a life lived 'from the inside'.[6] The principle thus arises that as long as people are capable of valuing their own lives, this fact by itself should be sufficient for considering their lives to be intrinsically valuable. The value of life is determined not by the fact that people value their lives for any particular feature but by the mere fact that they are capable of valuing it at all.[7]

Thirdly, and closely connected to the previous point, the liberal convention holds the belief that the status of persons is of primary moral concern. Persons are taken as moral agents, that is to say, as beings capable of choosing and acting upon their preference. This does not mean that 'nonpersons' fall outside the scope of liberal morality, but that they are only indirectly included in it. In some cases, such as the case of newborn infants, the inclusion of 'nonpersons' depends on potentiality. They will become moral agents in the future. In other cases, the inclusion of 'nonpersons' is taken to depend on the interests of their relatives. Such is the case, for example, with the profoundly mentally disabled. Furthermore, there is a specific case in which 'nonpersons' fail to be included even indirectly, i.e., that of the human fetus. This is why termination of a human fetus is not considered to constitute an act of homicide, as is reflected by the abortion laws of many Western democracies. At any rate, the moral views held by the liberal convention imply a dividing line between 'persons' and 'nonpersons' with regard to whom its core values pertain directly or only indirectly.

Fourthly, the liberal convention attributes high value to social and political equality. People ought to be treated equally according to their status as moral agents, which is grounded in their capacity to decide for themselves how they should live. This capacity as the ground for equality rules out unequal treatment on the basis of characteristics such as religion, class, race, and sex.[8] To treat people unequally on the basis of any of these characteristics constitutes a case of unjustifiable discrimination, which means that people do not receive due respect as agents. This antidiscriminatory stance implies a claim to public responsibility for the democratic state. The democratic state has an obligation to give equal consideration to the interests of every citizen while ignoring their characteristics other than that of citizenship.

Lastly, the liberal convention entails the belief that public morality should not address the issue of the relative value of different conceptions of the good. To accept a particular conception of the good as normative for how the members of our society should be treated is to treat them on the basis of convictions and beliefs that at least some of them do not share, given a widespread and deep moral diversity. There would be no harm in treating others on the basis of a conception of the good that is shared by the members of society, but with respect to the public realm in our society we cannot assume such a conception to be available.[9] The democratic state ought therefore to abstain from passing judgment on people's conceptions of what their lives should be about. It must abstain from holding any opinion on the good life for its citizens. Its goal is not to promote particular ends in life but to secure equal opportunities for its citizens to realize their own ends under the rule of law.

2.3 Implications of Starting with the 'Liberal Convention'

Introducing the liberal convention as the context of our discussion is obviously contestable because it entails convictions and beliefs that are not generally accepted. Many religious people, for example, will object to an agent-relative conception of the value of life as explained in the previous section. These people will probably argue that the value of my life is not necessarily what I think it is, nor is it given with the fact that I am capable of valuing my life. Instead they will say that the value of human life resides in the fact that it is a gift from God.

In view of this objection it is important to consider the implications of introducing the liberal convention as the context of moral debate in liberal society. Let me start with emphasizing once more that the convention expresses moral convictions and beliefs regarding how people in liberal society evaluate one another's actions from a public point of view. It expresses the moral views of a society in which different groups think and behave differently in questions regarding the human good. Even those who do not accept these moral beliefs as true and who nonetheless want to intervene in public debate will have to face the question of how to contribute effectively to that debate. That is to say, no strategy of argumentation aimed at public debate can ignore the question of its own rhetorical impact. In this respect public debate is not unlike academic debate. Contributions to academic debate can only be made by complying with its rules, including contributions regarding the question as to what these rules should be. Therefore, in discussing issues related to human genetics and the prevention of disability in liberal society, there is good reason to accept its moral idiom and use its public space as a moral battleground.

This methodological decision is not inconsequential, however. It will result in shaping the issues in terms of the core values and beliefs that the liberal convention embodies. From the point of view of public morality, many of us—including those among us who are religious—do believe that they ought to be free to make decisions about their own lives. It follows that accepting the liberal convention as a strategy of argumentation is anything but an innocent manoeuvre.[10] It tends to reinforce the narrow view on public debate by presenting the issue of genetics and prevention as as an issue about 'choice'. Decisions to prevent disabled children from being born are perceived as belonging to the private realm where we are free to decide for ourselves. If we face the risk that our offspring will be affected by genetic disease, we are free to seek medical help to see how this can be prevented. The decisions we make are between our doctors and ourselves. We do not have to justify ourselves in consulting a doctor. That is to say, seeking medical treatment for a bodily disfunction does not require special justification as long as it remains within the rights and duties of the medical profession and its clients. Consequently, a strong focus on the rights and duties of doctors and their patients in the debate on genetics and prevention is what we should expect in liberal society.

In this sense the moral context described as the 'liberal convention' reinforces some of the characteristics of the mainstream bioethical literature. It underwrites what Alasdair Macintyre has called 'the privatization of the good' because it refrains from raising questions about the substance of our moral lives.[11] Once it is clear that the introduction of the liberal convention tends to shape our discussion in a narrow way, however, the question is: Why accept it as a normative framework in the first place? There are two reasons that may be adduced. The first repeats what I stated concerning the persuasiveness of moral argument. Moral arguments are necessarily contextual in at least this sense that they need to address what people actually believe. Only in that way can they have a practical impact upon moral behavior. This is not to say that in addressing actual moral convictions and beliefs one also accepts them as justified, let alone as decisive. All one does and needs to do is to let them set the stage on which to develop one's argument. The second reason follows directly from the first. In discussing the issue of genetics and the prevention of disability we should ask whether liberal convictions and beliefs are adequate to say what needs to be said. As a matter of fact, my aim is to reveal that as far as questions about our responsibility for the disabled are concerned, public morality in liberal society is dependent upon substantial views that do not fit into its conceptual apparatus. The fact that it purports to be silent on questions of meaning and the human good creates an ethical vacuum in areas of social life where such questions cannot be ignored. The practices of caring for dependent human beings in health care provide an example of such an area. The fact that its conceptual apparatus renders our public morality impotent to support such practices does not mean, however, that it can silence the underlying questions of meaning and the human good. The ethical vacuum demands to be filled.

At this point it may be objected that the privatization of the good is not something optional, because it is a matter of moral principle. Even if it is true that public debate could address substantial moral questions about the human good—depending on what participants in that debate bring to the table—we should refrain from doing so for reasons of moral principle. What can or cannot be subject to public debate should not be made dependent on the particular moral identity of the participants. In this contention the narrow conception of public morality meets with political liberalism.[12] Public morality in liberal society requires that we strip ourselves of all our particular convictions and beliefs and retain only those that we can justifiably hold as citizens of the liberal democratic state. In other words, the objection argues that the recognition of ourselves as citizens rather than as people with particular conceptions of the good life is mandatory as a moral requirement in liberal society. There is, of course, a spate of recent literature on this aspect of contemporary liberal thought, known as "the liberal-communitarian debate." I will not try to review this literature here. Instead, I will discuss a philosophical theory that defends abstinence from issues about the human good as a matter of principle with respect to bioethics.

2.4 Morality among Strangers

The theory to be discussed in this connection is found in H. T. Engelhardt's widely acclaimed book *The Foundations of Bioethics*.[13] It offers an account of what people in liberal society can expect from one another from the point of view of public morality. Engelhardt holds the view that people in liberal society share certain moral convictions, but they do not share substantial conceptions of the good. They share only those convictions that are necessary for society to be minimally possible. Moral diversity with regard to the good is real in our society, according to Engelhardt, at any rate much more so than most bioethicists seem to realize.[14] Many arguments in bioethics proceed from substantial premises, he argues, regardless of whether these premises are held by those whom the arguments are intended to convince. Since there is no shared vision of the human good, there is no authority for moral demands other than the authority that flows from our own assent to agreements for peaceful cooperation. That is to say, the only authority available is one that is based on the 'principle of permission'.[15] Consequently, there is no moral absolute in Engelhardt's view other than the demand to abstain from the use of force.

Engelhardt's theory accounts for this state of affairs by introducing two pairs of technical terms.[16] On the one hand, secular society is constituted by the exchange between 'moral strangers' whose actions are governed by a 'procedural' morality, which derives its authority from the consent of the parties involved. On the other hand, however, there are particular communities constituted by relations between 'moral friends' who share a 'content-full' morality to guide their lives.[17] The difference between moral strangers and moral friends is that the latter have ways of settling moral disputes on grounds other than that of their mutual agreement. They are united by their adherence to a perspective or narrative that transcends their individual beliefs. Moral strangers, in contrast, lack this kind of authority because they do not share enough of a moral vision to reach substantial resolutions to their disagreements.[18] Not only do moral friends have more sources, but their sources for resolving moral controversies are also richer.[19] They can appeal to the authority of rational argument on the basis of commonly held premises and commonly recognized individuals or institutions.[20]

The peculiar characteristics of contemporary society in Engelhardt's view imply that its public morality is inseparable from the realm of politics. The *res publica* is what binds moral strangers inescapably together. Consequently, in this society 'public debate' is equivalent to 'debate on public policy', and 'public morality' is equivalent to 'general secular morality'.[21] The core business of public debate is to regulate the use of force for protecting persons who peacefully interact with one another.[22] The interaction between such persons may involve the pursuit of any project as long as it remains within the limits set by the principle of permission. Engelhardt concedes that the emerging picture of morality is a 'disappointing' one, but it nonetheless entails all that can be justified on general secular grounds.[23]

In view of this minimalist conception of public morality, the question arises as to why people should accept its authority unless it reflects a conception of the human good that appeals to them as attractive? Engelhardt retorts that the principle of permission creates moral space within which there can be cooperative action to establish institutions for the pursuit of common goods—"albeit in limited ways"—but he understands that his account of minimal morality leaves much to be desired. His own peculiar way of expressing these doubts is worth a lengthy quote:

Perhaps the reader hungers after unification of the genesis and justification of morality, as well as of the motivation to be moral, that can only be found with reference to the Deity. In terms of what the Deity is and wills, one can find an ultimate genesis of what it is to be right and what it is to be good and virtuous. . . . This coincidence of the grounds of knowledge and being, of the genesis and the justification of morality, as well as the motivation to be moral, all of which are so often sought in the philosopher's God, cannot be found in a generally justifiable secular account. Secular moral reflection cannot provide such a deep account of why it is rational and prudent to be moral. (*The Foundations of Bioethics,* xii)

Without an account of the moral vision that transcends the projects of strangers, however, how can they be motivated to behave morally at all? The question is pertinent since, in arguing for agreement and consent as the only available sources of moral authority, Engelhardt appears to accept that people behave morally because it suits their own purposes to do so. That is to say, he seems to accept that the demands of morality derive their binding force from the fact that people believe it to be conducive to their own interests. This is how he answers the question:

One is left with a polytheism of moral perspectives, none with the capacities sought from the univocal perspective of God. Still, secular moral reflection can offer the possibility of a secularly authoritative moral discourse as well as collaboration among moral strangers, despite the collapse of the modern philosophical project. If individuals are interested in resolving issues peaceably (i.e., without a basic reliance on force itself as authority), and even if the individuals do not hear God in the same way, and despite the fact that secular sound rational argument cannot establish a particular content-full moral vision, what is offered will still function to secure a general secular bioethics. Meager and contentless as it is, it is all that can be justified in general secular terms. In general secular terms, one cannot even show that it is good. (*The Foundations of Bioethics,* xii)

In other words, Engelhardt appears to be committed to the view that secular morality is capable of enforcing its demands on people because they have a stake in social cooperation and peace to further their own projects. This suggests an instrumental justification of public morality on the basis of enlightened self-interest. All his generally secular account can say about motivation is that, as moral strangers, we share an interest in controlled uses of force. This does not mean, of course, that moral strangers cannot be morally motivated by other reasons, but these other reasons can only be derived from the particular practices that they share with their moral friends. There may be reasons for being moral that are 'internal' to their deeper sources of meaning, but such sources cannot be tapped by secular philosophical reasoning. Engelhardt concedes that much more needs to be said on 'ultimate questions', such as the question of the nature of human existence and its limitations, but "a general secular bioethics cannot say it."[24]

With this account of public morality in secular society, Engelhardt belongs to a tradition of moral philosophy according to which morality is instrumental to social peace and civil order.[25] Among the main characteristics of this tradition is, first of all, its commitment to philosophical skepticism. There is no 'deep' truth about morality or its ultimate source to be discovered. Morality is a matter of invention.[26] It is a tradition within which morality is a social artefact, a tradition memorably represented by both Hobbes and Hume but long before them attributed by Plato to the sophist Protagoras.[27]

A further characteristic of this tradition is the fact that its main concern is to restrict the choices of action from the point of view of others whose interests are affected by these choices. Left to their natural inclinations, as Protagoras explains, human beings tend towards uncivilized behavior. Only because they have learned to keep the peace between them and maintain civil order can they survive. The Protagorean tradition thus understands the task of morality as teaching civic virtue to everyone because it is necessary for social life. The presupposition of this view is that unless they possess the 'art of politics' human beings would not know how to check their natural inclinations when acting in public.[28]

Thirdly, characteristic of modern versions of this tradition is the distinction that divides morality into two spheres. On the hand, there is morality in the narrow sense,[29] which is the morality of constraint aiming at social peace and civil order. On the other hand, there is morality in a broad sense, which guides people in their pursuit of their own conception of the good. This feature appears in Engelhardt's theory as a 'two-tier' conception of morality. The first tier is that of a procedural and empty morality found in modern secular society, which enables people with different conceptions of the good to coexist peacefully. The second tier is that of a content-full morality, which is found within the context of particular communities and which enables people to live and find meaning and direction in their lives. Engelhardt concedes that his account of a general secular morality presupposes the existence of these content-full moral visions and of communities where they are lived.[30] The important point about the distinction is, however, that the two tiers remain conceptually separated and that no appeal to convictions and beliefs acquired in the second tier operates in the justification of the first. The litmus test for failure or success of any such attempt, according to Engelhardt, is that one can account for the 'grammar' of secular morality without any reference to a particular moral tradition. In view of this test, let us see how his philosophical argument works.

2.5 Instrumentalism, Formalism, or Conventionalism?

Let me begin by pointing to a curious disagreement among Engelhardt's interpreters: some read his theory as belonging to the tradition of Hobbes and Hume, while others read him as he presents himself, namely as a Kantian.[31] The latter reading seems to follow from two observations. First, Engelhardt's principle of permission appears to be grounded on Kant's principle of respect for persons that says never use other persons merely as means, but always also as ends. Secondly, Engelhardt presents what he calls a 'transcendental argument' as a foundation of general secular morality that appears to be heavily indebted to Kant. Here I will mainly consider this second point. How does Engelhardt's transcendental argument work, given his view that secular morality unites moral strangers in a common enterprise of social cooperation and the peaceful resolution of conflict?[32]

After concluding that previous attempts to justify a content-full secular ethics fail, Engelhardt sets out to develop his alternative. It is important for my purposes to follow his precise wording:

> Because there are no decisive secular arguments to establish that one concrete view of the moral life is better morally than its rivals, and since all have not converted to a single moral viewpoint, secular moral authority is the authority of consent. . . . This basis for morality is available in the notion of ethics as a means of securing moral authority through consent in the face of intractable content-full moral controversies. *If one is interested* in collaborating with moral authority in the face of moral disagreements without fundamental recourse to force, *then one must accept* agreement among members of the controversy or peaceable negotiation as the means for resolving concrete moral controversies. This account of ethics and bioethics requires a minimum of prior assumptions. It requires only a decision to resolve moral disputes in a manner other than fundamentally by force. (*The Foundations of Bioethics*, 68–69, italics mine)

What can be clearly seen from this quote is that the argument starts with what Kant would have called a hypothetical imperative. *If* one is interested in making a moral judgment authoritatively, *then* one must accept agreement as the only means of conflict resolution. In other words, the argument presupposes a particular kind of commitment. Moral agents have to be committed to peaceful resolution of their conflicts with others. It requires "a decision to resolve moral disputes in a manner other than by force," as the author says.

The question now is: What are the grounds that make this decision a compelling one? There are two possible answers. The first is to say that people make this decision because they have a stake in peaceful cooperation. It is conducive to their interests to make agreements.[33] Let us call this the instrumentalist option. It says that the reason for moral strangers to accept the principle of permission is strategic. The second is to say that their desire to be moral is not induced by enlightened self-interest but by a genuine commitment to peaceableness as a moral value. Let us call this the conventionalist option. It is 'conventionalist' in the sense that the desire to be moral is inculcated by people's adherence to certain moral values that are shared in their society, such as the principle of nonviolent conflict resolution between individuals and groups in their capacity as citizens.

Faced with these two possiblities, Engelhardt may be expected at any rate to reject the latter. Not only would it prove his argument to be circular, since it would establish a moral principle by presupposing one, it would also commit him to the claim that moral strangers share a particular moral vision that has peaceableness and related values as its substantial core.[34] Consequently, his attempt to ground secular morality philosophically would fail for the same reason that he claims all other attempts have failed.

That leaves the first possibility, namely to accept that people engage in moral exchange for strategic reasons, which is in line with reading Engelhardt's theory as belonging to the Protagorean tradition. But to ground the justification of secular morality in enlightened self-interest is difficult, because one faces the possibility that people decide to cooperate conditionally and hold to their agreements as long as they think it profitable. Presumably with this weakness in mind, Engelhardt also rejects the strategic option as too shaky a ground for his foundation of secular morality:

> This view of ethics and bioethics is not grounded in a concern for peaceableness. *It is not based on an interest in establishing a peaceable community.* This view cannot be shown in general secular terms to be good, praiseworthy, or rationally to be desired. It should, instead, be recognized as a disclosure, to borrow a Kantian notion, of a transcendental condition, a necessary condition for the possibility of a general domain of human life and the life of persons generally. (*The Foundations of Bioethics*, 70, emphasis mine)

Clearly, in this statement, the author rejects both alternatives; not only does he deny that the decision to opt for peaceful conflict resolution is based on a prior moral commitment, he also rejects that it is based on prudence. Instead, he moves beyond the conventionalist and the instrumentalist to the formalist option.[35] Whereas he started with the claim that (1) abstaining from the use of force is obligatory *if* one is interested in peaceful collaboration, which was followed by the claim that (2) peaceful collaboration is in itself *not* a substantial moral value, he now seems to make the much stronger claim that (3) in dealing with others only on the basis of their permission we realize the very possibility of moral behavior, understood as "giving justified praise and blame."[36] Respect for others *qua* persons is the necessary condition for the possibility of justified blame and praise, Engelhardt argues, because the practice of blaming or praising others for their actions is meaningless unless one believes that they can act upon their own will.

However, Engelhardt then continues with a controversial claim when he says that the grounds for *morally* justified blame and praise are provided by the principle of permission.[37] This claim assumes that treating other persons with their permission is equivalent to 'morally right'.[38] What is the basis for this assumption? According to Engelhardt, the answer lies in the fact that his transcendental argument shows that the very possibility of morality is grounded in our character as persons.[39] But this is true only if one accepts the conception of personhood as endorsed by Kantians. The fact that I can act upon my own will does not provide you with a *moral* reason to think that I ought not be treated against my own will, unless you believe that my will is governed by the rules of reason *and* that reason represents the highest moral authority. Presumably, this is what Kantians believe, but why should others—for example, Augustinians—believe the same? The question is how this Kantian foundation of morality could not be part of a particular moral vision given the particular conception of personhood on which it is founded. I fail to see how Engelhardt could respond to this question otherwise than by reiterating his Kantian presuppositions. Consequently, we are left with the conclusion that the argument is compelling only for those who have already accepted what Engelhardt set out to establish, namely that secular morality is grounded in the moral authority of voluntary agreement between rational persons.[40] He has certainly not shown this on independent grounds, that is, on grounds that are independent of moral convictions and beliefs inherent to a particular moral vision.

If his formalist justification of the permission principle does not work, what about the instrumentalist option that occasionally appears in his text? Can it succeed where the transcendental argument fails? In order to see whether it can, we should look at what Engelhardt tells us about the position of 'outsiders', people who are not interested in collaborating with moral strangers but who nevertheless abstain from using force on the basis of their own content-full morality. In confronting such people, he says, "one has simply discovered a limit to a particular community or area of agreement, and not a warrant to force cooperation. It is here that one also has discovered a fundamental equality among all persons" (*The Foundations of Bioethics*, 70). But why should this follow if the confrontation with outsiders takes place beyond the jurisdiction of voluntary agreements? Why should parties to an agreement discover a "fundamental equality among all persons" when confronted by people outside that agreement who decline to join them? Surely their agreement *as such* does not warrant this claim, because it only regards those who are under its jurisdiction. Why should anyone who accepts the permission principle on the basis of an agreement to nonviolent conflict resolution accept to be bound by those who refuse to enter the agreement? In no way does an agreement to nonviolent conflict resolution generate an idea of equal treatment that extends beyond the parties to that agreement. Thus we can conclude that Engelhardt moves from the claim:

A *ought not to use force against* B *because they both agreed upon peaceable collaboration between them*

to a substantially different claim, namely:

A *ought not to use force against* B *because they both agreed not to use force against one another, therefore* A *ought not to use force against anybody who is peaceable.*

The inference in the second claim that *A*'s agreement with *B* implies a moral obligation toward all other peaceable people does not follow, however. This obligation only follows when the Kantian conception of the rational person has been shown to be a compelling one or when peaceable cooperation has been accepted as morally binding independently from any agreement. Apart from the fact that Engelhardt has failed to do the former, the case of peaceable outsiders also indicates that in accepting the Kantian conception of the person one renders the fact of the agreement irrelevant. People are to be treated with respect regardless of whether they have entered into the agreement.

Regarding the second possibility—peaceable outsiders are included because peaceableness has been accepted as morally binding independently from any agreement—we must conclude that this is what Engelhardt has already explicitly denied. It would clearly presuppose peaceableness as a moral value. By implication, it would clearly violate his strategy of argumentation. Not only does his transcendental deduction of the principle fail, the same is true of an argument based on the instrumentalist assumption that people engage in nonviolent conflict resolution because it suits their own purposes to do so.

In order to avoid the possible implication of wanton violence against non-collaborating outsiders, Engelhardt has no other option left but to assume that the parties to the agreement share the moral notion of a fundamental equality of all persons, including noncompliant outsiders. This assumption implies that, ultimately, the principle of nonviolent conflict resolution is based on the tacit assumption that moral strangers share certain substantial moral beliefs. That is, unless one presupposes a moral commitment to peaceable cooperation on the part of moral strangers there is no way of justifying the rights of innocent 'outsiders'. More importantly, at least for our present purposes, there is no way of justifying the rights of those who have a stake in peaceableness but who never will be able to participate in any cooperation whatsoever. The question of how 'incompetent' outsiders are to be treated is also a matter of agreement in Engelhardt's theory, but the fact of the agreement as such does not provide any guarantee for a morally acceptable answer.[41] In order to have minimal confidence in peaceful coexistence, incompetent stakeholders have to be sure that moral strangers actually understand their interest in peaceful coexistence as a *moral* rather than a strategic interest.

To conclude, we can be confident about the practical implications of Engelhardt's justification of general secular morality to the extent that it is shared by people who have assigned its values a prominent place in their own moral vision.[42] Historically, individuals who have been socialized in liberal democratic society are nourished by various moral sources, among which are the sources of previous moral cultures, such as, for example, the culture of Christianity. From this fact alone Engelhardt derives the tacit assumption that liberal society is made up of individuals whose lives display the moral values of peaceful coexistence and the abstinence of force. To the extent that liberal society is composed of such individuals, his justification of secular morality succeeds because it proves what people have already accepted. In other words, Engelhardt's foundation of bioethics is thoroughly conventionalist.

If correct, this is an important conclusion for the strategy of argumentation in the present inquiry. The narrow conception of public morality that is defended by Engelhardt is either circular or self-defeating. In order to make his theory work he must tacitly assume particular moral convictions on the part of moral strangers that commit them to substantial moral views. Consequently, he has not succeeded in showing that we can abstain from asking ultimate questions about the human good. Since I believe that Engelhardt's critique of previous attempts to ground secular morality on nonsubstantial moral premises is quite convincing, I see no reason to believe that further attempts will be successful. The more plausible conclusion is that the entire project rests on a mistake. If not only the formalist but also the instrumentalist justification of the permission principle fails, then Engelhardt has not shown that general secular morality is grounded in permission independent of substantial moral views.

This conclusion is particularly important for our discussion of moral practices of caring for human beings who cannot be considered as parties to any agreement, such as the mentally disabled. How we should live with these people and what we owe them as members of our society are questions that cannot be answered by appealing to procedural values such as are expressed by the notions of free choice and personal autonomy. This is not to say that such values have no meaning for our ways of dealing with the disabled, but only that they are insufficient to answer our most profound moral questions about them.

2.6 Beyond a Narrow Conception of Morality

Let me summarize the foregoing analysis of Engelhardt's views on moral justification in liberal society in the following way. Once one sees that the justification of secular morality cannot succeed without recourse to the moral convictions and attitudes that people bring to the public square by being the particular people they are, the conceptual and theoretical divide between 'procedural morality' and 'content-full morality' collapses. One can opt for the strategy of purifying ethical reflection from any vestiges of content-full moral sources in the way Engelhardt does. However, one can also opt for a strategy in which liberal moral views are presented as central to the context of public debate but are then shown to leave many elements of our moral culture unaccounted for. This second strategy is deployed in the present inquiry. Engelhardt wants us to realize unflinchingly the moral poverty of our public square. I would rather try to trace the remainders of its richer sources in order to remind our society that its moral fabric is much richer than liberal morality allows us to acknowledge. Our moral culture draws on moral sources very different from what the narrow focus of contemporary ethical thought is capable of articulating.

To close this chapter, I will tentatively explain this alternative strategy with regard to the main theme of this inquiry, the apparent tension between normalization and prevention of disabled lives as previously described. I take it that many people in liberal society are proud of the fact that this society, more than any other, proclaims its commitment to equal respect for individual human beings. Policies counteracting discrimination against people from minorities are implemented to exclude unequal treatment on the basis of religion, class, color, sex or age, and, recently, also disability. Disabled people, it is argued, ought to be free to shape their own lives according to their own potential and their values, just like anybody else. No doubt this liberal attitude has done much to support the paradigm shift towards the normalization of the lives of disabled persons.[43] However, the same attitude allows the strategies of prevention that point in opposite directions. On the one hand, liberal society takes pride in the fact that it respects each of its members on the basis of equality, at least as a matter of principle, which explains its commitment to normalization policy. On the other hand, however, its commitment to the equal freedom of individual citizens leads it to regard decisions about family matters as 'private', which explains its relative acquiescence with respect to using genetics for the prevention of disabled people from being born.

A crucial question for our discussion must be, therefore, whether our society can afford to continue its disregard for the coincidence of both developments—normalization and prevention—as if they occur in two separate worlds. In my view this question deserves serious attention. If we have reason to believe that the practices of prevention will have deleterious consequences for the position of disabled people in our society, what sources to counteract these effects, if any, are available? My suspicion is that the view of public morality embodied by the liberal convention will not give us much of a basis to counteract these effects, at least not without becoming self-contradictory. If so, it will do very little to safeguard the future of disabled people in our society. In that case we need to consider other sources than those that the narrow conception of morality allows us to acknowledge. One avenue is to tap the convictions and beliefs that sustain people in their commitment to care for their disabled children. The best contribution to the critique of procedural secular morality, it seems to me, is to investigate ways of living a human life, that include, rather than exclude, these children. In this way we may be able to sustain strategies of inclusion that the liberal democratic state has difficulty in sustaining if it is to rely strictly on proceduralist accounts of its own moral resources. We may desperately need to see the lights by which its citizens understand themselves as 'moral friends' and by which they live their 'content-full' moral lives.

Genetics and Prevention in Public Morality

It should be obvious that the attainment of a complete map and sequence of the genome will not provide a solution to human problems. Nor will it explain what makes humans uniquely human. But, the perception has been that the genetic is unchangeable, and that the problems of criminality, behavioral deviation, individual capability, even differences between sex, race, and general intelligence can be accounted for solely from within the domains of human genetics. Ultimately, *perception* is all that matters. If it cannot be persuasively dispelled, the application of genetic information in predictive and curative medicine and in practical human affairs will be problematic at best and could be dangerously attractive and destructive of cultural and moral interests.

Evelyne Shuster

3.1 Initial Distinctions

Recent developments in molecular biology and genetics have expanded our knowledge of disabling conditions considerably. In conjunction with other technological developments in the field of artificial reproduction and combined with the legalization of abortion 'on demand', this knowledge creates the option to decide whether, and if so, under which conditions, we should prevent the lives of disabled people. What are the moral grounds on which our society permits or even endorses the prevention of disability by means of genetic testing and screening? In this chapter we will consider some initial distinctions in order to fix the key terms in the discussion of this question from the point of view of public morality. Since the various terms of the question allow different readings, we need to make their meanings more explicit. For example, are we to

37

understand 'should' in the sense that prevention is a moral requirement—should prevention be endorsed as a matter of moral duty—or is the question meant to ask whether we have a right to do so in the sense that it is only permitted? Does it make a difference whether 'prevention' pertains to decisions regarding the lives of disabled children before or after conception? To whom is the question addressed: 'we' as individuals or 'we' as a political community? Are we considering the options for public policy or are we considering socially responsible choices by individuals? What sort of conditions are implied in the term 'disabled'? Does it include any limitations following from genetic disorders without further qualification as to their scope or degree? Does it refer to intellectual or physical disabilities or both? Are so-called 'late onset' diseases included or excluded?

Once we begin to ponder the various meanings that the question "Should we prevent the lives of disabled people?" may have, it dissolves into a wide range of more specific questions. The task of this chapter is to determine carefully what these questions are. This is not merely a matter of fixing terminology, for it involves the introduction of a set of distinctions that are not without normative implications. The language we use to discuss moral questions does not merely evaluate courses of action that are described non-normatively, but is itself value laden.[1] In order to determine the meaning of the terms needed to discuss the prevention of disability, I will specify the considerations that *public* morality in our society is most likely to generate in this connection. In doing this, I will again rely on the moral convictions and beliefs provided by the 'liberal convention', as explained in the previous chapter. That is to say, at many points I will make assumptions about what 'we' and 'many of us' or 'most people in our society' tend to believe or accept as moral truths. The idea is not to present a detailed account based on sociological data but to sketch an outline of what I take to be a dominant moral vision in contemporary society with regard to public responsibility in the area of health care and, in particular, of genetics and artificial reproduction. At this stage the aim is to describe the convictions and beliefs that inform the moral vocabulary used in discussing these topics in our society.

Allow me first to address one way in which our initial question—Should we prevent the lives of disabled people?—is obviously spurious. It cannot be understood as asking whether our society should engage in preventing those lives because that is what has already been happening for some time. There is no point in suggesting that we are on the brink of a new development and now have to decide whether or not we should move forward. Preventive gene technology is a well-established practice. The leading question, then, is not whether our society should move in that direction but how to frame questions and concerns about these practices, their prospects, their limitations, and their moral costs, if any, from a public point of view.

3.2 'Morally Permissible' and 'Morally Required'

Should we prevent the birth of handicapped children or is it morally wrong to do so? Medical uses of gene technology have been developed recently without significant moral debate beforehand and certainly without much awareness of their possible implications among larger segments of society. Apparently the scientists and doctors involved in this development did not question the principle of using gene technology for prevention. This suggests that the issue is not whether prevention as such is morally justifiable but rather to specify its moral limits and purposes. Presumably, living with a physical or mental disability is not a neutral fact for most people, one that is accepted with the same equanimity as the color of one's hair or the size of one's feet. The genetic disorders that are targeted by preventive medicine are generally considered to pose serious obstacles to one's opportunities in life. This is true not only for the individuals affected by these disorders but also for their families. When seen in this light, there seems to be at least one good reason to assume that the prevention of disabled lives cannot be *categorically* wrong, even if there are many 'ifs' and 'buts' to be considered. Given what people believe about the burden posed by such lives, it seems right for them to avail themselves of the means to prevent it when they can.

The other side of the coin is to ask whether the reverse could also be true. If it is implausible that prevention is categorically wrong, could it be that *failing* to prevent the lives of disabled people is categorically wrong? In other words, could there be a general duty to do so? Should this duty exist, then no one could be morally justified in accepting the birth of a handicapped child in case a decision needs to be made. Presumably, the claim to a general moral duty to prevent such lives would be just as implausible as its opposite.[2] Many people in our society tend to view the morality of prevention as ambiguous, confronting all who are involved with difficult issues. In some cases we will be reluctant to condemn the prevention of a handicapped child by means of abortion, while in other cases we will be equally reluctant to condemn the rejection of prevention as a moral option. Categorical judgments in this area will certainly not remain undisputed.

If these assumptions are correctly made, we can restate the initial question in terms of the distinction between what is morally required and what is morally permissible, i.e., between a moral *duty* and a moral *right*. Given the general moral climate of our society, most of us presumably would think that, other things being equal, to make the prevention of a disabled life a duty constitutes a serious violation of people's right to decide for themselves in private matters. Many would probably say that, at most, it can be morally appropriate to grant people a right to prevent the life of a disabled person. Because our society certainly would not be prepared to accept just *any* decision that people make with regard to their children, since some of these decisions may affect the interests of these children, their right to decide for themselves can hardly be an absolute right.[3] Consequently, the right to parental decision making will be justified provided the limits of what is permissible have not been transgressed.

Given these considerations, the burden of proof seems to fall on the claim that people never have a right to prevent the life of a disabled child and, conversedly, on the claim that people have an absolute right to do so. Moral experience in this area has various shades of gray. Determining the limits of what is morally required and what is morally permissible is a difficult task indeed.

3.3 Preventing Conception and Preventing Birth

So far I have been using the term 'prevention' quite generally, in contrast to common usage of the term.[4] There are several ways of preventing disabled lives. One way is to make sure that no child is conceived when there is a risk that it may be affected by a genetic disorder. Another way is to make sure that such a child will not be born, once it is certain that it will be affected in that way. In the sense in which the term is commonly used prevention applies only to the former situation in which the possibility of a genetic defect is anticipated in a given patient and based on a concrete calculation of risks.[5] For example, in the case of a woman who is a carrier of the disorder that causes hemophilia, it is absolutely certain that if the child turns out to be male, the child will be a hemophiliac. A 50 percent risk of conceiving such a child may be a sufficient reason to prevent pregnancy. But it may also may be a reason to accept a pregnancy 'conditionally'. This means that one takes the risk in order to find out, once one has become pregnant, whether the fetus is male or female. If it turns out to be male, one has the option of terminating the pregnancy. In this second sense, 'prevention' is in actual fact coterminous with 'abortion'. The difference between the uses of this term is, then, the difference between two kinds of situations. In the first situation the possibility of a disabled child is only anticipated, while in the second it is certain that there will be a disabled child, unless its life is terminated at an early stage of gestation.[6]

Given this distinction many people will think, presumably, that there cannot be anything wrong with the first situation. To prevent a life that has not yet been conceived does not constitute either an injury or a wrong. Very few people in our society actually believe that one should have as many children as physically possible. Perhaps even those who do believe this would be prepared to admit that a genetic risk constitutes sufficient reason to abstain from further procreation.

With regard to the second means of prevention, however, the situation is different. There is already a child underway. In this case, to prevent is to take a human life, even if we employ the term 'termination of pregancy' to describe such actions. In our society many people think—although not without strongly dissenting minorities—that a termination of pregnancy can be justifiable, even when it constitutes an act of taking a human life. Oftentimes this does not mean that they abandon the claim that human life ought not to be taken but rather that they regard the decision to have an abortion as lying with the pregnant woman. Many people who endorse the right to abortion 'on demand' believe that there is a moral pricetag attached to this right.[7]

Furthermore, the belief that abortion can be morally justified continues to raise another question: Is terminating 'fetal life' really an instance of killing a human being? As is well known, this question is the cause of deep controversy. It has generated a substantial amount of literature on whether or not the human fetus is a 'person'.[8] There are various ways of answering this question, but one of the most influential ways is so-called *gradualist* view. From conception onwards, the moral standing of beginning life is increasing, which means that the more the biological development of the fetus advances, the more it approaches human life in the full moral sense. The *conceptus* gains in moral weight in every successive phase of gestation. On the basis of this view, many people have concluded that the moral problem of abortion is less serious the earlier it is performed.[9]

As a matter of fact, a significant number of abortion laws in Western countries seem to be committed to the gradualist view. They determine a point in time after which fetal life has gained sufficient moral weight to become a good that warrants legal protection. Most of them declare termination of fetal life to be illegal beyond the beginning of the second trimester of gestation, notwithstanding the fact that exceptions are made, for example, in case of a diagnosis of a serious genetic disorder in the fetus. This state of affairs strongly suggests broad moral support for the claim that the problem of terminating life at an earlier stage of fetal development is a lesser moral burden for one's conscience.

The combination of these findings with those of the previous section leads us to conclude that a widely accepted limit on people's right to terminate a pregnancy takes into account the timespan within which this right can be exercised. The termination of a human fetus is considered unjustifiable beyond a certain point of time, other things being equal. Beyond that point, abortion is believed to require a much stronger justification than only the right to decide for oneself. This stronger justification may be provided by the fact that the future child will be affected by a serious genetic disorder. Assuming these claims to be widely supported in our society we can expect that many people will grant prospective parents a limited right to prevent the birth of a child with a genetic disorder by terminating pregnancy, depending on the stage of fetal development and on the nature of the disorder and its consequences for their child and themselves.

3.4 'Impairment', 'Disability', and 'Handicap'

Thus far I have used the term 'disability' and its derivatives such as 'disabled lives' to indicate the subject matter of the debate. This is the next term that demands clarification. In 1980 the World Health Organization introduced the International Classification of Impairments, Disabilities and Handicaps (ICIDH) that came to be widely recognized in the field. According to this classification 'impairment' is defined as malfunctions or malformations at the organic level, while 'disability' refers to limited capacities to perform certain activities on the personal level and 'handicap' refers to disadvantages due to such limitations on the social level.[10] The general feeling with regard to these stipulations is that the ICIDH rightly draws attention to the relation between individual capacities and their socio-cultural environment. People with disabilities have too often been identified with their condition as if it were essentially a personal trait. Without the suggestion that physical or psychological reality be ignored, it has been established that in many instances the social response to certain mental conditions caused more harm than these conditions themselves. The history of mental disability in particular has shown that many IQ tests were used to determine levels of cognitive functioning related to labor skills and, by extension, to the labor market.[11] To draw attention to harmful consequences of negative approaches by society toward people with limited mental capacities, the definition of handicap has been shifting from physical and psychological conditions of personal functioning toward the social consequences of these conditions.[12] In this connection it has been argued, however, that the restriction of the term 'disability' to mental functioning on the personal level is problematic for quite similar reasons. Limitations that count as disabilities are deviations from what human beings are normally capable of performing. The designation of a range of activities as 'normal' indicates that disabilities no less than handicaps are dependent on socio-cultural determinants.[13] For example, someone missing a leg who has received a well-functioning prothesis will, with some training, be capable of walking again, even though it will be impossible for this person to perform sports that require running. Given that many people with two legs who are not called 'handicapped' are also incapable of performing those sports—think of the elderly—we would have to say that a person with an artificial leg who is capable of normal social functioning is disabled but not handicapped. This usage is counterintuitive inasmuch as the concepts of disability and handicap appear to be coextensive. Therefore the distinction between disability and handicap as introduced by the ICIDH does not appear to be a very strong one.

This terminological exploration explains why the terms 'disability' and 'handicap' are used interchangeably in the present inquiry. For example, a given genetic disorder may or may not express itself in a way that has social consequences designated as 'disability' or 'handicap'. Consequently, the question "Should we prevent handicapped lives?" can be read in full as "Should we prevent the lives of people with a genetic disorder who as members of our society will be designated as disabled or handicapped?" I will stipulate that 'disability' is synonymous with 'handicap' and that the more important task, at least for present purposes, is to distinguish the meaning of both these terms from the meaning of the term 'disease'. The difference is that whereas disease refers to physiological, psychological, or anatomical disfunction, disability or handicap refer to the social consequences of such disfunction.[14]

To conclude these remarks on terminology, I will often write about 'the disabled' in general as if the population so designated were not as differentiated as the population of 'nondisabled' people. My usage of this term—and its derivatives—is directed primarily at the mentally disabled. This means that my arguments are always intended to refer to people whose disability or handicap has to do with mental functioning, even though they may apply occasionally to the population of disabled people as a whole. Lastly, I consider the term 'mental' in 'mental disability' to be preferable to the term 'intellectual' as used in 'intellectual disability'. The latter is often taken to include persons with psychiatric conditions. In this text 'disabled persons' refers always and only to persons who have developed a permanent and incurable problem at the level of cognitive, mental functioning.[15]

Having clarified the terms, we can now ask: What is it, if anything, that should be prevented by the use of gene technology? It follows from our stipulations that the extent to which a genetic disorder limits someone's opportunities in life varies a great deal with society's capacity and determination to remove or to accommodate these limitations. Apart from technological devices, such as artificial limbs or speech computers, there are social support systems that function as 'social prostheses' to realize, for example, independent living or job coaching for mentally disabled people. However, even if society is willing to provide these kinds of services for various types of disabilities, many people will still think that there is a considerable difference between a physical and a mental handicap. While physical handicaps imply a limitation to capacities such as motor skills, for example, they do not necessarily imply a limited capacity for living a life of one's own in the way that mental handicaps do. Whereas the first indicates a limited capacity for *carrying out* one's own conception of a good life, the second indicates a limited capacity even for determining one's own conception of the good life. Both types of handicaps are characterized by dependency as an unavoidable feature in the lives of those involved, but this dependency differs considerably as to scope and degree. Physical handicaps create dependency in the sense of requiring help in carrying out the way people want to live. Mental handicaps, in contrast, create an additional dependency in the sense of requiring help in determining what this way should be. The additional difference is a difference in capacity for competent judgment. Although individual cases of both types of handicaps may differ importantly in scope and degree, I take it that many people in our society would definitely consider a mental handicap the greater evil. If correct, the moral problem of terminating a pregnancy at an early stage if the child will be *mentally* handicapped, will not be perceived as very disturbing. Mentally disabled human beings do not function well as persons, that is to say, if we take 'persons' to mean what it often is taken to mean in liberal society: rational, self-conscious beings who are capable of determining their own plan of life. To prevent the lives of those who are lacking this capacity—or have it only in a diminished sense—is to prevent lives that in an important sense cannot succeed. Or so, many people in liberal society presumably believe.[16]

3.5 'Disease' and 'Disability'

There is a further clarification with regard to terminology that is crucial for my purposes. It is concerned with the distinction between 'disease' and 'disability'. We call genetic disorders 'disease' in the sense that they are physical, psychological, or physiological conditions that can be identified by means of warranted medical procedures. In the case of these disorders there is a direct link between a disease and a disability in the sense that a malfunction or malformation of a group of cells expresses itself in ways that have consequences for one's functioning as an individual. But even though disabilities or handicaps may be caused by disease, they need not coincide with illness.[17] 'Illness' refers to particular *clinical* symptoms of disease such as pain, fatigue, fever, or distress. One cannot by definition be ill and, at the same time, feel well. However, not every disease is characterized by the symptoms of illness at every stage. There are diseases, such as, for example, rubella, or cancer, that go without symptoms for a certain period of time. Illness cannot be separated from symptoms in this way. For example, pneumonia is a disease that is directly linked with illness, because one cannot have pneumonia without suffering from it (i.e., having a fever, feeling weak, being short of breath, and so on). Illness is constituted by a specific experiential state, which is not necessarily the case with disease.[18] The distinction between disease and illness holds for genetic disorders in the sense that in some cases they cause disfunctions but without the symptoms of illness, for example disorders that affect the process of normal growth such as Klinefelter's syndrome.[19] I will refer to genetic disorders of this kind as 'impairments', which signifies a subcategory of diseases that develop without the symptoms of illness.

These stipulations are not intended to secure a non-normative definition of disease but to make room for the suggestion that disabilities and handicaps caused by different kinds of genetic disorders designated as disease cause different kinds of moral problems.[20] In some cases people with genetic disorders will suffer from illnesses caused by these disorders at some point in time. These are the so-called 'late on-set diseases'. Diseases of this type need not be accompanied by illness at present though it is certain that they will later. Being infected with HIV is an example. In many cases genetic diseases are like that. Examples are Duchenne's muscular dystrophy, cystic fibrosis or Huntington's chorea. Each of these conditions can be diagnosed without the symptoms of illness.

There is another type of genetic disorder, however, that is not necessarily linked with illness. Examples are fragile X syndrome and Down syndrome. People with these disorders are disabled, but they are not necessarily ill or sick. Of course, they may suffer from medical complications that are caused by their genetic disorder. For example, people with Down syndrome have a 9 percent chance of suffering congenital heart disease, but it is not necessarily true that they suffer from Down syndrome. In contrast, people with genetic disorders such as Duchenne's muscular dystrophy will develop symptoms of illness that in many respects are very disabling indeed.

This distinction between diseases linked with disabilities and diseases linked with illness is important for our purposes, because it generates different considerations in thinking about the ethics of prevention. In some cases people suffer from disfunction because of illness. In other cases people suffer from disfunction because of limited capabilities. Given the fact that illness is necessarily a pathology, the appropriate response is medical care. But in cases of limited capabilities, the problem resulting need not be stated in medical terms at all. Limited capabilities are a source of human suffering depending on the social and cultural environment. In these cases, of which fragile X syndrome is an example, people suffer from a disabling condition, not because of illness but because of how this condition is socially evaluated. There are two types of considerations corresponding with these different cases. On the one hand, considerations pertaining to suffering from illness, and, on the other hand, the considerations pertaining to suffering from normality. Given this distinction, one can say, for example, that children with Down syndrome seem to be capable of living reasonably happy lives provided that their lives are not assessed in terms of the standards of normality.[21] It is not evidently true that the same can be said in the case of a disease that causes grave distress once its clinical symptoms have progressively developed, such as Duchenne's muscular dystrophy.

The aim of the proposed terminology is to suggest that, in principle, we can attack the consequences of a disease from two sides: not only by combatting the disease with the diagnostic and therapeutic means that medicine provides but also by changing the social and cultural environment that makes for the cause of a disability or handicap. The latter may be the objective of social and political reform rather than of medical intervention. The distinction between types of genetic disorders is important, then, because it generates different moral arguments. Preventing the birth of a disabled child because its life will be devalued as abnormal is surely morally different from preventing the birth of a disabled child that will suffer from a serious illness. Even if in both cases their lives may be burdened by distress to similar degrees, their distress is very different in kind. Furthermore, being devalued as abnormal in our society may be seen as constituting a case of discrimination, which means that prevention in that case takes on a completely different meaning. For it can be argued, given these different meanings, that in some cases prevention is a dubious response to a social evil. At least that is what I think many people in our society will believe to be true. Instead of confronting the agents of discrimination, one aims at preventing its victims from being born. Consequently, people in our society may be worried about preventing disabled children for reasons of abnormality, even if at the same time they may accept that parents decide not to have a mentally disabled child in order to avoid serious suffering due to illness. If the cause of the suffering is society rather than nature, the more appropriate response would be political rather than medical. This indicates in which sense disabilities and handicaps caused by different kinds of genetic disorders may raise different sets of moral questions.

3.6 'We' as Individuals and 'We' as a Political Community

When the question Should we prevent handicapped lives? is asked, to whom does the 'we' refer? Who is addressed by this question? In this connection the liberal convention requires us to introduce the distinction between people *qua* individual persons and *qua* members of a political community. This distinction helps to clarify the issues in yet another respect. In this distinction we regard ourselves in two different capacities of moral agency. In the capacity of individual persons we are faced with issues about our own private actions and the reasons we have for them. These issues are treated primarily in the context of the question What kind of life do I want to live? In our capacity as citizens we face issues from a public point of view. In the latter capacity the focus is on collective responsibility and public policy.

It should be noted, however, that many of the interactions between citizens belong to the private sphere but are nevertheless believed to constitute a legitimate area of public responsibility. For example, doctors providing medical services to the patients who are seeking their help in the process of dying are acting privately. But when we ask questions about the legitimacy of their private interactions from a public point of view we are entering a different sphere. Consequently, on many issues we will be confronted with a tension between two kinds of moral judgments. Even though we may personally abhor what some people ask of their doctors (for example, to terminate the life of a human being), we do not necessarily jump to the conclusion that they ought to be stopped by means of legal force. Thus the distinction between the 'we' in our capacity as private persons and the 'we' in our capacity as citizens marks a possible source of moral conflict. It is not a distinction between two types of action—individual actions as distinct from collective actions—but between two points of view. From one point of view we ask ourselves privately what should be done and why, whereas in the latter capacity we ask ourselves publicly what should be done and why. There is no reason to believe that our judgments on both questions will always coincide. As a matter of fact, people committed to the core values of the liberal convention will frequently experience that they do not so coincide.[22]

To explore this tension a little further let us concentrate on some aspects of individual freedom. Western society holds strongly to individual freedom in the private realm. Family life belongs to this realm and thus also the question of whether we want to have children, and when and how many. However, we all know that public policy will try to influence our private decisions in a variety of ways. For example, it may either provide or withhold child-care allowances, or raise or cut taxes for families. Given the pressures that rising or falling birthrates may exert on the national budget, the state has a legitimate interest in trying to influence the reproductive choices made by its citizens, notably their decisions regarding how many children they will have and at what age they will have them.

As a matter of fact, this kind of public interference with private decisions causes no major moral problems in our society. Everyone can see that our decisions to procreate interact with other people's decisions to do the same and that these interacting decisions collectively have demographic side effects with immediate consequences for social institutions such as education and health care. Specific policies in this area will seek to influence our private decisions. Since it is considered the legitimate business of public policy to control the effects of how we use our freedoms, it will necessarily deal with the social and economic effects of free reproductive choice. Consequently, not many people—apart perhaps from some orthodox groups—will object to the state developing policies to influence birth control.

The fact that this type of state interference is generally accepted indicates that most people do not regard it as an unjustifiable intrusion into their private lives. The explanation is, presumably, that however public policy may affect the conditions and consequences of our decisions, the decisions themselves are still ours. The latter is obviously what matters most to people who regard decisions about family life to be their own private affair. It does not seem to be troubling that our choices are conditioned in all sorts of ways—socially, culturally, economically, or fiscally—and that we are made to pay for their consequences in each of these ways. They still can be experienced as our own choices.[23]

If correct, it follows that many people in our society who believe in the right to free parental decision making would strongly object to the state directly intervening in individual reproductive choices. By 'direct intervention' I mean that the state goes beyond merely influencing the conditions and consequences of our choices and declares some of these choices illegal. This would be the case, for example, were the state to declare it illegal for a family to have more than one child. A legally enforceable termination of pregnancy in the case of every second child would surely count as a direct and very serious violation of individual liberty. Many people in liberal society would be horrified by public policies of this type—leaving aside the question as to whether they could be legal at all—even though they may at the same time accept tax laws that make a second child a costly affair. To be influenced in the material conditions of one's choices is one thing, to have one's choices outlawed is quite another.

If this reasoning reflects an important moral belief of many people in our society, then this will have important consequences for the question regarding the 'we' to whom the initial question of this chapter is addressed. Given this moral belief, people would definitely oppose large-scale policies of prevention such as, for example, making genetic testing and other kinds of prenatal diagnostics mandatory for every pregnancy. Supposedly, their opposition would be supported by the claim that citizens have a fundamental right to physical integrity. The democratic state is prohibited from prescribing that medical procedures be imposed upon its citizens unless there is a clear danger to public health, as in the case of epidemic diseases. As a matter of fact, a similar argument informed the opposition that forced many democratic states to remove from their penal codes laws prohibiting homosexual behavior between consenting adults. The same is true of laws that demanded the forced sterilization of 'genetically unhealthy' individuals.[24] The underlying principle for rejecting such laws is the right to physical and personal integrity.

If the assumptions in this section about the prevailing moral convictions and beliefs in our society are correct, then we can safely conclude that only very strong arguments, if any, will succeed in making a case for legal restrictions on reproductive choice.[25] That is, the state must adduce compelling arguments to declare illegal reproductive choices with regard to accepting or rejecting the birth of a disabled child. But to say that such arguments must be very strong is not to say that they are inconceivable. In fact such arguments may become quite conceivable if it were the case that unintended but harmful side effects can be anticipated from widespread genetic testing among the general population. If we can be reasonably sure that parental decisions regarding the birth of disabled children will have indirect consequences for the position of other people in society, then public policy may be called upon to address these consequences. In that case, to reconsider the range of reproductive freedom to which its citizens are entitled may become a conceivable option for the democratic state.

Let me summarize the argument in this section with the claim that, given some of our fundamental beliefs about individual freedom, the state does not have the right to enforce preventive strategies upon its citizens. Such would be an unacceptable intrusion into the private affairs of individual people. Furthermore, we may safely conclude that if the state does not have the right to enforce legal policies in this area, then nobody else in secular society has that right either. Combining this result with earlier ones we arrive at the following: from the point of view of public morality it is up to individual parents to decide whether they find it morally troubling to terminate the life of a fetus at an early stage of its development if the child is expected to be mentally handicapped. The right to reproductive freedom in junction with the widespread acceptance of abortion 'on demand' create the moral space to make these decisions.

3.7 Two Questions

Having spelled out how public morality specified by the liberal convention shapes our understanding of the moral issue of genetics and the prevention of disability, let me indicate how this inquiry will proceed from here. The various distinctions introduced in this chapter provide a more detailed background against which the argument will be developed. As was explained before, the inquiry will continue to argue from the point of view of public morality in our society and push the issue of genetics and the prevention of disability to the limits of what this public morality enables us to say about them. In the chapters to come we will investigate the kind of considerations that public morality in liberal society can bring to bear on answering the following two questions. The first is whether it can be argued that the proliferation of genetic testing may contribute to the discrimination of mentally disabled people and their families. The second question is whether or not such an argument, if it exists, is sufficiently strong to justify public policies aimed at the restriction of reproductive freedom. The analysis in this chapter suggested that (1) the option of preventing the birth of mentally disabled children in early pregnancy does not cause aggravating moral problems, given the convictions and beliefs of the liberal convention, but that (2) the restriction of parental freedom to exercise this option does create such problems. Sufficiently strong arguments to override parental freedom in this respect can only be generated by moral concerns that public morality in liberal society cannot possibly ignore. Eventually, the case for discriminatory side effects may warrant such a concern.

Before we start with the analysis of both questions, however, we will have to consider a preliminary objection. To suggest the possibility of discriminatory side effects one has to assume that genetic testing somehow sends a signal towards disabled people that their lives are valued negatively. Their kind of life being prevented because of its disabilities apparently means that their lives are not sufficiently worth living. But this assumption may be challenged. It is often denied that the practice of genetic testing is committed to negative evaluations of disabled people, particularly by medical people engaged in clinical genetics. "We are fighting genetic diseases," they say, "we are not fighting people with those diseases." Hence the objection that there is no relation whatsoever between the practice of clinical genetics and negative judgments on disabled lives. In the next chapter we will consider this preliminary objection in extensive detail.

FOUR

"The Condition, Not the Person"

> Any artificial attempt to split my child from his disability is dishonest, dissociatively psychotic, or without any knowledge of my child. It is like saying, "I like your child; its just his body, mind, and spirit that I don't like." David's disability is global. It is part of him just as much as his species or gender. It affects every aspect of his existence. It is not like a pair of shoes that he can take off. Without it, he would be a total stranger to me.
>
> *Dick Sobsey*

4.1 The Charge of Negative Evaluation

The diagnosis of a genetic disorder is often seen as entailing the prospect of a burdensome life. This indicates the moral meaning that modern medicine ascribes to it. People with disabilities and their families are believed to face a life that is filled with disappointment and distress, if not suffering and grief. Given this perception, using genetic testing procedures for reasons of prevention appears to be morally quite appropriate. Conception can be prevented, or, if a child has already been conceived, the option of terminating pregnancy presents itself as a 'last resort'.[1] If the test result is positive—indicating that there is a genetic disorder—the affected fetus can be aborted.

This approach to the use of gene technology is sometimes seen as a cause for alarm within the disability community. Advocacy organizations such as Inclusion International fear that using gene technology for reasons of prevention may reinforce negative attitudes toward disabled people in our society.[2] Likewise, feminist authors have argued that, apart from jeopardizing the reproductive rights of women, widespread genetic testing will affect the position of disabled persons in society.[3] Those who oppose its further proliferation fear that specific groups, such as the disabled, will suffer exclusion. They criticize the genetics approach to disability for having possible discriminatory effects.[4] In contrast, supporters of clinical genetics underscore the opportunities that the new technology offers to enhance reproductive choice and the quality of choice by means of more accurate information.[5] Their moral claim is that the prospect of a disabled child can justifiably be considered as dreadful if the disease will cause prolonged suffering for the child and the family.[6]

Despite the opposite conclusions of both these groups, the interesting point to notice is that both their positions are based on the same assumption. The assumption is that a genetics approach to disability is somehow committed to a negative evaluation of the lives of disabled people as lives full of suffering. The ethical debate on gene technology thus far has not paid much attention to this assumption.[7] This need not be a regrettable omission, however, because one can argue that the issue is not suffering but individual choice. That is to say, the question of how to respond to the risk of a genetic disorder is a question that concerns individual patients, their families and their physicians. The decisions these persons have to make are ones that affect their own private lives and the lives of their families. They do not involve the lives of other people, such as the disabled who are currently living in society. On this view, the supposed negative evaluation of disabled lives can be discarded as a red herring, because clinical genetics in no way is committed to this kind of judgment. There is no link whatsoever between the genetics approach and the view that it would be better if disabled people did not exist. Genetic counseling and screening are not about devaluating the lives of disabled people but about helping people who seek medical assistance with respect to reproductive choice.

This objection to the charge of negative evaluation—which has been briefly considered in the opening chapter[8]—raises a number of interesting questions that deserve careful analysis. Several of these questions focus on whether 'being disabled' is a medical condition or something else and perhaps much more. Even if it is argued that people in clinical genetics seek only to enhance the quality of reproductive choice by giving people reliable information rather than good advice, it remains true that the parameters of this information are dominated by medicine. From a medical perspective, the lives of disabled children appear as a problem that is to be treated. Thus it is not implausible to argue that, in one way or another, the practice of clinical genetics presupposes negative evaluations of disabled lives, regardless of whether individual counselors are making such judgments.[9]

One way to acquit the practice of clinical genetics of the charge of negative evaluation is to say that it is directed at the disabling results of genetic disorders. Preventing genetic disorders at a fetal stage is quite different from devaluating disabled persons once they exist. To suggest that it would be better if disabled people did not exist because of the suffering and grief in their lives is not to suggest that disabled people, once they exist, have no right to exist. Doctors do not combat disabled people, but they do combat genetic disorders that cause disabling conditions. This is how the Canadian bioethicist Eike H. Kluge makes the point:

> Saying that something is a handicap or saying that it would be better if we could prevent people from suffering from a particular handicap instead of trying to find ways to deal with after it has occurred, is not to say that those who suffer from the handicap are worthless as persons. Nor is it to brand them as second-class citizens. To say that something is a handicap is to say just that: that it is a handicap. This is not a comment about the person who suffers from the handicap but about the condition of that person.[10]

We thus encounter an argument that is based upon the distinction between the condition and the person. It says that genetic counseling and screening is directed at disorders and not at the persons living with these disorders. In the course of this chapter we will discuss several versions of this argument in order to see which of them, if any, succeeds. My conclusion will be that, although clinical geneticists may be right in rejecting the charge that they personally think negatively about the lives of disabled people, they are mistaken in the belief that the distinction between the person and the condition is sufficient to acquit their practice of this charge.[11]

4.2 The DPC Argument

Let me begin by returning to the distinction between disease and disability that was introduced in the previous chapter. The former is distinct from the latter, I stipulated, in that a disease is a physiological, psychological, or anatomical disfunction, while a disability (or handicap) signifies the social consequences of a disease.[12] Furthermore, disease is distinct from illness. An illness is indicated by the presence of clinical symptoms such as pain, fatigue, or fever, which is not necessarily true in the case of a disease. Finally, impairment was defined as a disease that has clinical symptoms but does not develop into an illness.

These distinctions, one should remember, allowed us to separate two types of cases. While all genetic disorders are to be classified as diseases, some of them will develop into illnesses, while others will only develop into impairments. Conditions in both classes can—and often do—have social consequences that amount to a handicap or disability. But this occurs for quite different reasons. In some cases the disability stems from the fact that the person is incapacitated due to illness. She is simply too weak or too frail to participate in social activities such as education or employment. In other cases, however, the disability stems from a different source, namely a lack in capacity for 'normal' social functioning. The person in question, though in reasonable good health and condition, is incapable of performing certain tasks that are valued in our culture. In this type of case the disability is informed by the standards of normality maintained in society. This conceptual point enables us to distinguish between two different moral questions regarding the issue of genetics and the prevention of disability. The first is: Should we prevent lives that will be handicapped because they suffer from severe illness? The second question is: Should we prevent lives that will be handicapped because of societal standards of normal functioning?[13]

It is important to see that, in pressing the charge of negative evaluation, people often appear to have in mind disabled lives characterized by impairment rather than illness. That is, they seem to argue from the type of case where the limitations posed by the disability is not caused by suffering from pain or exhaustion. People with impairments can actually feel quite well and enjoy their lives. A well-known example is presented by people from the deaf community who say that for them being deaf is a part of their personal identity which they value positively.[14] Their argument is that to prevent deafness is to prevent people whose identity is shaped by their deafness.[15] This view can be extended to other conditions as well. For example, Down syndrome is a condition with which one can learn to live, particularly when supported by so called 'early intervention programs'. It is quite possible for people with Down syndrome to have a happy life if society provides them with the means to do so. To prevent the life of a child with this syndrome is—on this view—to express a desire for a 'normal' child, one that is capable of normal functioning.

Apparently the critics of the genetics approach to disability argue from a different type of case in which genetic disorders are seen as analogous to conditions such as, for example, schizophrenia. Schizophrenia creates schizophrenics. It is not possible to suffer from schizophrenia without being a schizophrenic, that is, without having the personality of a schizophrenic, as one can suffer from pneumonia without being a 'pneumoniac'. In cases such as schizophrenia, the one implies the other. In the same way one cannot have Down syndrome without having the particular characteristics of people with that syndrome. The advocates of clinical genetics, in contrast, seem to argue from cases in which genetic disorders do create a life full of suffering, as, for example, cystic fybrosis. In this type of case it can be plausibly argued that the patients suffering from these disorders experience a seriously diminished quality of life.

The point of this analogy is to suggest that these examples help us to see how the controversy is fueled by different moral perceptions of genetic disorders and their relation to diseases and disabilities. The claim that is advanced by the critics of the genetics approach—a disability is not a disease—indicates the evaluation of genetic disorders from a social perspective regarding the 'normal' and the 'abnormal', rather than from a medical perspective regarding illness and disease. From their point of view the genetics approach reflects and reinforces the medicalization of disability. Accordingly, the International League of Societies for Persons with Mental Handicaps writes:

> There is a danger that genetic research and new reproductive technology could frustrate the progress made in achieving rights for people with disabilities by diverting attention away from handicapping social and systemic barriers. When a disability is detected in a fetus through prenatal diagnosis, abortion is frequently the recommended *therapeutic* course of action. The view of disability is so negative and knowledge of the capacities and abilities of people with disabilities so limited that the presence of a disability is seen to overpower any positive qualities there might be in living with a disability. (*Just Technology?*, 14–15)

Having prepared the ground for the discussion let us now turn to the argument against the charge of negative evaluation of disabled lives introduced in the first section. The argument says that, because of the distinction between the person and the condition, combatting genetic disease does not entail a negative evaluation of someone with that disease. Clearly, the argument has a strong intuitive force. At least, it seems that the distinction between the person and the condition is generally accepted with regard to other medical conditions. We fight cancer; we do not fight people with cancer. If research to eliminate cancer does not imply an attitude that supports discrimination against persons who suffer from this disease, why should clinical genetics be different? Like all other diagnostic and therapeutic interventions, clinical genetics is also directed at the condition and not at the people suffering from it.[16] We use diagnostic tests to detect heart failure caused by coronary arterial sclerosis, but no one takes this to imply that in using these techniques we are devaluing the lives of persons suffering from coronary disease.

Let us call this argument the 'Distinction between the Person and the Condition' (DPC) argument. The DPC argument is important particularly from the point of view of the medical profession. Doctors and other professionals working in genetics fight diseases, they do not fight people. Accordingly, clinical geneticists are dedicated to alleviating conditions of suffering. The charge of negative evaluation is completely unjustified, therefore. It is based on the false identification of persons with their conditions. Is this a valid argument?

4.3 Actual and Future People

There is an obvious rejoinder to this argument which states that the analogy between conditions such as cancer and Down syndrome does not work. We use diagnostic tests in oncology to detect and combat cancer, but killing a lethal tumor with chemotherapy is not exactly the same as killing a fetus with Down syndrome.[17] While the former is adequately called a malignancy, the latter is no less adequately called a potential human being. Furthermore, the fact that in previous times people with Down syndrome were called names such as 'moron' or 'idiot' is in itself sufficient to suggest that they have been perceived as a particular kind of people. Even if such labels are rejected as inappropriate, it is still the case that a large majority of people with Down syndrome are viewed as sharing the same kind of personality.[18] Finally and most importantly, the DPC argument can be rebutted by claiming that, with very few exceptions, the genetic diseases that are currently known can be 'treated' only by eliminating the fetuses that are affected. In actual practice the distinction between persons and their conditions remains inconsequential, therefore.

Apparently the DPC argument requires further explanation if it is to be accepted as valid. One attempt to do so is to invoke the distinction between future people and actual people. Clinical geneticists work with people who have to decide about their future children. Since these children do not yet exist, the use of technology to prevent them from being born can in no way affect their lives. Nor can it affect the lives of people with the same disorders who already exist. These people are persons with a name and a personal history who are included in the social networks that constitute the lives of individuals in society. Nothing of the sort can be true about future people. Decisions about such people are decisions about admittance to life; they are not decisions about lives already underway. Accordingly, a decision to abort a fetus affected by Down syndrome has no implications whatsoever for existing children with that syndrome. Nothing follows from that decision with regard to the issues of mainstreaming these children in education, job coaching, independent living, or respecting their rights as citizens. The conclusion must be that existing persons with disabilities are in no way involved in the use of gene technology for prevention.

This explanation indicates a second version of the DPC argument, which runs as follows. The genetics approach to disability cannot logically imply negative evaluations of the lives of disabled people. The reason for this is that genetics is directed at the prevention of diseases in people who do not yet exist. Existing people cannot be the target of prevention, while nonexisting people cannot be the object of negative evaluation. The genetics approach aims at preventing disorders of future people, it is not directed at actual people with those disorders who already exist.

4.4 Evaluating Other People's Lives

Insofar as clinical genetics aims at prevention, the lives of actual people cannot fall within the range of that objective. So much is clear. But this explanation will not silence the worries of the critics of clinical genetics. Even when the lives of actual people with disabilities are not the object of prevention, this does not at all mean that the lives of these people are not implicated. The second DPC argument appears to overlook the reasons in favor of decisions to prevent the birth of a disabled child. Let us take as an example trisomy 21, the chromosomal abormality that causes Down syndrome. Let us consider someone who faces the decision whether to accept or reject a child with that syndrome. Clearly, anybody who faces this decision needs some basis for arguing for or against having a such child. Obviously, the required basis is provided by a judgment about what one believes life with Down syndrome or with a child with this syndrome to be. It seems that the only way to arrive at this judgment is to look and see what such a life is like. In other words, one needs to be informed about what one can expect from living such a life or from living with a child with Down syndrome. The question then is: What source provides the required information and how can that source be established as adequate? The answer to this question must be that—unless one is satisfied in relying on myth and prejudice—there is no other way than to look at the lives of actual people with Down syndrome and then ask oneself whether or not one would want to live that kind of life or be involved in it.

This indicates why the second version of the DPC argument is unconvincing. The question is on what basis do we decide to prevent a life with a particular genetic disorder if not on the basis of information about the lives of actual people with the same disorder? In that sense it must be true that a decision to prevent a life with that disorder exemplifies a negative view of the lives of people who are actually living with it. Without such a view this decision would fail to make sense.

This is not the end of the DPC argument, however, for there is yet another line of defense. It is similar to the second version in the sense that it is also based on a distinction between two different modes of being. Only this time the difference is not between actual and future but between me and other. It can be argued that we can only judge our lives from 'the inside'.[19] If this is true, there must be some mistake in the rationality of the decision to accept or reject a child with Down syndrome, as it was presented above. Since we cannot subjectively know what the lives of other people mean for these people themselves, we are mistaken in thinking that *their* account of *their* lives gives *us* a reason to decide about our *own* life or that of our children. Evaluations of the meaning and value of life are necessarily 'first person'. Reasons for preventing the birth of a disabled child are internal to what people think about their own lives. They cannot—logically cannot—be reasons inferred from other people's lives.

Does this attempt to defend a modified second version of the DPC argument hold? It does not, because there is no need at all to make the move that is criticized by this defense. We do not need to presuppose insight into what other people's lives mean to them. Let me explain. In order to judge the life of person P I need not be able to step outside my own first person point of view and step into the other person's shoes and see what P's life means to *her*. The relevant question is not what the life of P means to her but what her kind of life would mean to me if it were mine. In evaluating a life like P's, I am not evaluating it from her own perspective, nor am I trying to assess it in any objective manner. I make a judgment from my own point of view, based on what I know about her life. Consequently, the judgment is not at all based on a comparison between x seen from the 'first-person' point of view of P_1 and x seen from the 'first-person' point of view of P_2. The comparison that matters is a different one. It is a comparison between two different versions of *my* own life, that is, a comparison between x and y both seen from the 'first-person' point of view of P. The question I need to ask is what I would judge my life now to be and what I judge my life to be were it to have the relevant features of the life I am evaluating.[20] The question of which features to select as relevant depends on what I take to be crucially important in my present life. A negative evaluation of particular features of the life of P is the necessary condition for the conclusion that I do not want a life like hers or to have a child with that kind of life.

Even if the above is true, however, it still does not seal the fate of the DPC argument. The distinction between persons and their conditions may reappear in yet another version. The following example may serve to suggest how. Fragile X is a genetic disorder that causes mild to severe developmental disabilities.[21] The genetic location of this disorder is well known, but as yet there is no therapy available even though theoretically the principle of such therapy has been clarified. Removing the gene (DNA) that induces the production of the deficient protein and injecting the appropriate material so that the right protein is produced in the right amount would count as a genetic therapy. If this therapy could be used, one would no longer have to choose between accepting a child with fragile X or having the fetus aborted. Instead, one could choose to have the same child, genetically speaking, but without the syndrome. Who would not want that?

The third version of the DPC argument thus amounts to this. It cannot be denied that preventing children with a genetic disorder from being born by aborting them in their fetal stage is, in a sense, killing potential people with disabilities. This is only true, however, because of the use of gene technology in combination with abortion. But this combination is not necessary. Once scientists become successful in developing gene therapy, the situation will change dramatically. At that time, the analogy with other diseases, such as cancer, will finally obtain. We will then be able to eliminate genetic disorders without eliminating the persons whose lives are affected by these disorders. In other words, the moral evil resides in abortion and not in clinical genetics. The distinction between the person and the condition will at last hold for all those genetic disorders for which therapeutic treatment is conceivable in the future. Here is how this view was expressed by an American NIH task force more than twenty years ago:

> The techniques of prenatal diagnosis are not, except in very few instances, associated with any medical therapies for the alleviation of the diagnosed disorder. Many leaders in the development of this technology recognize this as unsatisfactory. They affirm that studies of the etiology of genetic and hereditary disorders are of the greatest importance and that, based on knowledge of etiology, therapeutic measures must be developed. Thus, prenatal diagnosis, while presently most often associated with the choice of abortion, is not intrinsically linked to abortion.[22]

When gene therapy becomes a real option, the charge that the use of gene technology for prevention implies a negative evaluation of disabled persons will no longer obtain. Children treated with gene therapy will remain genetically the same, but without their disabilities.

4.5 Disability and Identity

This third version of the DPC argument looks very strong, but there is a remaining worry. To see what the worry is, we need to switch from a first-person to an impersonal point of view. Suppose someone were to ask us how we would feel about having a disabled child as opposed to having a nondisabled one. From an impersonal point of view, it is clear that people would prefer the latter. Thus we would say, "Of course, I would rather have a healthy child!" The point here is that from this impersonal point of view there cannot be a personal relation between ourselves and the imagined child. If the question is asked in general— "Would you rather have a child with or without a genetic disorder x?"—then the answer appears to be fairly obvious. Personal relations being absent, it is rational to prefer a child without a genetic disorder. But this preference becomes much less obvious once we shift back to the personal point of view of parents who are actually living with a disabled child. To them, the question means something different, namely: Would you rather have your own disabled child or a child without her disabling condition? The difference between the two questions can best be explained by a point about the connection between disability and identity.[23]

In this connection parents of disabled children often express the following dilemma. On the one hand, they claim that they would not want to miss their present child because of what it has to give, not in spite of, but with its disability.[24] On the other hand, they say that had there been a choice before their child was born, they probably would have decided not to have it. As a parent of a disabled child one appears to be caught in the paradox of not wanting to miss a child that one nevertheless would not have chosen.[25]

On a closer look, however, we will see that there is no real paradox here. The first thing these parents say is that had they been given the choice without knowing who this child would be, they probably would have chosen not to have it. The second thing they say is that now that they know about their life with this child they do not want to miss it. This suggests that the fact of sharing the life they live together makes all the difference. Accordingly, the remaining worry about the third version of the DPC argument is that it reduces the parental perspective on a disabled child to an impersonal point of view.

To explore this suggestion, let us consider the case of James, who is a young man with fragile X. Suppose we put this question to James's parents: If your son could be cured, would you not prefer to have him without fragile X? What could James's parents say by way of response? Not much, I am afraid. A reasonable answer would be that the question is not only hypothetical but also false. Of course they would want to have James without fragile X, except for the fact that he then would no longer be James. James is who he is because of his fragile X syndrome. His identity cannot be distinguished from the bodily existence that is characterized by his genetic condition. It is therefore mistaken to suggest a hypothetical choice between James with and James without fragile X. His parents cannot step outside their relationship with James and ask themselves whether they would have preferred *this boy* without his disability. They cannot possibly answer this question without denying their relationship with him, that is, without denying who they actually are. For them, it is a question without an answer.

To this rejoinder the defender of the DPC argument has a subtle response, however. He may say that the mistake stems from the fact that we put the wrong question. We should have asked James's parents this: Had there been a choice at the time *before* James's birth, would you have chosen to have him without rather than with fragile X? To this question his parents would have no problem answering what appears to be a perfectly sensible question. Their answer would be that, of course, they would have chosen a child without fragile X. But it should be noticed that this alternative question presents them with a very different choice. The question of whether they would have chosen a child without rather than with fragile X prior to James's birth is a question about *any* child. It cannot possibly be a question about James because they could not possibly have chosen James at that point of time. It follows that the alternative question cannot corroborate the version of the DPC argument that we are considering here.

To conclude, the third version of the DCP argument states that with the arrival of gene therapy the distinction between persons and their conditions will hold true in clinical genetics, just as it does in other medical disciplines such as oncology. As the analysis in this section has shown, however, this claim raises a problem about the connection between disability and identity. From the personal point of view of parents whose identity has been shaped by their lives with a disabled child, the two cannot be so easily separated. One cannot expect these parents to answer questions as to whether they would rather have had *their* child without a disability without alienating them from *that* child.[26] From an impersonal point of view, on the other hand, one may expect parents to say that, of course, preceding any relationship they would have preferred a life without a disabled child. If they were to apply this judgment to their present lives, however, then they would in fact do what the DPC argument wants to deny. For in that case they would be rejecting their life with their present child because of what that child is.

4.6 The Fallacy of Geneticization

There is a final point to be considered. The analysis in the previous section supported the notion of a connection between disability and identity. Put more generally, this notion presupposes an inextricable link between mental and physical aspects of our personal identity. In answering questions such as Who am I?, Who is she?, and so on, we do not only refer to mental states. Persons are not only their minds but also their bodies. Much of what we think about ourselves is rooted in the kind of bodies we are. Personal identity does not even begin with mental states. It starts to develop in the context of our physical existence from the moment of our birth. We become who we are because of the bodies we are, that is, because others respond to our bodily existence in its subsequent stages. In the response of others, starting with our mothers, we become caught up in the web of socio-cultural meanings that constitutes the world in which we grow up. From the very beginning these meanings are produced in the interaction between ourselves as bodies, on the one hand, and our socio-cultural environment, on the other.

It is in this context that the genetics approach to disability provokes the issue of the so-called fallacy of geneticization. Geneticization is a cultural process in which the expanding knowledge about genetic dispositions reinforces the strength of biological and medical paradigms in the explanation of social phenomena.[27] Let me quote once again the ILSPMH: "In its application to people with disabilities, geneticization may perpetuate and reinforce the traditional view of disability as a medical concern. Language such as 'defect', 'abnormality' and 'congenital malformation' is sometimes used to describe fetuses in which a disability has been detected. This frames disability in the context of individual pathology, rather than in a social context" (*Just Technology*, 11). In previous times the fallacy of geneticization—or biological derterminism—has led people to believe that socially and culturally based differences between human beings could ultimately be explained by genetics. As Robert Proctor has observed:

> Among all the potential dangers of human genomics, to my mind the most all-encompassing is the danger of its confluence with a growing trend toward biological determinism. Biological determinism is the view that the large part of human talents and disabilities—perhaps even our tastes and institutions—is anchored in our biology. . . . Genes have become a near-universal scapegoat for all that ails the human species. Even where genetic influence is well established, critics worry that aggressive promoting of genetic testing may generate fears out of proportion to actual risks. In the rush to identify genetic components to cancer or heart disease or mental illness, the substantial environmental origins of those afflictions may be slighted.[28]

The mistake of geneticization is to infer from the claim that our identity develops on the basis of our genetic makeup the further claim that our identity must therefore be an expression of our genes. This inference is false because personal identity in the sense used in this connection is a psychological and social construct *in response* to our bodily features, which are caused by our genetic dispositions. This is not to deny that our genes determine many of our prospects in life, but this fact cannot be separated from the further fact that we can respond to them in different ways.[29]

The question is whether the DPC argument in its third version can be said to commit the fallacy of geneticization. If the argument is that gene therapy will eventually give people the option of having their child cured of a genetic disorder while remaining the same child, then that argument would be fallacious, because social responses to the conditions in each case would have been very different. One could not even argue that they would remain genetically the same, because some of the genetic makeup would have to be changed in order to remove the disabling condition.

Presumably, defenders of the DPC argument will argue that I am overlooking a crucial point here, which is the fact that gene therapy would be carried out at the fetal stage. Since James in that case would not yet be a member of the social world, he could not have developed a personal identity that extends beyond his biological characteristics. Consequently, the fallacy of geneticization does not apply. This response is fair enough, but unfortunately it takes us back to the point of the previous section. As we saw there, the DPC argument failed because none of our hypothetical questions to James's parents could make the distinction between the person and the condition in any significant way. We could have asked them (1) Would you rather have had James than another child even if that child would have been another person? To this question they may respond negatively, assuming their personal point of view ("We would not want to have missed our life with this boy"). Or they may respond positively ("We regret the life we had to live with this disabled child"). In neither case is there a distinction between the person and the condition. We also could have asked them an alternative question, which is (2) Would you rather have chosen a healthy child rather than a child with fragile X syndrome? This question could not possibly refer to James but only to an unidentified child, indicating again that the distinction fails. While the first question makes a distinction between a known person and an unknown one, the second makes a distinction between an unknown healthy child and an unknown disabled one. However, what we cannot—logically cannot—ask is (3) Would you rather have James with or without fragile X? This third question does make use of the distinction between the person and his condition, but it fails to make sense from a personal point of view. Neither James nor his parents exist as the people they are outside their relationship with one another. Given that the question about James with or without his genetic disorder does not make sense, the conclusion must be that the DPC argument in its third version fails.

Clearly, this conclusion does not settle in any definite way the issue of whether the use of genetic testing for reasons of prevention presupposes a negative evaluation of disabled lives. It does so only provisionally. Since the various versions of the DPC argument seem to present the strongest case against this presuppostion, however, the burden of proof is once again on those who reject it. The remaining conclusion must be that any attempt to distance the practices of prevention from negative judgments about the lives of disabled people is bound to fail, because it deprives such practices of the only rational grounds that people can have for pursuing them.

4.7 What Are Clinical Geneticists Doing?

Let us move onward to consider the moral implications of what has been argued so far. Are those involved in prevention rightly accused of judging negatively about the lives of disabled people? The answer to this question must be yes and no. The reason for the affirmative answer has already been given: the genetics approach to disability is inevitably based on evaluative assumptions regarding disabled lives, otherwise there would be no rational grounds to justify the strategies of prevention that it produces. Presumably, people involved in clinical genetics will argue that I have misrepresented their practice, because in principle it has nothing to do with prevention. Clinical genetics is primarily about reproductive choice. Its most important aim is to enable people who are at risk to make responsible decisions with regard to their own offspring by providing them with adequate diagnostic information and risk assessment.[30]

I will respond to this objection by saying that the justification of clinical genetics cannot possibly succeed only on the basis of the principle of reproductive choice. Society does not allow us absolute freedom in any area of social life. Individual freedom is necessarily balanced against other goods. Even in the case of highly personal decisions, such as the decision to have an abortion, our freedom to decide for ourselves is restricted (e.g., to a particular stage of fetal development). Free choice, therefore, is always restricted to publicly acceptable uses of freedom. The claim to reproductive freedom by itself is not sufficient, just as the wish to have one's pregnancy terminated is not sufficient.[31] Consequently, if society accepts the prevention of disability as justified, it is because and only because it is regarded as a legitimate use of individual freedom. Since freedom cannot be the sufficient reason, there are other reasons that explain why prevention is the publicly accepted goal of those who make use of the services offered by clinical genetics, even if it is not the professed goal of those offering these services. It is difficult to see how these other reasons could be independent of the judgments about disabled lives. Our society considers prevention to be morally acceptable.

Having looked at this side of the issue, we now have to consider the other side. From the point of view of the medical profession, the charge of negative evaluation is clearly unjustified. Doctors can rightly complain that their moral integrity is violated by this accusation inasmuch as they are committed to helping people to combat disease. Obviously the intention to help is not an intention to do wrong. Needless to say, members of the medical profession who deserve public esteem for the intention of helping their patients are entitled to that esteem.

To make the point philosophically, we need to think about how intention is involved in an account of what doctors are doing. A doctor who provides a pregnant woman with a prenatal test that enables her to decide for herself whether or not to have a handicapped child can be doing a variety of things. That doctor is carrying out her medical duty, earning a salary, combatting a disease that causes her patient to suffer, pursuing a career, using medical equipment, serving her client, performing an experiment, respecting the patient's right to decide, contributing to cost containment of medical care for disabled persons, trying to expand her hospital's share of the market, and so on. Obviously, some of these descriptions are more relevant to a moral evaluation of what this doctor is doing than others. However, no morally relevant description of what an agent does can ignore what the agent herself intends to be doing without undermining the very possibility of moral agency. Assuming this to be correct, professionals who intend to help their patients are justified in saying that their integrity is violated by the charge of negative evaluation of disabled lives. Since the notion of integrity necessarily refers to reasons on the basis of which we act, the reasons clinical geneticists have for doing their work cannot be irrelevant. Their practice is justified within the context of the doctor-patient relationship. Disabled people in society are not part of that relationship. From the point of view of the medical profession, therefore, the charge of negative evaluation can arguably be rejected. But seen in the wider context of a society that allows, if not endorses, its practices—a context that includes existing people with disabilities—this charge is not invalid and needs to be addressed.

This conclusion takes us back to the point where we left the argument at the end of chapter 3. As we proceed, the tougher questions regarding this wider social and political context cannot be avoided. Not only will we have to think for ourselves about decisions to prevent the life of a disabled child which other people think are morally justified, but also about how we think the state should respond toward decisions that we believe to be morally unjustifiable. Does the right to reproductive freedom imply that we as a political community may accept choices that we as individuals may believe to be morally objectionable? In other words; do we accept the right to do wrong? Or do we as a political community want to impose limits regarding what is morally permissible upon the right to parental choice, and if so, what are these limits and how do we justify them?

My own suspicion is that our public morality—which is the political morality of liberalism—will have a hard time providing adequate justifications for the restriction of reproductive choice, even when it has strong reasons for considering such a policy. Among the more curious aspects of our public morality with regard to disabled persons is its apparent incoherence. On the one hand, it supports full citizenship for the disabled in order to realize their inclusion in society. This commitment is justified by one of the pillars of liberal morality, e.g., the right to equal opportunity. On the other hand, it is committed to the right to reproductive freedom that includes the freedom to prevent a child with a disability from being born. It is not easy to see how public morality in liberal society can keep the balance between both of these commitments. While one can see why they both can be considered morally justifiable when taken separately, it is not so easy to see how they can be considered thus when taken together.

FIVE

Disability, Prevention, and Discrimination

If a society were even partially successful in "eliminating" retardation, how would it regard those who have become retarded? Since retardation was eliminated on grounds of being an unacceptable way of being human, would the retarded who remain live in a society able to recognize the validity of their existence and willing to provide the care they require? Of course it might be suggested that with fewer retarded there would be more resources for the care of those remaining. That is no doubt true, but the question is whether there would be the moral will to direct those resources in their direction. Our present resources are more than enough to provide good care for the retarded. That we do not provide such care can be attributed to a lack of moral will and imagination. What will and imagination there is comes from those who have found themselves unexpectedly committed to care for a retarded person through birth or relation. Remove that and I seriously doubt whether our society will find the moral convictions necessary to sustain our alleged commitment to the retarded.

Stanley Hauerwas

I desire to be understood and recognized, even if this means to be unpopular and disliked. And the only persons who can so recognize me, and thereby give me the sense of being someone, are the members of the society to which . . . I feel I belong. My individual self is not something which I can detach from my relationship with others, or from those attributes of myself which consist in their attitude towards me. Consequently, when I demand to be liberated from, let us say, the status of political or social dependence, what I demand is an alteration of the attitude towards me of those whose opinions and behaviour help to determine my own image of myself.

Sir Isaiah Berlin

5.1 Negative Side Effects?

Assuming that negative evaluations of disabled lives cannot be denied as a necessary presupposition for employing genetic testing for reasons of prevention, the next question is how this affects the position of the disabled in our society. Reasons for avoiding the birth of a handicapped child will refer primarily to what we think such a life will entail for the child or for its parents and other siblings. In either case a rational justification involves passing negative judgments on lives characterized by similar handicaps. The question to be considered in this chapter is whether the fact that genetic testing presupposes these judgments contributes to the discrimination against the disabled. We need to ask whether using genetics for reasons of prevention may affect the social position of the disabled in such a way that their interests are seriously damaged either now or in the near future.

Introducing this question indicates that in this chapter we will consider the effects of genetic testing on 'third parties'. In many areas of social life the decisions people make affect other people's lives in ways that may be neither intended nor foreseen but are nevertheless a matter of serious concern for public policy. Recent legislation against smoking in public areas as well as against advertisements for tobacco products are examples of this concern. That people who smoke in public areas may inadvertently damage other people's health as well as their own is considered a sufficient reason for restricting the freedom to smoke in public. Advertisements for tobacco products aim at converting smoking adults to a new brand of cigarettes, or so it is argued by the industry, but at the same time these advertisements may induce young people to become smokers. In having this side effect advertising for tobacco can be potentially damaging to their health. Consequently, public policy infringes upon the freedom of tobacco companies to advertise. The negative side effects of our actions upon other people may induce public policy to restrict our freedom. By analogy we can ask whether or not the use of procedures for genetic testing may have side effects that make it an appropriate matter of public concern.

The analogy with legislation against the tobacco industry is useful because it reminds us of the fact that society has accepted the principle of assigning responsibility for side effects that affect other people both directly and indirectly.

Advertising tobacco products by using culturally established symbols is a way of influencing people's choices. In contrast, blowing smoke into their lungs does not influence their choice but directly damages their health. The proliferation of genetic testing may have similar effects as advertising in that it influences people's reproductive choices. Even if this is still a far cry from showing that genetic testing for reasons of prevention betrays discriminatory behavior, the analogy suggests that we look at the possible indirect side effects of the prevention of disability and see whether or not they should be a matter of concern for public policy. Once it is clear in what sense and how these side effects may occur, the question as to their practical implications cannot be avoided.

In pursuing the issue of discrimination I will distinguish between discriminatory attitudes that are expressed in personal and informal social relations, on the one hand, and discriminatory actions in the context of institutions such as health care insurance and the labor market, on the other. Discriminatory attitudes cause the victims to feel that they are not respected. Such attitudes reflect a cultural atmosphere that divides people into them and us. It is in this kind of atmosphere that the seeds are sewn for discriminatory actions that infringe upon institutional rights and opportunities. With regard to the context of informal social relations, I will start by developing a distinction between two types of reasons to which people may appeal in passing judgments on disabled lives. This maneuver may appear to be a cumbersome detour, but I hope to show that it is not. Discrimination is grounded conceptually in the fact that particular people are treated differently for particular reasons. But not all ways of treating people differently are sufficient to warrant the charge of discrimination. To preclude people from jobs requiring high technical skills because they lack these skills is not discriminatory in a morally relevant way. Precluding them because they belong to a particular ethnic minority is discriminatory because ethnic membership per se does not affect their job performance in the way that the lack of skills does. Consequently, discriminatory behavior is connected with the reasons people have for their actions. Therefore we will have to ask what reasons we can have for passing judgments on the lives of disabled people.

5.2 Two Types of Reasons

In facing reproductive decisions of the kind we are considering, to what sorts of reasons do parents appeal to ground their decisions? Clearly, this question must be addressed before we can say anything about the discriminatory aspects of the use of genetic testing. Parental decisions aiming at prevention can be grounded in two distinct types of reasons. In facing such situations, parents may ask how having a disabled child will affect the quality of their lives. But not all people believe that this is the appropriate question to ask. Grounding parental decisions in reasons based on 'quality of life' is only one possibility. The other is to ground them in reasons based on moral standing. Let us refer to these types of reasons as QL reasons and MS reasons respectively.[1] There are a number of differences between these two types of reasons, the most salient of which is the fact that QL reasons are prospective, whereas MS reasons are classificatory. The former are based on what parents expect life with a genetic disorder will entail for their child and for themselves as the parents of this child. These reasons concern the question of when a human life qualifies as a good or meaningful life. QL reasons are reasons that refer to states of experiences such as satisfaction and disappointment or joy and sorrow. In contrast, MS reasons do not refer to states of experiences in which we may find ourselves but to classifications relative to conceptions of what kinds of beings are worthy of our moral consideration. Their classificatory nature serves the function of inclusion or exclusion. Put somewhat crudely, reasons based on moral standing tell us whether or not particular beings should be included in our moral lives. MS reasons are expressed in statements such as; "handicapped or not, it is still your child," "people incapable of self-consciousness are vegetables, not real human beings," or "whoever is born of a human being is a human being."

Statements such as these reflect people's moral convictions and beliefs about the standing of disabled children. To act upon such beliefs is what Derek Parfit calls 'to act subjectively rational'.[2] QL reasons are not rational in that same sense. They are objectively rational, that is, they are derived from states of affairs expected to become true at some point in time. People who decide to prevent the birth of a disabled child on the ground of QL reasons may think, for example, that having such a child will lead them into a state of misery during the years to come because of the constant worries about the child's medical condition. They do not think that they will *believe* themselves to be in a state of misery at that time. In this sense QL reasons are grounded in judgments concerning expectations of future states of affairs. Such reasons are prospective. MS reasons, in contrast, do not concern future states of affairs but matters of moral belief. They tell us where and how to draw the boundaries of our moral community. Such reasons do not refer to states of experiences but assign moral 'titles'. This function implies that reasons of this type are categorical. A judgment of the kind "disabled or not, it is still your own child" demands either confirmation or rejection. Reasons based on moral standing reflect a moral taxonomy that guides us in discerning the proper 'nature' of the case, which explains why they do not leave room for something in between.[3]

To clarify a bit further the distinction between these types of reasons, we can ask how are they related. For example, QL reasons do not merely concern future states of affairs but also signify preferences about these states of affairs.

Parents not only express what they expect from the future but also what they hope or fear. How are these preferences related to MS reasons? Let us proceed to answer this question by means of an example. Suppose a religious woman who has had a prenatal test is now facing the prospect of giving birth to a child with Down syndrome. She strongly believes that children are a gift from God and that this also includes children with this disorder as well. However, she is aware at the same time of the many difficulties that living with such a child may entail. Given her preference for a happy future with a healthy baby, is there a way to decide rationally between her religious moral belief and her preference for a healthy baby? One way is to take her belief as just another preference and try to balance the weight of the one against the other.[4] Suppose that she stands back, reflects calmly upon both preferences, weighs the odds and then arrives at the conclusion: "I feel less miserable about abandoning my belief than about the prospect of having to carry the burden of living with a child with Down syndrome." If we assume her religious moral belief to be both firm and honest, however, the most likely result is that her decision will produce in her a feeling of remorse. To treat one's convictions and beliefs as preferences seems to betray a lack of integrity. Accordingly, we might say that a moral belief that is weighed as if it were a preference cannot have been firm and honest in the first place. The choice in this example is different from the choice between, say, staying at home with your lover or going away for a trip to the mountains with a friend. Facing this choice you may decide that, since you feel more attracted to the former, that must be the stronger preference. Of course, you may regret that you cannot do both, but this is simply how things are. But suppose that you had in fact promised your friend that you would join her on a mountain trip. It is unlikely that you could decide with the same equanimity to stay home with your lover, assuming your belief that promises ought to be kept. In the same sense, it is unlikely that the woman in our example could decide with equanimity to override her religious belief and have her pregnancy terminated. Assuming, as we do, that her belief is a firm and honest belief, she will not merely feel regret, but remorse or even guilt.[5] If she decides to override her belief, she will incur a value judgment upon her own act that does not signify a missed opportunity of preference satisfaction but she will blame herself for her failure to act according to what she deeply believes to be true about the moral standing of disabled children.[6]

5.3 Discrimination and Exclusion

Having distinguished these two types of reasons, I will now turn to the issue of discrimination. In view of the proliferation of genetic testing in our society the issue arises in at least two different contexts. The first is the context of insurance and employment. Once genetic information becomes available to insurance companies and employers, will people who are predisposed to genetic disease be barred from access to medical care and the labor market? This question evokes a discussion of institutional frameworks and regulations for just distribution to which we will turn in the next section. Here I will address the second context, which is that of personal and informal behavior. Husbands who treat their wives in a degrading way are charged with discriminatory behavior, as are students who exclude colleagues from ethnic minorities from their peer groups. Discriminatory behavior of this kind does not affect people's opportunities in a direct sense, as is the case in the institutional context of insurance and employment. But it does betray an attitude that is experienced as degrading by those who are discriminated against. Discriminatory attitudes make us feel as if we are outcasts, as people whose feelings about themselves do not matter. Discriminatory behavior in this sense is often implicit and inarticulate—not so much a matter of policy as a matter of attitude. Is this kind of discriminatory behavior relevant to the use of genetic testing for reasons of prevention?

In answering this question we will first consider reasons based on moral standing. If parents are considering the prospect of having a disabled child, reasons based on moral standing inform us about how they view such a child. MS reasons justify judgments about whether disabled children are regarded as 'normal' or 'abnormal', that may have exclusionary force. The question of whether the use of genetics to prevent their existence is one further way of excluding them from the moral community must be taken seriously, therefore. The fact that we are concerned with the prevention of *mentally* disabled children in particular makes consideration of this kind of reason all the more important.

Throughout human history people with mental disabilities have been victims of discrimination and exclusion in various ways because they were regarded as 'abnormal'. Any major struggle against discrimination in recent history has been a struggle against judgments grounded in reasons of this type. Discriminatory views inappropriately justify instances of unequal treatment of particular people. Presumably, many people in our society do consider mental disability to be a characteristic that appropriately warrants unequal treatment. Given the ideal of independent living as grounded in the capacity for individuality that is strongly disseminated in liberal culture, many people with mental disability fail to live up to that ideal because they are incapable of pursuing their own lives without guidance by other persons. In view of this ideal, these people must appear as defective agents who are permanently 'incompetent'. That is to say, they do not qualify as members of the class of competent agents that constitute the moral community of free and independent human beings. If the characteristic of mental disability is a sufficient warrant for this judgment, we seem to have a moral reason for the justification of unequal treatment.

Of course, the fact that many people in our society subscribe to this view on mental disability—if that is a fact—is not by itself sufficient to settle the issue of discriminatory attitudes. What we need is a normative account about the moral standing of the mentally disabled as members of our community, not merely a descriptive one. However, the observation that they do not fit easily into the description of the moral ideal that many people in contemporary liberal society hold about themselves as competent agents suggests a serious problem. Indeed, as we will see in chapter 7, the framework of liberal morality does encounter a serious problem in this respect.

Pending the discussion of that problem, however, let us for the moment simply assert that the liberal convention provides us with the claim that people deserve equal concern and respect as a minimal requirement of just treatment.[7] This is not an implausible claim, given that there is a well-established list of characteristics deemed morally inappropriate for unequal treatment in liberal society that includes disability. Religion has been on that list for the last two centuries, whereas race and sex have been added about a century ago. Age and disability have been added to it only recently. This can be inferred from the fact that discriminatory acts and regulations based on age or disability have been declared illegal.[8] The liberal convention as presented earlier allows this type of legislation, let us say, on the ground that society ought to pay equal respect to all its members. Presumably, that is what antidiscrimination laws to protect disabled citizens seek to establish.

If correct, we can conclude that the failure to pay equal respect to these people will constitute a clear case of discrimination at least from a legal point of view. Rightly so, I believe. The suggestion that disabled people fail to qualify as normal in the full moral sense of that term contrasts strongly with the goal of accepting them as equally respected members of our society. To obtain this goal society has implemented legal and social policies of integration and normalization. In view of these policies, classifying mentally disabled children as somehow 'defective' is at odds with the moral convictions and beliefs that underwrite them.

A further indication that lends plausibility to this claim can be found in the language used to label mentally disabled people. Labeling occurs in order to see whether particular people fall under particular regulations or should have access to particular services. In the area of mental disability we can observe a continuing change in labels considered appropriate in public policy. Labels such as 'idiots' or 'morons' are no longer accepted, of course, but more recent terms such as 'mentally retarded' have also been expelled from public use.[9] Even if one is inclined to discard such changes as merely responding to political correctness, they nevertheless testify to the upward mobility of the disabled in the public frame of mind. To change a label such as 'mentally retarded' is to indicate that in using it one betrays a lack of respect for the people so designated. Shifting terminologies are indicative of shifting patterns of inclusion. This is true even though the continuing change in labels is largely a matter of political correctness, since it shows what the publicly accepted standard is: disabled people ought to be treated with equal respect. Every human being has an interest in being treated with equal respect, including the mentally disabled, inasmuch as everyone has an interest in being included as a respected member of society.

5.4 Discrimination and the Value of Life

Reasons based on quality of life may seem to be different in this respect. They are reasons that ground decisions about what prospective parents can expect from their future lives with their children. These decisions may be such that the prospect of sharing their lives with a disabled child does not fit in with what they expect from life. Why should they be accused of discriminatory attitudes in expressing their own preferences for a certain kind of life, even if in doing so they reject the kind of lives others are living?

One might think that such decisions are morally wrong because as human beings we have no right to judge the lives of other human beings. That this claim is doubtful, however, becomes clear as soon as we realize what it means to value our own lives. In valuing my own life I implicitly or explicitly apply some sort of standard. Let us call this my personal standard of the good life. No doubt other people can be quite satisfied with their lives when valued in light of their own standards, but this does not exclude the possibility that from my point of view their lives appear to be quite shallow. Of course, I need not make such judgments explicit because I may not even be aware of what I think about their lives. As soon as I find myself reflecting upon the matter, however, it will become apparent that in valuing my present life I am bound to pass a judgment on the value of other people's lives. This is even more so when, in reflecting upon the matter, I have to focus explicitly upon the lives of other people in order to find out whether I would want to live that kind of life, as happens in the case of reproductive decisions regarding disabled children. Consequently, the claim that we have no right to judge the lives of others appears to be false, since it seems to imply that in that case we can have no right to judge our own lives either.

To clarify this, let us proceed again by way of example and consider the case of people with the neural tube defect called spina bifida. Suppose I participate in a panel discussion on genetics and reproductive choice broadcast on public television. Suppose further that I state as my personal opinion that I would prevent a child with spina bifida from being born were I informed that my future child would have this disorder. Would viewers who live with this condition be justified in accusing me of discrimination? Or suppose that one of the panel members herself was a person with that disorder. She responds, "You are telling me that if you had been my prospective father, I would not have existed." Would she be justified in accusing me of showing lack of respect to her as a person?

The complicated answer to this question is, it seems to me, yes and no. The affirmative part of the answer is grounded in the importance of self-esteem, in which every member of society has an interest, including the handicapped.[10] I cannot possibly think of my life as worth living without self-esteem. Self-esteem, however, is a social concept in the sense that my self-esteem is based upon the fact that other people share it with me (at least partly) for the same reasons. In other words: self-esteem needs to be confirmed by others. Without such confirmation, my self-esteem will be undermined.[11] If someone tells me that she does not want my kind of life because she does not think it worthwhile to live that kind of life, that surely will be an assault on my self-esteem. Given our nature as social beings, it is simply too hard to say: "I think my life is great and I don't care what other people say about it." Self-esteem is of social origin and that is why the negative judgment of the panelist cannot be experienced in any other way except as offensive by the woman with spina bifida. It is hard to see how she could ignore with equanimity such an unfavorable opinion about her kind of life, particularly when this opinion is aired by someone who is apparently sufficiently respectable to appear on public television. Publicly disseminated negative judgments about disabled lives can only be offensive to people living those lives. To the extent that these judgments imply that their kind of lives are not worth living, they express discriminatory attitudes.

At the same time, however, the answer to our question cannot only be affirmative but must be negative as well. If the panelist on the TV show states his view about a life with spina bifida, he is talking about his *own* life. He does not criticize the standard of people living with that disorder. In other words, he does not pass a judgment about what their lives mean to them.[12] He only says that he would not want to change places. Of course, this does not mean that the person with spina bifida will not be offended by his views. Confronted with the charge of discrimination, however, the panelist can simply say that he does not intend to offend anyone but is merely stating his own views on the value of life.

The question about discriminatory attitudes as expressed in judgments about the quality of disabled lives, then, shows us two sides of one and the same coin. The practices of prevention look different to the disability community than to doctors and patients who engage in genetic testing. Since the latter will consider the confrontation with genetic disorders from a medical point of view, their focus will be on the limitations that a disabled life may bring. From the point of view of both the users and providers of these medical services, the crucial issue is free reproductive choice for people who want to protect themselves and their children against suffering. Granting this interest is insufficient, however, to evade the charge that discriminatory attitudes may be implied. Reproductive decisions have ramifications far beyond the medical context of individual patients consulting their doctors, even if they tend to regard their decisions as private. From the point of view of disability advocates, the issue is to resist the growing impact of genetics on social and political barriers against full participation in society. Inasmuch as the genetic approach to disability is based upon negative evaluations, it will not help to eliminate these barriers. Instead, it may well threaten the gains of normalization that have been made in recent decades in their public appeal. Apparently, in considering the issue of discrimination on the level of personal and informal behavior we once again stumble on the undeniable fact of two opposing tendencies in our moral attitudes toward mental disability.[13]

5.5 The Social Position of the Disabled

Discrimination against people affected by genetic disorders may take another form in the context of institutional regulations and requirements. Such people pose a particular kind of risk to institutions that have somehow accepted responsibility for them. Insurance companies that have accepted these people as their clients will have to pay costs of medical care once the disorder actually develops into a disease. Something similar is true for employers who cannot simply fire their employees once they get sick. Both the insurance and the labor market are therefore sensitive areas for genetic information because it is in the interest of insurers and employers to minimalize financial risks. Whenever these topics are discussed in the literature, the issue of discrimination is discussed in connection with two other issues, namely privacy and social justice. Between them, the issue of privacy oftentimes takes priority. The reason is not difficult to imagine: "If certain types of information make you vulnerable to institutions on which you are dependent, keep it to yourself!" Thus the question arises of whether genetic discrimination can be prevented simply by protecting the privacy of genetic information. Society may have mixed views on privacy in this connection, however. On the one hand, to deprive people with genetic disorders access to insurance and jobs will lead to genetic discrimination. People will be barred, through no fault of their own, from social opportunities that are vital to them. On the other hand, it is not immediately clear that the financial risks adhering to their medical condition should be accepted by other members of society. Even if we are held responsible for one another, that does not and should not eliminate our individual responsibility.[14]

The problem with the focus on privacy—on keeping information about one's future health status to oneself—from a disability perspective is clear: one cannot hide the presence of inoperative functions in one's body, be they physical or mental. The issue is not merely how to prevent people with genetic disorders from becoming a separate class of citizens—'the new pariahs'[15]—because to some degree such is already the case for people with mental disabilities. That is why we have legal statutes and regulations explicitly designed to protect them. Governments have repelled discriminatory laws so as to protect their civil rights and enacted new laws to allow them access to the community. Also, financial support has been regulated to assist people with 'special needs' in order to allow them to reenter, and participate in, society. From the point of view of the disabled the primary issue is not the formation of an underclass of people with 'bad genes', therefore, but the reemergence of the medical model that may undermine these policies.[16] Now that legal discrimination in the sphere of civil rights has been abandoned, it must not be followed by genetic discrimination in the socio-economic sphere. To see whether this is a real threat we have to ask how the proliferation of genetic testing will affect the position of disabled people in society.

Following the strategy deployed in previous chapters, let us again proceed from certain convictions and beliefs that can be inferred from contemporary moral culture. In other words, let us once again look at the liberal convention. One of the strongest convictions in liberal morality in this context—if not *the* strongest—is the belief that reproductive choice is primarily a matter for individuals to decide. Consider the way in which this conviction is expressed in Lee Silver's recent book *Remaking Eden*. Referring to Aldous Huxley's famous novel, Silver claims that Huxley's imagination had the science right but the politics wrong. That is to say, the picture of a new world in which people are in control of their own reproduction is becoming a reality, but Huxley misjudged the goals for which these new powers were going to be used and by whom:

What Huxley failed to understand, or refused to accept, was the driving force behind babymaking. It is individuals and couples who want to reproduce themselves in their own images. It is individuals and couples who want their children to be happy and successful. It is individuals and couples, . . . *not governments*— that will seize control of these new technologies. They will use some to reach otherwise unattainable reproductive goals and others to help their children achieve health, happiness, and success. And it is in pursuit of this last goal that the combined actions of many individuals, operating over many generations, could perhaps give rise to a polarized humanity more horrific than Huxley's imagined Brave New World.[17]

I take Silver's view to be a fairly adequate expression of what many people would say. Deciding whether or not to have children and when and how many is our own, and not the government's business. But the question of whether individual choice requires public regulation cannot be discarded so easily, however. Silver seems to overlook the fact that liberal society not only believes in individual freedom but also in the equal distribution of freedom. Individual freedom is restricted in many areas of social life. We accept the restriction of freedom for the sake of coordinating actions of individuals, as in the case of traffic regulations, as well as for the sake of protecting individuals against the freedom of others, as in the case of legal restrictions on the private use of firearms. There may be a similar reason to consider regulating reproductive freedom as well. The proliferation of 'reprogenetics' in society may have dramatic, unintended, long-term effects upon people's lives. Even if it may not be the government's business to interfere in reproductive decisions made by individuals consulting their doctors, the possibility of these decisions having side effects that negatively affect disabled people would make it difficult to deny that this *is* a matter for public policy.

To explore this matter we need to speculate about social and cultural responses to the new technology. Speculations of this kind are a dangerous enterprise, since the possibility of checking one's imagination is limited. The subject of human genetics stimulates thought experiments about all sorts of different scenarios of either utopian bliss or catastrophic disaster for humankind, hampering our ability to see clearly. Speculations about social and cultural responses are even more doubtful than predictions about scientific developments in the field of molecular biology. Nonetheless, I think that we should engage in this exercise in order to raise public consciousness about the question of how the new technology will affect the lives of future people. Could the proliferation of genetic testing have damaging effects on the social security of disabled people? How might these effects come about? What reasons do we have to think that their position in society may be undermined by the continued development of human genetics? The speculations that answer this question amount to something like the following: (1) the growing knowledge of genetic disorders will increase the awareness of the possibility of preventing the birth of people with those disorders; (2) the increased area of reproductive choice will mean that reproduction will be perceived as a matter of choice, including parental responsibility for the birth of disabled children; (3) the argument claiming social support for children with special needs will be considerably weakened if there is a question of parental responsibility for their existence; (4) the rising pressures on national health care budgets demand that individuals be held responsible for risks they take with regard to their health; and (5) decisions to allow the birth of a disabled child will be seen as a decision for which people should be held personally accountable. Taken together, these assumptions suggest that people with disabled children have reason to be worried about their future in our society. But this is only true of course to the extent that my speculations are plausible.[18] Let us see whether they are.

5.6 The Future of Disability

The continued development of new technology suggests that in the near future genetic testing will proliferate among the population.[19] The expectation is that new testing procedures will be marketed as relatively inexpensive 'testing kits' for private use. If correct, this assumption justifies the further assumption that more and more people in society will have access to such tests. The area of reproductive choice will not only be increased, it will also be popularized in the sense of becoming less dependent on medical intervention. People can perform a test to discover that there is no risk or, if there is one, they can decide not to have children. If they decide to take the risk, they can conceive a child, and seek medical assistance to see whether the fetus is affected and, if so, decide to have their pregnancy terminated. They can then repeat this procedure or else choose to engage in some form of artificial reproduction. In other words, the emerging procedures for genetic testing will shape control of reproduction in a degree similar to the way contraceptives has shaped birth control since the sixties and seventies. A majority of people in our society will be acquainted with these procedures and regard their use as a 'normal' ingredient of reproductive behavior. Since the late fifties people have grown accustomed to the idea that, if one wants to prevent an unwanted pregnancy, one should take adequate precautionary measures. Given the availability of inexpensive 'testing kits' for private use, it is plausible that many people will also grow accustomed to the idea that, if one wants to prevent a child with a genetic disorder, one should take precautionary measures.[20] This is the first speculation.

The second is closely connected with the first. If the means to control reproduction expand and are used by an increasing number of people in an increasing number of cases, reproductive choice will become identified with the possibility to control the undesirable.[21] An increasing range of options with regard to our offspring implies an increasing range of choice. This is not necessarily an increase in the range of positive choices in the sense that we will be able to order the child we would like to have but in the opposite sense that we do not have to accept what we do not want.[22] Of course, people have known for a long time that procreation is a human affair, even if they believed that children were a gift from God. Before the explosion of contraceptives in the sixties, the conception of a child was also a personal decision, in a sense, but in recent times the notion of reproductive choice has gained prominence in the public mind. What follows is that in the future people will tend to believe that their children are the products of their own choice.[23] If so, they will also tend to think that the birth of a disabled child falls within that same category as well, if not in a positive then at least in a negative sense: parents who conceive such a child will have failed to act in a responsible way, just as 'unwanted pregnancies' used to be the result of irresponsible behavior. This concludes the second speculation.

The intense discussion on the welfare state that has occupied public debate in many Western societies over the last twenty years has resulted by and large in the victory of a neoconservative critique. Even if there is considerable disagreement about the cure, there is much less disagreement about the disease. The transfer of social responsibility from local communities and mediating institutions has created a new 'underclass' of people who do not know how to govern their own lives in a responsible way. The expansion of welfare programs in the sixties and seventies went hand in hand with the expansion of the state bureaucracies that administered these programs. Consequently, the welfare state needs to be dismantled and replaced by a social 'safety net' that is much more cost effective and at the same time stimulates people to take responsibility for their own communities. All Western democracies have their own versions of this argument. It has inspired political change with a curious mix of economic and moral motives. National governments are pressing for budget cuts on welfare and health care, which means—among other things—that access to social services is tightened and that people are required to contribute financially for using health care provisions. If this picture is adequate, as I think it is, it is plausible to assume that the emphasis on personal responsibility for reducing social costs will affect the area of reproduction as well.[24] The general attitude will be that people with special needs should be legitimately entitled to social benefits but that it is fair to withdraw such benefits as soon as these special needs are no longer a matter of misfortune but can be attributed to personal responsibility and 'choice'. Philip Kitcher makes the point as follows. Democratic societies, he says, are grounded in the rights of their citizens to fashion their own lives as they choose, as long as they do not infringe upon the equal rights of others. If the actions of one group threaten the opportunities of another group to shape their lives, those who are threatened ought to be protected unless there are special circumstances. In specifying which circumstances he has in mind, Kitcher arrives at the view that my third speculation expresses:

> Occasionally the circumstances are special. Conflict between groups may result from decisions that people have made freely in the past, in full awareness of the consequences, so that they are now vulnerable to the loss of something

important for the shaping of their lives. Perhaps higher premiums for health insurance are justified when the applicants have voluntarily overindulged all the
wrong habits, knowing the medical effects. (*The Lives to Come*, 134)

The right to be protected against medical costs can be forfeited if people fail to
take sufficient precautionary measures to promote their own health and that of
their families. I should add that Kitcher rejects the view that risks imposed by the
'genetic lottery' should be relevant to the costs of health-care insurance. On the
contrary, he claims that a morally acceptable arrangement would strive to protect the genetically unfortunate and offer them *lower* insurance rates.[25] But he
admits that especially in the United States such proposals are very controversial
while at the same time under attack in other countries as well. The important
point, however, is the suggestion that society will only be prepared to support
people burdened by genetic disorders as long as these burdens are imposed by
natural hazards.

 This is where the fourth speculation comes into play. 'Through no fault of
their own' will be important in the way the public regards support for families
with disabled children. Once the perception is widely established that a disability is no longer a condition of natural misfortune, the public mood will
change. Especially if economic pressures on national health-care budgets continue to increase—as they most likely will in view of an aging population—the
demand of personal responsibility for health care expenditures will become an
important issue. When a disabled child comes to be associated with the notion
of irresponsible behavior, then the erosion of political support will occur in only
a matter of time. The least that can be expected in this connection is a shifting
burden of proof. Families with handicapped children will most likely have to
face questions about why they have these children.

 · These speculations complete the scenario of how side effects of the proliferation of procedures for genetic testing in society may affect the position of mentally disabled people. Under the condition of expanding health care costs and
deminishing resources, combined with an increased range of reproductive
choice, the existence of disabled people will no longer be taken for granted and
their families can expect to be interrogated about their personal behavior. The
legitimacy of social support will be subjected to the clause of individual responsibility. If the current trend in rethinking the moral basis of social security continues, it seems utterly naive to think that shifting perceptions about the nature
of reproduction in the public mind will not affect the social position of the disabled and their families.

 There are at least two moral grounds to challenge the legitimacy of this scenario. First of all, in many cases the presence of a disability will not be due to
the failure of 'responsible reproductive behavior' at all. This means that families

with disabled members may face obstacles in obtaining social support without any fault of their own. Secondly, and much more important than this, is the obvious fact that disabled people themselves can never be held responsible for their existence, even if their parents failed to take precautionary measures. If the scenario described above will become a reality, it means that in a number of cases disabled people will be discriminated against in the sense that they will face more than average difficulties in obtaining social support because of a disability resulting from a genetic disorder. The crucial point in considering the possibility that this may occur is not whether political authorities accept the views on which the scenario is based. It is rather that these authorities will have a hard time—given the way that representative democracy works—in resisting the perception of the public that the presence of disabled people in society is 'unnecessary' and that the burden of their existence should be on the shoulders of those who bear the responsibility for their existence.[26] The argument on the strengths and weaknesses of democratic control of reprogenetics is ultimately based on the issue of whether or not disabled citizens should be protected against this public perception and its possible political consequences.

5.7 No World without Disabled People

One response to this scenario deserves to be considered here. Assuming that the speculations I made on the basis of current developments are not implausible, should this not lead to the conclusion that the proliferation of genetic testing may turn out to be very effective? Should we not expect decreasing numbers of disabled people among the general population such that none of the foreseen side effects will seriously harm them? Whatever the costs of health care for these people may be, it will be negligible compared to the costs of other categories of consumers. To combat the scenario depicted in the previous section, the best option seems to be to make genetic testing for reasons of prevention as effective as possible. Welfare and health care services will have fewer disabled clients to serve.

Let me conclude this chapter by considering the force of this response. It is based entirely on the supposition that the number of disabled people *can* be significantly decreased. There are, however, at least four reasons to think that this supposition is mistaken. First, consider the fact that both the concept of an impairment and the concept of a disability or handicap are 'open-ended'. Apart from the fact that the indogeneous causes of quite a number of genetic disorders are unknown, some of these conditions have also exogenous causes, some of which are environmental. Given the complexity of such environmental variables it is most likely that these conditions will remain unexplained within the foreseeable future. The fact of exogeneous causes is by itself sufficient to expect that further changes in climatological, ecological, chemical, and pharmacological conditions may produce new genetic disorders. However, these new disorders can be identified only when they become manifest on a certain scale. It follows that people with these disorders must already exist before their condition can be eventually recognized as falling within the range of genetic testing.

Second, mapping the human genome does not necessarily mean mapping all the genetic disorders that are possibly regarded as the cause of a disability. The reason is, as we already saw in chapter 3, that the concept of a disability or handicap refers to normal social functioning. To explain its content is to explain what people are expected to be capable of doing in a particular society. The moral meaning of genetic disorders is therefore connected to patterns of expectations of normalcy. Given the fact that these expectations are culturally mediated, we can infer that the moral meaning connected to genetic disorders is a cultural variable. A dependence on mobility by wheelchair in an easily accessible urban area is different from the same dependency in a rural mountainous environment. If there are such real differences between different areas in one culture, they will be even more likely to occur between cultural shifts over time. For centuries there was no reason for distinguishing intellectually disabled people from other socially 'deviant' types. It is only since the time of general public education that these people were classified as mentally retarded. Cognitive functioning did not always have the meaning it has in our society. This indicates that we should not be too confident about our insights into which conditions in the future will be viewed as handicaps.[27] This is an additional reason for thinking that we will continue to have people with handicaps among us even if we could be successful in trying to prevent all the handicaps with which we are currently familiar.

The third reason stems from the obvious fact that handicaps occasionally stem from traffic accidents. Furthermore, there are, of course, also the handicaps and disabilities that are accidentally caused at birth when there was no foreseeable risk. Consequently, we cannot succeed in eliminating handicaps and disabilities even if our society were to embark on large-scale screening policies covering all pregancies. In all the cases mentioned in this section the result would be the same: there would be disabled people in our society who, for one reason or another, escaped our comprehensive prevention scheme, assuming that we have one. Given the limits to our powers of prediction, it appears that the presence of disabled people will be beyond our control.

There is, however, a final reason why a comprehensive policy of prevention would most likely fail in preventing all, or nearly all, disabled lives, even if we were able to predict the occurrence of each of them. This reason has to do with a most happy inconvenience of liberal democracy, i.e., the fact that it breeds public dissent and opposition.[28] Given a strong belief in the moral value of individual freedom, it is utterly implausible that all citizens would comply with any compulsory large-scale screening program. People opposed to total reproductive control by the state would more likely try to give birth to their children illegally. These considerations lead to the conclusion that there will always be a considerable number of disabled people among us, whether we like it or not. This conclusion reinforces the claim that we cannot evade the question of what we, as a political community, are going to do about the side effects that preventive strategies may have upon the lives of these people. This is the question for the next chapter.

SIX

Restrictions on Reproductive Choice?

In a society that values individual freedom above all else, it is hard to find any legitimate basis for restricting the use of reprogenetics. And therein lies the dilemma. For while each individual use of the technology can be viewed in the light of personal reproductive choice—with no ability to change society at large—together they could have dramatic, unintended, long-term consequences.

Lee M. Silver

6.1 *'Free Choice' in Human Reproduction*

The paramount value of individual freedom indicates that liberal morality is strongly oriented towards the preferences and ideals of individual agents. The freedom of individuals to live their lives as they please comes first, and concern for the public good comes second. Or, one should say, the latter is defined in terms of the former. The morality entailed in the liberal convention is a morality that governs social interaction between people who are primarily interested in their own projects, not in the sense that they are egoistically self-interested, but in the sense that they want to pursue their own conception of the good.[1] The paramount value of freedom in liberal society implies an important restriction on public justification, particularly with regard to public policies that affect individual freedom in a negative way. Policies of this kind can be justified only by giving reasons that can be shared by those whose freedom is involved. Since people are entitled to their own conception of the good, no moral claim can be grounded in the authority of an 'external' conception of the good. When no generally accepted conception of the good is available substantial questions about the good life can have no other answers than those given by individual members of society.[2]

In this political culture reproductive choice will be an important element of public morality. Robert Edwards, the intellectual 'father' of in vitro fertilization observed that "the desire to have children must be among the most basic of human instincts, and denying it can lead to considerable psychological and social difficulties."[3] Accordingly, the moral framework laid out by the liberal convention includes a right to reproductive freedom. The decision to start a family—when, where, and with whom—is among the most private decisions that people can make. Such decisions belong to the domain of individual freedom if anything does, which will make many people in our society very reluctant to endorse coercive policies in the area of reproduction.

The question to be addressed in this chapter is whether or not the liberal democratic state has a case for the restriction of reproductive freedom for reasons of protecting its disabled citizens. If the foregoing considerations ring true, any argument favoring such restrictions must be very strong. The question as such is unavoidable, however, once it is established that the proliferation of procedures for genetic testing may have negative side effects in the sense that some people are harmed indirectly by other people's actions and decisions. In such cases the issue of protection arises 'naturally' for liberal democracy, given its commitment to balance individual freedom against equality of opportunity. Individual freedom as the paramount moral value of liberal morality is not an absolute value, but is limited by the protection of equal freedom. Moreover, in order to make individual freedom effective, liberal morality endorses 'equality of opportunity' as a necessary side constraint on individual freedom. This commitment to equality of opportunity has in recent times induced many Western democracies to support participation of disabled people in society by means of public policy. In the era of genetic testing the commitment to equal opportunity faces another challenge, however, namely the possibility of discriminatory side effects. If there is reason to believe that reproductive decisions will affect social opportunities for disabled citizens in the future, does this create sufficient ground for the restriction of reproductive freedom? Public policy could be designed in order to limit free access to genetic testing and to curtail the free distribution of testing procedures by the market. Is there an argument sufficiently strong to justify this kind of public policy because of the negative side effects that prolific use of genetic testing procedures may have?

In this chapter we will consider the strength of the argument that our discussion in the previous chapter produced. The argument in question consisted of two parts. The first part was that since the lives of disabled people are negatively evaluated in decisions to prevent the birth of a disabled child, such decisions are vulnerable to the charge of reflecting discriminatory attitudes. The second part of the argument was that following the rapid proliferation of genetic testing, the birth of a disabled child will raise the suspicion of irresponsible behavior on the part of its parents. Under the condition of cost containment in health care and welfare, the perception of irresponsible behavior will press the question as to whether society should pay the price. This concern may well undermine the position of the disabled in society, which at that point means that genetic discrimination is a fact. Both points raise the issue of public responsibility to protect citizens with 'special needs' who are dependent upon social support. Side effects of individual decisions made by people using their reproductive freedom, though unintended, can collectively have very damaging effects in society. The question then is whether the proliferation of genetic tests should be restricted and whether such restriction is sufficiently justified on the grounds of the unintended but harmful side effects of large-scale use of such tests.

As we will see, the answer to this question will proceed in two stages. First, it will be argued that the case for protecting the disabled appears to be relatively strong but, second, that it is not at all clear what kind of policy can be implemented with respect to that objective. The instrument that presents itself is a restriction of distribution and access to prenatal testing procedures based on the principle that what remains undetected cannot be prevented. But the implementation of such a restriction would be fraught with all sorts of practical difficulties. As an analysis of these difficulties will show, restrictive policies in this area are most likely to backfire on public attitudes toward disabled citizens. Instead of securing their position in society, the result may rather be counterproductive in that social stigmatization is reinforced. The conclusion drawn from this analysis will be a disquieting one from the perspective of liberal morality. Given the moral attitudes and beliefs that support the legitimacy of its protective policies, the liberal state has strong grounds for controlling genetic testing in order to protect equal opportunity for its disabled citizens now and in the future. But in trying to do so by restricting reproductive freedom, the liberal state will run into insurmountable difficulties.

6.2 Restriction of Reproductive Freedom?

Before we consider the strength of the case against genetic discrimination as presented in the previous chapter, let us consider a preliminary objection against setting the issue as an issue of restricting individual freedom. Given all that has been said about the overriding value of individual freedom, the suggestion of restricting individual uses of genetic testing by means of public policy will appear highly implausible. Why should we concentrate on the restriction of negative rights, people's rights to free choice, rather than on the creation of positive rights for the disabled? Why should we not discuss social justice as the heart of the matter? Why not tackle the issue of genetic discrimination—assuming that there is one—as a problem of equal distribution of resources, as the liberal convention would allow us to do? These questions arise from the fact that the liberal convention as I portrayed it combines the moral values of freedom and equality, which creates the possibility of different rankings between them. Given my focus on individual freedom as the paramount value, it may be objected that I seem to interpret the liberal convention from the perspective of libertarians, such as Engelhardt rather than from the perspective of egalitarians, such as, for example, Ronald Dworkin. As indicated, the objection is that instead of focusing on the problem of curtailing individual rights, an egalitarian perspective invites us to focus on the creation of positive rights for people in socially disadvantageous positions.

I propose that we deal with this objection by looking at the egalitarian argument against genetic discrimination as presented by Philip Kitcher. In making this move I intend to show that egalitarian arguments in this context are very likely to slide back to arguments about individual freedom. But let me first lay out Kitcher's argument. A key assumption of this argument is that genetic information will be available about each of us, which means that we all are potential victims of genetic discrimination. This assumption is not uncommon among scientists. The detection of genetic 'defects' is developing on such a scale that it is expected to change the very nature of medicine. Here is how Francis Collins, director of the National Center for Human Genome Research, perceives the ubiquitous role of genetics in future medicine: "Given that virtually all diseases have a genetic component, and that we all carry predispositions to certain illnesses, the hope of a healthier future through genetic research is not restricted to a rare individual here and there; it applies to all of us."[4] Assuming this to be the case, Kitcher seems right in suggesting that genetic discrimination is something for all of us to worry about. Aside from the possibility of false information, we can be reasonably sure that many of us will be classified as falling within the defined categories of risks, some of which will make us very unattractive as applicants for insurance or jobs.[5]

In the context of a largely market-driven insurance system, according to Kitcher, the position taken by many insurance companies and consumers will be to argue that those who are likely to make greater claims should pay higher premiums. Kitcher rejects this position because it could easily lead to 'crippling high premiums' that would effectively deny particular groups of people any access to any kind of health care. His counterargument hinges on two presuppositions. The first is that health is a basic good that is crucial to human lives. A society that values the rights of citizens to shape their lives as they choose cannot refuse them the possession of this good. The second is that a genetic disorder is a condition with which one is born and which one cannot change. People ought not be penalized for characteristics they cannot change.[6] Given these presuppositions, Kitcher claims that a democratic and just society cannot allow insurance companies to pursue more profit at the expense of barring some people from the opportunity to maintain their health. The complete adjustment of premium to risk would surely mean that many applicants could not afford to pay the costs of health insurance. The most obvious arrangement designed to avoid this inequality, according to Kitcher, is a system that provides universal coverage for all citizens and that is funded by progressive taxation. Although the author is aware of the fact that public opinion in the United States has not been very favorable to proposals of this kind, he nevertheless maintains that this is what social justice demands:

> The principle that all citizens should have health care coverage at costs determined by their ability to pay is indeed fundamental, and we should not be tempted to compromise it because of panegyrics to the free market. Justice requires that we do not secure whatever advantages accrue from competition by sacrificing the well-being of those who have already been unlucky in the distribution of genes and the distribution of wealth. (*The Lives to Come*, 136)

The argument Kitcher provides in order to justify his principle bears a strong resemblance to John Rawls's famous thought experiment of choosing principles of justice behind a veil of ignorance. The idea of hypothetical choice is meant to make sure that we cannot curtail justice to serve our own interests. Likewise, Kitcher presents a thought experiment suggesting that we are at the eve of 'the great unveiling'.[7] We do not as yet know what our genetic dispositions will be, but we will know shortly. In the mean time we have to make up our minds about the following options. Tomorrow 10 percent of the population will discover that they are genetically at a significantly higher risk for serious disorders than the remaining 90 percent. Given that we do not know if we will be among that 10 percent, we are invited to decide between two methods of managing health-care coverage. The first way assigns premiums on the basis of risk and the second does so on the basis of wealth. Tomorrow, when we know the facts, we will discover that 90 percent of those who have chosen the first method will be somewhat better off than those who have chosen the second. They happen to be the genetically fortunate who chose the method that was more profitable for them. The remaining 10 percent of those who chose that same option will be significantly worse off up to the point where they have no health coverage at all. This is what we will know tomorrow, but we have to decide now: Which method of managing health coverage are we going to support? The answer will depend, of course, upon what we know about our private income. People with sufficient wealth may be prone to gamble, accept the risk that they will be among the genetically unfortunate, and still choose the option of risk-adjusted insurance premiums. To reduce this temptation, however, Kitcher adds the further factor of economic uncertainty. Even if not very plausible for ourselves, economic depression may decrease the wealth of our children and grandchildren. Given this presupposition, how would we choose on their behalf? The rational answer, Kitcher suggests, must be that in a world in which the great unveiling is about to begin and genetic testing can make victims of all of us, it no longer makes sense to reject a system of universal coverage based on progressive taxation:

> There have long been many excellent reasons for viewing a system of health care coverage as a cooperative venture in which the fortunate help to support those who have been victims of circumstance. Because genetic testing can make victims of us all, its advent may help to undermine the glorification of self-sufficiency that has so far blocked appreciation of those reasons. After the great unveiling, any of us—or, more probably, any of our descendants—may be vulnerable. (*The Lives to Come*, 138)

As is the case with all moral arguments based on a hypothetical reduction of information, Kitcher's thought experiment shows a weakness as soon as it is applied to ordinary life where the condition of reduced information is absent. His argument is based on the moral principle that in choosing schemes of just distribution we should adopt—as Rawls has taught us—an 'omni-personal' point of view.[8] In order to make people accept this formal principle, Kitcher provides them with an argument to do so from the point of view of their own interests. But this is a risky strategy because to make arguments about justice dependent on enlightened self-interest, as Kitcher's experiment does, is to invite people to consider what their best interest tells them to do. If they do consider the issue from that point of view, they may infer from what they know about their current wealth status and from what their family history tells them about their genetic dispositions that egalitarian proposals for a just scheme of health care coverage is not at all in their best interest. In other words, the attempt to justify an egalitarian position on grounds of a hypothetical choice argument that is based upon enlightened self-interest is counterproductive when people are as a matter of fact self-interested. This conclusion can only be avoided when people *actually* accept the egalitarian belief that different socio-economic assets and natural endowments should remain outside the justification of distributive justice. However, the assumption that people in the real world do not accept this belief was the reason to construct the hypothetical choice argument in the first place. Seeking to establish arguments for distributive justice on the ground of enlightened self-interest by means of hypothetical choice theory, is either inconsistent or self-defeating.[9]

Furthermore, it appears that the notion of being burdened by blind fate is crucial to Kitcher's argument. As long as people continue to believe in this notion, they will be susceptible to the claim that blind fate may strike anybody. However, as soon as they are aware of the potential of reprogenetics, the force of his argument will wither away. Many will be inclined to believe that they can interfere with the genetic lottery and take the responsibility of preventing themselves and their families from being burdened by genetic disease. In other words, Kitcher can hope to convince people only because he abstains from thinking about the future implications of the notion of 'responsible reproductive behavior'. This is a further weakness in his argument. Just as many people already believe that the distribution of wealth is largely a matter of individual responsibility, they may come to believe the same with regard to the distribution of genes. If correct, this implies once more that Kitcher's invitation to consider the plight of genetically affected people in the light of enlightened self-interest is a self-defeating strategy. Once the assumption of individual responsibility for the reproduction of 'bad genes' is firmly in place, people will be wary of sharing the costs of health care services for people with special needs whose existence they believe to be caused by 'irresponsible reproductive behavior'.

To sum up, there are two flaws in Kitcher's argument. First, in order to make his argument for universal coverage work, he cannot but presuppose that people already accept the egalitarian premises that the argument is designed to establish.[10] That is, they will accept his proposal if and only if they already believe that people with special needs should receive social benefits because in a democratic and just society all members are entitled to a fair equality of opportunity regardless of their differences in socio-economic assets or natural endowments.[11] Second, the more people believe in the option of reproductive control, the less they will be prepared to share the burden of people who failed to use that option in order to take responsibility for the genetic condition of their offspring. Only by ignoring the possible impact of this belief Kitcher can hope to persuade us with the suggestion that genetic disorders distributed by blind fate may strike us all.

However, suppose Kitcher is right. Suppose that the issue of genetic discrimination can be effectively dealt with by a scheme of universal health-care coverage. This would mean that nobody would have to worry about health insurance or access to services, but it would also mean a significant increase in national health-care expenditure. As a consequence, many people would face an increase in income tax, which would in fact be a tax for other people's bad genes. Given the unpopularity of increasing income tax, this is a very unattractive prospect indeed for any government. Even in case our government is willing to provide social security for people with special needs, it will at the same time be very interested to increase cost containment and cost effectiveness in our health-care system. In that situation the prospect of expanding genetic testing to prevent as many genetic disorders as possible would be very appealing. Although the authorities may want to keep a low profile on the issue of prevention to avoid charges of genetic discrimination, their political opponents will surely expose the causal link between a 'tax for bad genes' and the 'irresponsible reproductive behavior' of particular people in society.[12]

These considerations suggest that, for both theoretical and practical reasons, the issue of social justice in connection with genetic discrimination will most likely slide back into an issue of individual responsibility and reproductive freedom. This may happen in two different ways. According to one scenario, implementing social justice by means of universal health-care coverage would most likely be accompanied by rising pressures to contain the costs of health-care services, which, in turn, may lead to an increased demand for 'responsible reproductive behavior' in order to prevent as many disabled lives as possible. In order to justify the necessary increase in income taxes, political authorities would be under strong pressures to promote prevention schemes. This would surely amount to a policy of genetic discrimination, since it would be to prevent disabled people from coming into existence for political reasons. According to another scenario, the danger that part of the population is going to suffer from genetic discrimination may induce the state to counteract the cause of that danger. To the extent that this cause lies in the expansion of reproductive control used for reasons of prevention, the state may consider a policy of restricting the option of reproductive control; hence the question of whether our government should curtail the freedom of individual citizens to use that option in order to protect particularly vulnerable groups of people in society. To discuss this second scenario I will consider the argument of the previous chapter. Individual citizens may use their freedom in such a way that their decisions collectively have negative side effects on the lives of disabled people. Though unintended, these collective side effects of individual actions can constitute a reason to take measures for the sake of protecting others.

6.3 The Charge of Discriminatory Attitudes

The argument for considering a policy of restricting reproductive freedom, it will be recalled, consisted in making two points. Decisions to abort genetically 'defective' fetuses selectively entail negative judgments about the kinds of lives that are to be prevented. These judgments can be experienced as reflecting and reinforcing discriminatory attitudes toward disabled people. This was the first point. The second point was that, because of the rapid proliferation of genetic testing, the cause of disability will be viewed as irresponsible behavior rather than as natural misfortune. Given the interest in cost containment and cost effectiveness in health care, this perception may undermine social security for the disabled and their families. Both points have been analyzed in terms of negative side effects of the development of human genetics in general and of clinical genetics in particular. Here again, it may be objected that scientists and medical doctors working in this field have no other goal than to help patients and families as best as they can. The knowledge produced by geneticists is used to serve the goals of medicine. In this respect, the objection claims, there can be no moral questioning of what they are doing.

As I argued in the previous chapter however, medical practices do not evolve in a social and political vacuum. These practices thrive on cultural meanings about normal human functioning, about lives worth living, about unbearable suffering, and so on. Not only do these practices thrive on such beliefs, they also tend to reinforce them. In bringing further aspects of our bodily existence under control, human genetics adds new dimensions to these cultural meanings. Therefore society cannot ignore the kind of question that is raised here, even though the question itself will appear as inappropriate when regarded from within the practice of clinical genetics as such.

Let us therefore consider the force of the first point about discriminatory attitudes. Clearly, restrictions on genetic testing to protect disabled people from discriminatory attitudes would mean a serious infringement of individual freedom, but infringements of individual freedom as such are not uncommon in the context of medicine. In the United States, for example, patients do not have the freedom to choose physician-assisted suicide. Another example, more directly connected with our theme, is that the freedom to reproduce oneself by means of cloning does not exist. Even if it is true that individual freedom is the core value of public morality in liberal society, this does not mean that in the case of conflicting values freedom always trumps other values. Therefore, even if people ought to be free to make decisions regarding their own lives on the basis of their own conception of the good, the state can still be justified in limiting their freedom on other grounds.

Is the argument about discriminatory attitudes sufficiently compelling to justify any such policy? In my view it is not. To explain why, let me briefly recall the two types of reasons for deciding to prevent a disabled child from being born, that have been discussed before. Although reproductive decisions stemming from reasons based on moral standing constitute a strong case against genetic discrimination, given their implications of inclusion or exclusion, such reasons are not likely to come up in the context of clinical genetics. In that context, the relevant reasons will much more likely be reasons based on quality of life. People will be primarily interested in how a genetic disorder in their family will affect their future lives. As we saw, however, decisions against accepting a disabled child based on this second type of reason are at best morally ambiguous. Even if the lives of people with the same disorders are negatively implicated in these decisions, it does not follow that these implications are intended. Consequently, there is no clear-cut case against genetic discrimination in these cases. If a couple after having had a prenatal test decides to abort the fetus because it is affected by Down syndrome, they can justify this decision by referring to what they think they are capable of in raising a family. The fact that their decision may be informed by culturally mediated images of people with Down syndrome does not render it illegitimate. The argument here, again, is an argument about intention. Even if we know that cultural images about Down syndrome depend on cognitive frameworks that reinforce negative attitudes toward people with that disorder, it does not follow that prospective parents should know about them, or that they should understand how their own attitudes are shaped. People who decide in this way may simply and honestly be worried about their own future.

This ambiguous state of affairs is not uncommon in the public life of liberal society. People from minority groups are often confronted with negative views of themselves that offend their sense of self-esteem, even if the people who are expressing these views do not in the least intend to be offensive. Consider the case of homosexuality. It is surely possible to treat homosexuals with respect and, at the same time, to regret the homosexuality of one's own child. Even if disappointment about this fact may be misguided, and even if homosexuals may be offended, one is still entitled to one's opinion without the intention of being offensive. Unintended offense is the price that minority groups in liberal society pay for the value of allowing its members to express their own conceptions of the good.

A similar Janus-faced argument holds for clinical genetics and the people who are involved in it. From their perspective, its goal is to help people make the right reproductive choices. The criterion for right, according to the professional ethos of clinical geneticists, is found in what their clients want for themselves. What they want for themselves can be guided by cultural ideals that are unfavorable to people with disabilities. Even then it is difficult to see how a restriction on their freedom of choice could be justified on so weak a basis. The charge of discrimination, should it be leveled against them, can be rebutted by saying that citizens can act respectfully toward people with disabilities and their families, even if they would do anything to prevent themselves from having a disabled child.

6.4 Restrictive Policies against Selective Abortion

To consider the force of the second point of the argument, let me briefly recall the chain of assumptions about empirical and conceptual trends that—in combination—yield the prospect of genetic discrimination in health-care insurance and welfare programs. In a few generations the idea of deciding to have a genetically screened baby will be quite normal.[13] Once a large majority of citizens are familiar with testing for an expanding number of genetic disorders, the birth of disabled children will raise suspicions about people's reproductive decisions, indicating a shifting burden of proof. The myth of reproductive control may put social pressure on parents to explain that they did not behave irresponsibly.[14] Should this scenario be a realistic one, then the future of disabled people in our society does not look very reassuring, assuming that a substantial number of disabled lives can neither be predicted nor prevented. If individual responsibility becomes an important issue, the idea of reproductive control—spurious though it may be—will most likely undermine political support for people with special needs.

If this set of assumptions creates the strongest possible argument for subjecting the proliferation of genetic testing to restrictions on free choice, the question arises whether the argument is strong enough. I will approach this question indirectly, namely by asking which instruments for carrying out the suggested policy, if any, are feasible. The idea behind this strategy is a version of the rule 'ought implies can'. Unless we can identify feasible instruments for implementing restrictions on reproductive freedom, there is no point in arguing for such policies.

Let us grant that, as a matter of principle, there can be no objection to acquiring foreknowledge about our own offspring. People were doing this already long before they knew anything about genes. Aristocratic families carefully selected spouses for their sons in order to make sure that the next generation would also be of excellent breeding. The fact that at present people have the same interest in breeding healthy children is not the problem. The problem is that the development of reprogenetics is closely connected with the practice of selective abortion. This connection suggests that one option for the state to pursue might be to reconsider the legitimacy of abortion on demand.[15] The abortion debate that ravaged Western society in the last decades has largely been a debate on the conflict of interest between a woman's right to free choice and the fetus's right to life. The main controversy concerned the basis on which the law could be used to protect the one against the other. The debate on *selective* abortion, however, includes a third-party interest, thus raising a new question, i.e., that of whether selective abortion should be restricted to protect the interests of people with those disorders that are subject to prevention.[16]

Suppose we would consider this kind of policy, what should be the general principle for revising existing abortion laws for the protection of these interests? Apparently something like the following: abortion is not permitted on the basis of just *any* genetic indication. Abortion laws revised according to this principle would add a further restriction to existing ones, but it would be a restriction of a new type. Existing restrictions regard the developmental stage of the fetus, to the effect that abortion becomes illegitimate beyond a certain point in time. Furthermore, they regard how the decision to have an abortion is reached. Women are required to state before their doctors the reasons why they want to abort. They are also required, according to some laws, to take a leave of absence after having contacted an abortion clinic to reconsider their decision for a fixed period of time. The additional principle of restriction suggested here is different in that it rules out a particular class of reasons, namely, those grounded in the prospect of a genetic disorder that falls within a clearly defined set.

Obviously, this suggestion entails some very serious problems as a feasible policy option. Leaving aside the objection from the point of view of women— the arguments here would be largely the same as in the abortion debate[17]— there is the objection that it is implausible to rule out *every* indication of genetic disorder, given the fact that some disorders result in conditions that are irreconcilably hostile to human life, such as, for example, Lesch Nyhan disease.[18] To meet this objection some distinctions between disorders causing 'profound', 'severe', and 'mild' conditions are needed. There has to be a clearly defined set of conditions to which a revised law should apply. Assuming such distinctions to be possible, one could then argue that, for example, the prevention of 'profound' disabilities is legitimate, that the prevention of 'mild' disabilities is illegitimate and that the prevention of 'severe' disabilities would be a matter of co-operative decision making between families and doctors in each case.

Before engaging in a discussion as to how to develop these distinctions, however, let us consider a practical problem that leaps to mind immediately when we think of what implementing this principle as a matter of public policy would mean. First of all, the principle would effectively exterminate the legality of abortion on demand. Anyone who wants to have a selective abortion to prevent a disabled child from being born could circumvent legal prohibition by arguing that her pregnancy is unwanted.[19] The expectation that the child will be disabled creates other reasons, such as anxiety for a life fraught with unbearable burdens. Women do not need to justify their decision by giving reasons of the first kind rather than the second. If women have no freedom to decide about their own reasons for having an abortion then there is no basis left for free abortion. In other words, it is difficult to see how one could implement a ban on some kind of selective abortion without at the same time banning abortion on demand. I do not think that any government in the Western world will attempt this option, not even the United States, given the rampant divisiveness over the abortion issue. If correct, this implies that a ban on selective abortion would be ineffective as far as the interests of disabled people as third parties are concerned. This conclusion implies that this is hardly a feasible option for public policy in dealing with the negative side effects of reproductive freedom.

6.5 Restrictive Policies to Control Genetic Testing

Perhaps there is a different way. Perhaps we should focus not on what people can prevent but on what they can find out. Arguments against selective abortion propose outlawing certain choices that individuals may want to make. Curtailing individual freedom does not necessarily proceed in that way, however. It need not mean that citizens are no longer free to make reproductive decisions according to their own standards. But it could mean that the range of what people are allowed to find out about their own genetic dispositions is limited. Under such a policy the price would be deliberate ignorance rather than unacceptable use of information. The principle would be "what one does not know, one cannot prevent."[20] This principle focuses on access to prenatal testing procedures.

In this connection it seems that access to these procedures takes shape in one of two different ways. It can be left to the mechanisms of supply and demand, which means that health care insurance schemes will channel what genetic industries produce for consumers. Or else, to the extent that inexpensive testing kits will be available that can be used without medical assistance, the market will largely operate without mediation of insurance companies. In either case, the question is whether or not limiting access to prenatal testing is a feasible option for the liberal state. Restricting people's freedom in this way does not mean that the state has control over the choice they make, but that it controls the range of conditions from which they can choose at all. This option is not without serious difficulties, however. To begin with, the state would face the problem that we encountered in discussing the option of a revised abortion law, namely the problem to identify disorders that are to be excluded from diagnostic practices. Can there be a so-called black list? If so, which genetic disorders should be on that list and why? What is the standard on the basis of which this list should be determined?

A first attempt may be to base such a standard on the condition that prenatal testing should be related to health problems. Consider the example of prenatal testing for reasons of sex selection on nonmedical grounds. Parents are occasionally desparate to know the sex of their child in advance without any medical reason. Clearly, being a boy or a girl is not a health problem, although it may create a cultural or socio-economic problem for a family.[21] Suppose a pregnant woman wants to know the sex of her baby because she does not want a girl. Suppose we deny her the option of a prenatal test by saying, "being female is not a disease." Now, this woman could reply that of course being a girl is not a disease, but as a matter of fact girls in her culture are devalued and she does not want to expose her baby to that culture. Being female is not a disease but it can surely be a handicap.

Clearly there is an analogy with mental disability in this case. Parents expecting a mentally disabled child may make the same argument. Because their child will be disabled, it may face a devalued existence to which they do not want to expose it. Regarding such cases, one could argued that to allow genetic testing for reasons of beliefs about normality rather than health problems should be rejected because it reinforces cultural prejudices. In the previous chapter I identified such reasons as reasons of moral standing and showed how prevention for these reasons constitutes a case of genetic discrimination. Assuming that argument to be valid, we may conclude that the standard of health problems appears to be a viable option to exclude such discriminatory grounds as being female or being disabled.

How to identify health problems? Given the distinction between disabilities resulting from impairments and disabilities resulting from illnesses, one class of genetic disorders may be excluded in this way. A child born deaf will develop the handicap of being a deaf-mute. But does the fact that it cannot hear and that it has difficulties with speech render being a deaf-mute a health problem? It does not appear so. Deafness is a condition that results in an impairment and not in an illness. One is not sick from being deaf. The handicap of being a deaf-mute relates to adaptations in social functioning, but not necessarily to problems with health conditions. Blurring the distinction between differences in social functioning and health problems would render conditions such as being female or being homosexual in certain cultural contexts health problems as well. Intuitively, therefore, the option of developing a standard of health problems does not look hopeless.

The question now is how to establish such a standard. Apparently, one way to do so is to defer the identification of health problems to the medical profession. After all, identifying illness and disease is what medicine is all about. But clearly this will not work. Developments in modern medicine as well as in medical ethics have changed the role of patients into clients. Medical professionals offer their services to people who want to pay for them. Consequently, caring for the sick is more and more framed within a business perspective. The question of what counts as a health problem is more and more subject to the mechanism of supply and demand. In pursuing the projects of their private lives people stumble on obstacles and limitations, some of which they simply have to accept as a fact of life while others may be overcome. Their different projects reflect different rankings of goods, about which there need not be a consensus among them. Adhering to different views on human life, they have no shared views on how to live or what makes their life worth while. Consequently, they lack a common standard for deciding which obstacles and limitations to accept as naturally given and which to define as health problems. If true, this implies that conceptions of health and disease are thoroughly conventional. In a society governed by the conventions of liberal culture, the medical profession has lost its prerogative to define the content of these concepts. There is no sufficient moral justification for the prolongation of its traditional role.[22]

But obviously, if the medical profession does not have the moral authority to define the notion of health problems, neither does the state. Who is the state to decide whether or not I have to accept a given obstacle as part of my life instead of using professional help to remove it? Suppose my wife and I come from families in which most males lose their hair in their late twenties. Since I have spent a fortune on various aids to stimulate hair growth and hair transplants without much success, I want to know the sex of the child that my wife is expecting, because if it is a boy, we would seriously consider having it aborted. Let us suppose that the response would be that surely baldness is no disease. Obviously, this response may fail to impress me because it completely ignores my restricted chances at finding attractive girlfriends, my diminished opportunities for careers that have a representational aspect, and my being stigmatized as an early aging person.

Outrageous as the example may seem, the question is on what grounds the state can justifiably deny me access to genetic testing procedures to detect 'juvenile baldness', should they be available. In terms of my question in this section, on the basis of which conception of the good life can the state argue that baldness is to remain outside the scope of medicine? And if the state does not have this conception, how could it hope to establish a standard of health problems for deciding which genetic disorders to exclude from prenatal testing? If it is true that our society is beyond the point where a canonical standard of medicine has moral authority, as I believe is the case, then the standard that we are looking for cannot be enforced with sufficient justification. The concept of health problems has been replaced in modern medicine by the concept of health desires. Medicine will include whatever problems people define with regard to their own bodies as health problems and are prepared to pay for.

6.6 Degrees of Seriousness?

The distinction between 'profound', 'severe', and 'mild' disabilities suggested above may be more helpful than the distinction between 'health' and 'disease'. Not all genetic disorders have consequences of the same degree of seriousness with regard to people's lives. We may not have very strong grounds for arguing, for example, that in contrast to juvenile baldness Klinefelter's syndrome is a disease, but we surely have strong grounds to argue that living with Klinefelter's syndrome is significantly different from living with Tay Sachs.[23] If so, a standard for restricting access to prenatal testing grounded in degrees of seriousness looks more promising.

Nonetheless, difficult problems remain. Even if we think that a certain range of agreement might be possible, we can safely predict that this agreement will concern the class of profound rather than mild disorders. The logic here is that the further a given condition is from the average condition of human life as we know it in our society, the less contested the assessment of that condition will be. Conversely, the closer a given condition is to the average condition, the more disputed will be the question of whether or not it should be prevented. Klinefelter's syndrome produces boys with underdeveloped male attributes whose performance in social functioning is only a little below average. While the question "What is wrong with boys with underdeveloped male attributes?" may leave room for dispute for people who are particularly keen on sons with male attributes, the question "What is wrong with Tay Sachs?" will leave much less room, if any, for dispute.[24] Following this logic, we may hope to identify some genetic disorders that cause health conditions so severe that hardly anybody in our society would reject the option of preventing the birth of children with those disorders.

There are other problems, however, that make the possibility of operational distinctions rather questionable. For example, the problem of degrees of certainty. Not only is it often unclear what the degree of handicap will be (fragile X, spina bifida), it is also unclear how the burdens posed by these handicaps will be assessed. In the eyes of some people the condition of Down syndrome is compatible with a reasonably happy life, while for others this is an appalling view. There are both empirical and normative differences in assessing the future condition of children with specific disorders. Perhaps with some exceptions, these differences make a fixed list of genetic disorders that are to be excluded from prenatal testing a hazardous undertaking.

Are these two points sufficient to rule out this option? Let us consider the example of Down syndrome somewhat further. People with that condition have a higher risk of congenial heart failure (about 9 percent), their life expectancy is between forty and fifty years of age. At that age a number of these people develop Alzheimer's disease (about 40 percent). Are these figures sufficient to conclude that Down syndrome should be on the list of conditions that qualify for selective abortion? I do not think this conclusion follows. What follows is only that among the conditions that cause people with Down syndrome to suffer from disease are heart failure and Alzheimer's. But this does not at all mean that those who suffer from such conditions suffer from Down syndrome. In certain regions in Western society a considerable number of females are a high-risk group for developing breast cancer. In these regions does that make being female *in itself* a condition to be prevented? If not, why can Down syndrome not be viewed in the same way? If organizations of parents and self-advocates within the disability community assure us that the condition of Down syndrome as such is often compatible with a happy life, why not accept their testimony as sufficient reason to exclude this condition from prenatal testing?

The answer to this question must be, again, that all depends on what one takes a reasonably happy life to be. I do not suggest that there can be no argument about our views on the matter, but that is not the point. The point is that the liberal democratic state is in a very weak position to act upon any such argument. Even if I personally accept the argument that the prevention of Down syndrome is based on cultural standards of normality, and that, therefore, the failure to meet these standards is not a sufficient reason for the prevention of people with this disorder, this does not at all imply that the state can adopt the same argument in order to justify a policy to that effect.[25] The argument only works if one accepts that (1) people with Down syndrome are capable of reasonably happy lives, (2) medicine should not be used, in principle, to cure suffering that results from socio-cultural standards of 'normality', and (3) the task of curing this kind of suffering demands policies of integrating the disabled in society and giving them the opportunity to participate. In accepting these points one implies a normative conception of health care and medicine that is limited to traditional conceptions of disease and illness. As was suggested above, however, our society is beyond the point where such a normative conception can be imposed upon people who want to use health care for whatever problems they think medical professionals can solve for them. Given the inevitable problems in justifying from a public point of view the value judgments underlying the distinction between 'profound', 'severe', and 'mild' conditions, the democratic state will unlikely succeed in this policy option.[26]

6.7 The Weakness of the Liberal Convention

The principle of state intervention to counter negative side effects of how citizens exercise their freedoms is applied in liberal society in a number of ways. The state interferes with smoking in public in order to protect the health of others by means of designating certain areas as smoking areas. The state also interferes with the distribution of jobs across different segments of society in order to counter discrimination by means of preferential hiring. Furthermore, it intervenes in the distribution of students from different ethnic minorities in schools and colleges. There is no initial reason why the state should not consider intervening also in how people use their reproductive freedom if it can thus protect equal concern and respect for disabled persons.

As we have seen, however, there are serious problems with the *public* justification of this kind of policy in liberal society. All of these problems basically stem from the same source. To justify restrictions on reproductive freedom, the state must identify a range of disorders that it wants to exclude from prenatal testing combined with selective abortion. Arguments in support of any proposal to that effect cannot but appeal to normative conceptions that are based on particular rankings of the good. Consequently, they fail to meet the crucial requirement for public justification in liberal society. None of the normative questions that we have been considering in this chapter is without a sound and reasonable answer, but in each case these answers are based upon particular convictions and beliefs that belong to what Engelhardt calls 'content-full moralities'. In other words: the answers that we can provide go beyond what the liberal convention enables us to argue with moral authority. Surely a liberal framework leaves us with the moral space to exchange substantial moral arguments about the good in our capacity as private citizens. But it does not provide us with grounds that are based upon these arguments to demand the implementation of coercive public policies curtailing other people's freedom. Hence, the conclusion must be that public morality in liberal society *does* provide us with an argument against genetic discrimination that may result from the proliferation of genetic testing procedures, but it does *not* provide us with arguments for particular policies to counter this tendency, such as the restriction of reproductive freedom.

If this is the main conclusion, what is its point? The point is an important lesson with regard to the liberal convention as a moral framework for thinking about ethics and the prevention of disabled lives. It teaches us something about the relative weakness of public morality in liberal society concerning its disabled members, particularly those who are mentally disabled. Liberal society takes pride in its stance of equal respect toward all of its members. But how strong can the claim to equal respect for mentally disabled people be if it has to compete with the paramount value assigned to free choice? That the threat of genetic discrimination as a result of the proliferation of genetic testing among the population at large will become a serious issue is more than likely. That the most effective way of dealing with that issue will be a socialized system of health-care insurance is an argument that has much to say for it. But even then the issue of genetic discrimination will reenter from a corner where it may be even more frightening, i.e., as an instrument of governmental policy to lower the costs of the health-care system. One way or another, people with disabilities run the risk of paying the price. Why then should we not place the proliferating genetic testing in chains? Because the liberal state will not find publicly justifiable methods to that effect. Despite its commitment to equal opportunity among its citizens, there is reason to doubt if the liberal democratic state will be capable of maintaining this commitment with regard to the disabled. The answer to this question may for the most part depend on the moral will and imagination of those who are themselves committed to care for disabled persons. To the extent that these advocates will succeed in inspiring other citizens to share their point of view, liberal democracy may hope to avoid the threat of genetic discrimination.

Part Two

SEVEN

The Inclusion of the Mentally Disabled

One determines quite reasonably that it would be *unfair* and *unjust—exploitative*—to exclude certain humans from the scope of equal consideration simply because they lacked the capacity for moral reciprocation. Indeed, that such exclusion would be unfair *is*, I submit, the judgment of common moral consciousness.

Edmund N. Santurri

Modern conceptions of justice emerged in conjunction with the idea of a social contract. Justice is applicable to and binding upon rational, responsible parties. . . . Justice is responsive only *after* the question is answered as to who is a recognizable participant. Thus the sensitivities carried by the value of justice miss the most critical and precarious moment in the politics of enactment.

Stephen White

7.1 The Moral Standing of Disabled People

In this chapter we will discuss the problem of how to account for the inclusion of mentally disabled people in our society as a moral community. As will become apparent in this connection the moral standing of the mentally disabled is particularly relevant because they do not neatly fit the moral conception of the individual as it occurs in liberal theory. The question as to why they are nonetheless included in our moral community poses an awkward problem for liberal theory. The conception of the individual presupposed in that type of theory is based on the capacities of human beings *qua* moral agents, e.g., the powers of reason and free will. Assuming that the mentally disabled lack these capacities, liberal theory faces a problem.

To discuss this problem I will proceed from the conclusion reached in earlier chapters with regard to the issue of genetic discrimination. It said that, given certain empirical assumptions about the proliferation of genetic testing procedures among the general population, the liberal democratic state has strong reasons for protecting disabled citizens against discriminatory side effects of genetic testing, but it lacks feasible options for implementing policies to do so. In that connection we considered two options: one tackling the issue as one of social justice in order to defend protection against genetic discrimination as required by the principle of equality of opportunity. It was argued that given certain beliefs about individual responsibility for the genetic condition of one's offspring, this option is most likely to slide back to an issue of curtailing individual freedom. The second option was to tackle the issue directly as one of curtailing freedom for the sake of protecting disabled people from negative side effects of other people's actions. The conclusion—the state should do something, but does not know how—was taken to indicate that liberal democracy is quite weak when it comes to protecting its disabled citizens against the negative side effects of gene technology. In this chapter we will inquire into the source of this weakness. Why is it that liberal morality that takes pride in equal respect for each individual and that objects strongly to discrimination, is left empty-handed when it comes to the genetic discrimination of disabled people?

Obviously, part of the answer has to do with the prospective character of the argument. As the speculations that I made on the possibility of unintended side effects of prevention by means of genetic testing indicated, the strongest case against discrimination regards the social position of disabled people *in the future*. Whether or not these side effects will actually become manifest is still an open question. Hence, the argument may have a certain plausibility—as I claim it does—but its force must remain a matter of dispute. I do not think, however, that the relative weakness of the case against genetic discrimination is fully explained by its prospective character. It is important for my argument that we arrive at a more complete understanding of the problem. Discrimination is morally objectionable in liberal theory because it fails to give due respect to other persons. To discriminate against other persons is to ignore their capacity as human agents by treating them unequally on grounds of morally irrelevant characteristics such as race, sex, religion, or age. Since the characteristic of being mentally disabled affects one's capacity for human agency, this theory of discrimination appears to exclude the mentally disabled from its protection. That is to say, people with mental disabilities do not seem to qualify as human agents in the sense presupposed by the theory: they do not possess the powers of reason and free will; they oftentimes cannot give an account of why they do what they do, nor can they make plans for the future, given the fact that they lack a sense of time. Consequently, their behavior hardly counts as human action understood as intentionally directed and guided by reason. For all of these reasons, human agency is incompatible with the more profound varieties of mental disability. If so, the liberal theory of discrimination as outlined above also fails to apply. As the issue of discrimination is an issue about the moral justification of differential treatment on the basis of individual characteristics, it appears that, according to liberal theory, 'mental disability' *is* a relevant characteristic allowing such treatment because of the limited capacity for human agency that it involves.

Assuming this to be correct, we cannot but admit that in the context of liberal thinking the charge of discrimination is misguided whenever the capacity of agency fails to apply. This suggests that the relative weakness of the case against genetic discrimination is not only a matter of the prospective nature of the argument, but also that it results from the moral standing ascribed to the mentally disabled in liberal theory. To explore this suggestion in this chapter, we will look in detail at liberal solutions for this problem. If the concept of human agency as intentionally directed and guided by reason is as crucial to the liberal frame of mind as it appears to be, then to give an account of the moral standing of mentally disabled people in liberal society will face serious difficulties. To see whether this claim holds, I will engage in a lengthy discussion with John Rawls and H. Tristam Engelhardt Jr., two philosophers whose accounts are in surprising agreement at this point, given their otherwise diverging theories of liberal morality. My aim in spelling out their views on this issue is that they reveal a pattern of argumentation that I take to be unavoidable for any theory that regards itself as liberal.

In order to understand their views on moral standing, we will have to sketch their theories in some detail. I will first return to Engelhardt's theory of secular morality, as developed in *The Foundations of Bioethics,* and then look at the work of John Rawls, as presented in both his seminal book *A Theory of Justice* and his more recent *Political Liberalism.*[1] As we will see, both authors think that people who are permanently incapacitated should be included in a theory of moral standing, but their attempts to include them fail. Confined within the frame of liberal thought these attempts reveal a pattern of argumentation that fails to generate strong reasons for the moral standing of the mentally disabled. If this is true, it helps one understand more fully the relative weakness of liberal morality to protect disabled citizens against the negative side effects of genetic testing. Liberal morality does not have much strength, if any, to generate moral arguments for the protection of people who do not possess the powers of reason and free will.

7.2 Persons in the Social Sense

The fact that disabled people pose a problem for Engelhardt's conception of secular morality should not surprise us. Once the principle of permission is taken as central, the question arises of what to say about those who are incapable of giving or withholding permission: "Not all humans are self-conscious, rational, and able to conceive of the possibility of blaming and praising. Fetuses, infants, the profoundly mentally retarded, and the hopelessly comatose provide examples of human nonpersons. They are members of the human species but do not in and of themselves have standing in the secular moral community" (*The Foundations of Bioethics*, 138–39). The crucial concept in this connection is the concept of the person. In Engelhardt's theory persons are defined as "those entities who can establish by their agreements a web of moral authority for their collaboration, or who can refuse to be involved with others." Only they are "active participants in the morality that can bind moral strangers."[2] Although from the perspective of a 'content-full morality', this concept of the person looks very impoverished indeed, it presents the only view that can stand the test of authoritative justification in what Engelhardt calls 'general secular morality'.

What about those human beings to whom this concept does not apply? Engelhardt answers the question in terms of what he calls 'the social sense of persons.' Even if secular morality does not grant disabled people moral standing per se, this does not necessarily mean that they are deprived of it. One can find certain practices that recognize these human beings as persons for 'social considerations.'[3] Within these practices people assume a particular role that weaves them into the fabric of communal life. This role grants them the standing in the fabric of secular society that—as a matter of moral principle—only 'real' persons can have. According to Engelhardt, most societies have such social roles. Newborn infants, for example, are included in a community through a ritual that marks the transition to the status of membership. Since the social roles of persons created in this way are clearly not generated by secular morality, they depend on the existence of 'particular communities' and their moral practices. Persons in the social sense receive the standing they have for reasons inherent in the morality of these communities.[4]

Obviously, this account of the social roles of persons does not succeed in justifying the moral standing of nonpersons from the point of view of secular morality. Any justification in secular morality that is generated by moral views belonging to a particular community is invalidated by Engelhardt's own criteria. Since the social roles of persons are generated in this way, we are still left without a valid solution for our problem, which is how to account for the moral standing of nonpersons in liberal morality. Furthermore, the fact that

Engelhardt's account of liberal morality in general secular terms has no use for cultural forms such as rites and rituals implies that the inclusion of nonpersons can be justified only by giving *reasons*. So the question remains, What sort of reasons are available within general secular morality for assigning the social role of persons to people who are not persons?

To answer this question and make room for the moral standing of non-persons, Engelhardt suggests that we follow a lead provided by Kant. If including such beings in our public morality will strengthen respect for its core values, then that is a reason for doing so.[5] Interestingly, Kant is called upon here to provide a consequentialist reason for acting toward nonpersons *as if* they were real persons.

> Since this [social] sense of person cannot be justified in terms of the basic grammar of morality (i.e. because such entities do not have intrinsic moral standing through being moral agents), one will need rather to justify a social sense of person in terms of the usefulness of the practice of treating certain entities as if they were persons. If such a practice can be justified, one will have, in addition to a strict sense of persons as moral agents, a social sense of persons justified in terms of various utilitarian and other consequentialist considerations. (*The Foundations of Bioethics*, 147)

This indirect justification implies, however, that the moral standing of non-persons can be ascertained only through substitution. To treat the disabled as if they were persons has no basis in these people themselves but is justified by reference to other persons. In other words, the standing of nonpersons in Engelhardt's theory is not something we owe to disabled people as such but is indirectly derived from the value that secular morality places on the protection of real persons. This means that Engelhardt resorts to what looks like a form of indirect utilitarianism. According to this theory the act of killing the innocent, for example, is not condemned for its intrinsic features but for its overall utility when adopted as a general moral rule. Analogously, the social sense of person is defended not on the basis of the intrinsic characteristics of disabled people, but also on its overall usefulness for the protection of real persons.

7.3 Justice and Beneficence

How strong will this indirect justification in the actual practice of secular morality turn out to be? The answer to this question is found where it can always be found in utilitarian theories, namely at the point where it comes to weighing conflicting interests. Engelhardt is very clear on this point:

These practices of assigning rights to humans who are not persons will not be absolute, at least in general secular terms. When a set of considerations shows that suspending the practice will achieve a greater balance of benefits over harms, such an exception will be justified. . . . The obligations imposed by others in terms of the social roles of persons will thus at best in general secular morality be prima facie obligations, which can in particular circumstances be set aside. (*The Foundations of Bioethics*, 148)

Social practices that include nonpersons in a scheme of rights can be suspended in particular circumstances if such is of greater benefit. What sort of circumstances could these be? Engelhardt mentions the case of parents who want their handicapped newborn infant to die painlessly. In claiming that they should be allowed to make this decision, they are not imposing any burden on other persons nor do they demand cooperation from others against their own will (they can look for doctors willing to carry out their wish). Given these considerations, there is no reason for not granting them the right to make this decision. The justification of their claim does not violate the rights of other persons. Nor do they impose "undue financial and psychological burdens" on other persons.[6]

Drawing on Engelhardt's theory, this example can be multiplied by many others. Eventually it can be very beneficial for real persons when new types of drugs are tested on other human beings before being admitted to clinical practice. Suppose that proxys of disabled people consent to their being used in drug experiments, what could be said against it? Not very much, it seems, provided that the proxys are not forced to consent. Only when the side effects of such practices would be harmful to real persons—it may undermine a general respect for the right to bodily integrity, for example—would there be grounds to prohibit these experiments.[7] However, this type of constraint—call it a reason from 'public fear'—does not solve our problem. If the maintenance of respect for the right to integrity among the public is the only reason for prohibiting experiments with 'nonpersons', the good of adequately tested drugs can still be achieved by keeping these experiments out of the public eye. If public knowledge of such practices is what creates public fear they should be kept secret, which would solve the problem without any moral problem remaining.

This may appear an unduly formalistic account of Engelhardt's theory because apart from the principle of consent it also has room for the principle of beneficence. Would the simple fact that drug testing may cause significant suffering not be a sufficient reason to prohibit it on grounds of beneficence? One does not inflict the risks of drug experimentation on other creatures because of what it does to their well-being. As it turns out, however, the principle of beneficence, insofar as it can be justified from a secular moral point of view, has only formal content. It tells us no more than to do good and avoid evil. To specify its content more substantially, Engelhardt maintains, one has to rely on a particular 'moral sense' that a general secular morality cannot provide. Weighing the goods implied in conflicting interests cannot be carried out by secular moral reasoning, because rankings of goods depend on particular moralities. "The bonds of beneficence, if they are to be established, must be framed through mutual understandings, both implicit and explicit, which establish both content and authority. Only in particular social contexts, within the embrace of particular moral communities, can one discover what are in fact the bonds of beneficence" (*The Foundations of Bioethics*, 112). When applied to our present example we may take this to mean, presumably, that what counts as 'significant suffering' or 'inflicting acceptable risks' in connection with drug testing cannot be specified with authority by general secular morality. Nor could it be argued that we cannot use disabled people interchangeably with animals for drug experiments, provided that consent is obtained and that our moral community has no problem with this.

The formal nature of beneficence in secular morality leads Engelhardt to conclude that in general secular terms "the problem of justifying any particular view of beneficence is under such circumstances insuperable."[8] Such justification depends on the 'web of sympathies' that characterizes communities of 'moral friends'. If the prima facie duties of beneficence in particular cases cannot be justified in general secular terms, what about the principle itself? Engelhardt develops his answer—again—in reference to Kant. Kant attempted to justify the principle of beneficence by arguing that to reject it one would inescapably become involved in a contradiction of the will. Having rejected sympathy for others as a moral duty, one cannot will others to be sympathetic toward oneself. Since everyone can foresee being in need of other people's sympathy in the future, one cannot without contradiction will to reject beneficence as a moral principle.

Engelhardt criticizes Kant's argument as insufficient in that it seeks to show that the justification of beneficence has the same source and structure as the justification of respect for persons. In both cases Kant seeks to make justification dependent on coherence. The principle of beneficence, however, is not as 'inescapable' in the way that the principle of consent is, because "one can act in nonbeneficent ways without being in conflict with the minimal notion of morality."[9] Nevertheless, he proceeds, Kant's argument has 'heuristic' meaning in that it reminds one of what the moral life can be about. The principle of beneficence "can at least *suggest* that it would be good to benefit persons in need" by creating "webs of sympathy" by way of "providing goods to fellow persons in need."[10] Consequently, rejecting the principle of beneficence leads to an essential impoverishment of the moral life.

It occurs to me that this argument fares no better than Kant's, however, if only for the reason that a suggestion is not a justification. If one can coherently be 'moral' in a secular sense without adopting a principle of beneficence, as Engelhardt suggests, then there is no *moral* reason—in his sense of the term— to adopt one. The only reason for adopting one can be found on the ground of a substantial view of what the moral life is about, which is beyond the scope of liberal morality understood in general secular terms. This conclusion shows what I will call the parasitic nature of liberal morality as Engelhardt understands it. It allows moral strangers to legislate anything they want as long as they assent voluntary to the agreement. Any claim exceeding the limits of consent between strangers—for example, claims regarding the interests of third parties not included in their transactions—can only be justified by the moral sense of these agents in their capacity as 'moral friends'.

To this criticism, Engelhardt may want to respond that this is what he has been saying all along, since he has repeatedly argued that secular morality has no content by itself and that it draws its content from particular moralities.[11] Even if this response is correct from the perspective of his theory, it hardly makes this theory commendable to those who remain skeptical about it. Particularly when Engelhardt insists that in general secular morality "the principle of permission always trumps the principle of beneficence," we seem to be ill-advised to rethink moral issues in health care on its terms, as Engelhardt suggests we should do.

> The world of general secular morality is quite different from what many think or hope it might be. It presses a fundamental reappraisal of what moral strangers can share as moral judgments regarding the status of fetuses, infants, the profoundly mentally retarded, and the severely brain-damaged. The full implications of secular morality in this area are yet to be realized in health care policy. (*The Foundations of Bioethics,* 140)

One fails to see the necessity of giving priority to finding out what moral strangers *can* share when all the weight seems to rest on what in fact they *do* share. Engelhardt may respond that he has no problem accepting that public morality in our society is actually richer than his empty formalism suggests. 'Moral strangers' can agree on whatever they want—he might say—provided they do not violate the principle of abstaining from illegitimate force. But this response does not alter the conclusion that the moral standing of nonpersons is a question on which public justification in secular morality has very little, if anything, to say. Even though it does not *rule out* that people hold substantial views on this matter, it does not *require* such views either.

At the end of his argument Engelhardt assures his readers that he does not intend to weaken the status of nonpersons but to offer "the strongest grounds, justifiable in terms of general secular arguments, for the moral standing of humans."[12] As has been shown, however, he has not provided *any* such ground because whatever grounds there are do not have secular morality as their source. Freely choosing agents may assign any moral standing to nonpersons—varying from 'full' to 'zero'—as long as they settle the issue in agreement and as long as their moral friends let them get away with it. In other words, for their moral standing in society, nonpersons such as the mentally disabled are completely dependent upon the good will of their moral friends. Secular morality, if it is what Engelhardt tells us that it is, has nothing to say on their behalf that does them any good.

7.4 Recipients of Justice

John Rawls's philosophy of liberalism has dominated much of contemporary thought on public morality. I therefore must ask for some patience with the presentation of yet another account of his views, but we cannot avoid providing a short outline to set the stage for the question I want to raise, which is what Rawls as a leading liberal theorist has to say about the moral standing of the disabled.

Rawls starts with the observation that, given the fact of pluralism, a theory of justice cannot proceed from a conception of the good life for human beings. People in pluralist society will not accept their common affairs being governed by rules of justice derived from a particular conception of the good. They will only agree upon principles of justice that are reached as conclusions of a fair procedure. This methodological requirement leads Rawls to turn to the tradition of contract theory. The question for Rawls is, "What are the conditions under which the parties to a fair contract are reasonably bound to accept the principles of justice that it generates?" He answers this question by developing his own version of contract theory as a hypothetical choice theory.

Notwithstanding the fact that Engelhardt rejects Rawlsian contractualism,[13] there are some striking similarities between their theories. Given Rawls's methodological requirement, the question of the moral standing of nonpersons for Rawls appears as difficult as it proved to be for Engelhardt. As we will see, there is a remarkable similarity between the ways in which they resolve this problem. I will present Rawls's solution in two stages that mirror the two crucial claims of Engelhardt's theory. In *A Theory of Justice* Rawls resorts to the consequentialist type of argument for the moral standing of nonpersons that we already encountered in Engelhardt. In his more recent *Political Liberalism* he resorts to the moral views that people hold on the basis of their comprehensive doctrines. Thus the Rawlsian conception of public morality in liberal society is as parasitic on comprehensive doctrines as Engelhardt's solution is on the morality of particular communities.

The principles of public morality will be accepted, according to Rawls, once it is made clear that the conditions under which they are chosen are fair to each and everyone. Each of the parties to the social contract has the same procedural rights, which secures their being treated equally as moral persons. In order to secure strict impartiality, however, Rawls adds a further characteristic of the contracting parties. They are not only defined as moral but also as rational persons. Each of them will accept those principles of justice that advance his or her own interests more than any alternative. Subject to the condition of equal procedural rights, their tendency to maximize self-interest does not violate the idea of fairness. Within a fair procedure of contracting, everyone can seek to further his or her own interest while disregarding the interests of others.[14] This characterization of the contracting parties in hypothetical choice, Rawls claims, secures the possibility of mutual advantage. It follows that, choosing under the conditions of a fair procedure, all have an equal interest in choosing principles of justice as a scheme of 'reciprocal advantage'.[15] To maximize one's own goods, under the constraint of recognizing the equal rights of others to do the same, is to engage in a scheme of social cooperation that is for the best of all parties concerned.

At this point the question of the moral standing of nonpersons in Rawls's theory begins to raise difficulties.[16] If the principles of 'justice as fairness' are accepted because they are mutually advantageous for persons capable of mutual respect, then the question must be asked to whom the principles of justice apply.

The natural answer seems to be that it is precisely the moral persons who are entitled to equal justice. Moral persons are distinguished by two features: first they are capable of having (and are assumed to have) a conception of their good (as expressed by a rational plan of life); and second they are capable of having (and are assumed to acquire) a sense of justice, a normally effective desire to apply and to act upon the principles of justice, at least to a minimum degree. We use the characterization of the persons in the original position [the Rawlsian condition of hypothetical choice] to single out the kinds of beings to whom the principles chosen apply. After all, the parties are thought of as adopting these criteria to regulate their common institutions and their conduct toward one another; and the description of their nature enters into the reasoning by which these principles are selected. Thus equal justice is owed to those who have the capacity to take part in and to act in accordance with the public understanding of the initial situation. (*A Theory of Justice*, 505)[17]

However, assuming that the condition of being a moral person is sufficient for being a recipient of justice, is it also a necessary condition? What about people who lack the capacity of "persons capable of mutual respect"? Rawls suggests the question can be left undecided "since the overwhelming majority of mankind fits the description." With regard to those who do not, "it would be unwise in practice to withhold justice on this ground. The risk to just institutions would be too great."[18] Rawls does not explain this claim any further, but it apparently means that to exclude nonpersons from justice would be unwise because it would undermine the respectability of democratic institutions in the public eye. Citizens advocating for specific groups of nonpersons may lose faith in a society in which their protégés have no equal standing. Rawls argues at length that the advantage of justice as fairness depends, among other things, upon its tendency to strengthen the respect for just institutions.[19] Excluding certain segments of the population from being the recipients of equal justice may undermine this tendency.

The Rawlsian argument for the moral standing of nonpersons, then, is strikingly similar to what we found in Engelhardt. Since justice as fairness does not generate any reason to include nonpersons directly, one needs a reason to include them indirectly.[20] The reason that Rawls suggests is that the contracting parties should be impressed by the risk of undermining public respect for just institutions, because these institutions are designed to work for their mutual advantage. The price of excluding nonpersons may be too high when it turns out to have destablizing effects.

Obviously, this argument makes the case for the standing of nonpersons entirely dependent upon political perceptions. For example, if there is little to fear of public outcry about neglecting the disabled, there is no reason to be troubled by their unequal standing. To insure stability, Rawls argues, "men must have a sense of justice or a concern for those who would be disadvantaged by their defection, preferably both."[21] Since the sense of justice installed by Rawlsian justice as fairness does not necessarily include such a concern, we are again left with the conclusion that there is a gap to be filled. That is, if the sense of justice nourished by Rawlsian principles does not generate direct reasons for granting equal moral standing to the permanently incapacitated, we need other sources to install "a concern for those who are disadvantaged by their defection." Rawls admits this much when he points out the limits of a theory of justice: "A conception of justice is only part of a moral view."[22] Other domains of morality should install "duties of compassion and humanity" to guide our conduct toward creatures to whom justice is not owed, strictly speaking. Such duties are "outside the scope of a theory of justice," however, so that other branches of philosophy are needed to elaborate them.[23]

7.5 Public Morality as Overlapping Consensus

In discussing the main differences between his first book and *Political Liberalism*, Rawls argues that he has shifted from a moral to a political conception of justice. In *A Theory of Justice* his conception of justice as fairness is developed as a comprehensive moral doctrine.[24] People are supposed to accept it on rational grounds, that is, as serving their best interests as free chosing agents. However, the attempt to justify justice as fairness in terms of rational choice theory is abandoned by the later Rawls and replaced by the "idea of an overlapping consensus." Modern democratic society is characterized not merely by pluralism, but by a variety of reasonable comprehensive, moral, philosophical and religious doctrines that are nonetheless incompatible. Political liberalism is capable of answering the question how modern society characterized by a reasonable pluralism can be stable. Rawls's answer: it can because it can be justified as a "freestanding view" that can be supported from within any of the comprehensive doctrines to which citizens adhere. The grounds provided for this justification are political. That is, they are derived from premises that 'reasonable' agents will accept, as distinct from the premises that 'rational' agents will accept. The main difference is that reasonable agents regard themselves and their actions from a public point of view, whereas 'rational agents' do so only from an individual point of view. "Reasonable persons, we say, are not moved by the general good as such but desire for its own sake a social world in which they, as free and equal, can cooperate with others on terms all can accept. They insist that reciprocity should hold within that world so that each benefits along with others" (*Political Liberalism*, 50). Since reasonable persons regard themselves as free and equal, they are not motivated by rational self-interest but by the social world as cooperation "for its own sake." Of course, they hold the social world to be beneficial to all, but they do not calculate its benefits on the basis of their own individual interests. In other words, the 'reasonable' is not derived from the 'rational' as its foundation.[25]

Given this difference between Rawls's earlier and his more recent thought, however, one of the arguments regarding the moral standing of nonpersons in his earlier theory no longer works. It can no longer be argued that our society should include nonpersons in its scheme of just distribution because the destablizing effect from the failure of doing so would be disadvantageous for the contracting parties. This kind of appeal to rationality is abandoned.[26] What remains is the other argument for inclusion, namely that justice cannot resolve all questions, and that some questions are dependent for their solution on other parts of morality. The shift in the Rawlsian conception from rationality towards reasonableness explains why this second argument gains prominence in *Political Liberalism.*

Rawls uses this argument with respect to the problem of the moral standing of the permanently incapacitated. Considering this problem he concedes that in their case it is more than a problem of extension. Whereas the duties of justice can be extended to those who will enter the scheme of social cooperation at some point of time (future generations, children, the temporarily ill, other nations), such duties cannot be extended in the same way to those who are *permanently* nonpersons.[27] In pondering ways to resolve this problem Rawls concedes that a theory of justice cannot answer all our moral questions. We should acknowledge its limitations and not expect justice as fairness to cover the entire field of morality: "political justice needs always to be complemented by other virtues."[28]

In order to explain these limitations, we need to pay attention to the concept of public reason, which is a crucial concept for political liberalism according to Rawls. In giving an account of what public reason entails, one also determines the range of moral questions that can be answered on its basis. In a democratic society public reason is the reason of equal citizens who exercise political and coercive power in enacting and amending laws. The idea of public reason is not independent of but rather part of a political theory of justice.[29] The range of questions that can be resolved include such questions as who has a right to vote and who is to be assured fair equality of opportunity or to hold property. In other words, public reason is capable of dealing with moral questions regarding policies that affect citizens who are subject to the principles of justice.

Questions that this conception of public reason cannot answer, says Rawls, are the ones that deal with such issues as the protection of the environment, preservation of endangered species, funding of the arts and sciences, and so on. In deliberating on these questions, Rawls concedes, we do not reason as citizens but as members of communities and associations such as churches or universities. Philosophical, moral, and religious views have their appropriate role to play here, according to Rawls, because they are part of the "background culture" that is vital to political liberalism.[30]

Surely it would be worthwhile to analyze how Rawls exactly determines the relation between his conception of public reason and his notion of a background culture, but for our purposes it is sufficient to see how his argument affects the issue of the moral standing of the mentally disabled. Given the range of questions that can be addressed on the grounds of public reason, the problem emerges as to how Rawls's theory can allow advocates for the mentally disabled to defend the inclusion of these people in the realm of citizenship. If the rights of citizenship are justified by a political conception of justice and if this conception defines persons as 'political persons' in the way Rawls does, then public reason does not seem to entail any grounds on which the inclusion of the mentally incapacitated can be justified. If, in advocating their inclusion, we are not allowed to appeal to considerations derived from nonpublic reason, then it appears that we are left with no justifiable reasons at all. Not unlike Engelhardt, Rawls also defends the limits of public reason by claiming that the political values that it expresses are highly important and should not be easily overridden.[31] That is, the justification of public policy cannot appeal to values that are non-neutral between different conceptions of the good. But the problem is not only that of adjudicating competing claims between contending parties in the public sphere. It is also, or rather, a problem of justifying why nonpersons are recognized as contending parties in the first place. Why, after all, should 'nonpersons' such as the mentally disabled be recognized as citizens? *Public* reason as construed by Rawls's political liberalism cannot provide us with any ground for doing so.[32]

7.6 The Parasitic Nature of Liberal Morality

I have singled out the theories of liberal morality as presented by Engelhardt and Rawls to discuss the moral standing of mentally disabled people, because these theories suggest a pattern in the liberal solution to this question. I classify their theories as liberal because of two claims that I take to be characteristic for any liberal theory. First, public morality in their view should be guided by a conception of public justification that rules out conceptions of the good that are derived from particular moralities or comprehensive doctrines. Second, the moral content of their basic principles is in their view strictly derived from a conception of the human person as a free and equal being endowed with the powers of reason and free will. These claims cause the problem of justifying the inclusion of the mentally disabled in our community in a direct way because they are not included in this conception of the person, while at the same time their inclusion cannot be justified on the grounds of some 'content-full' or 'comprehensive' conception of the good.

The strategy to solve this problem consists of two steps. The first is to include the disabled on indirect grounds in terms of the enlightened self-interest of other persons. That is, the 'full' members of our community will be better off by including 'defective' members because it will foster general respect for the institutions of liberal democracy, which is to the advantage of everyone. As we saw, however, this consequentialist argument may not be very reliable. Given the assumption that in distributing burdens and benefits the liberal state will have to allow trade-offs between conflicting interests, the equal standing of defective citizens may fail to hold the line. For example, whether or not there will be sufficient support for granting equal rights to health-care services and welfare may come to depend on how the calculation of gains and losses turns out. Should maintaining these rights be considered too costly, the health-care and welfare benefits may become subject to budget cuts. In other words, should this consequentialist line of argument be accepted, the disabled may find public support for their rights to be wanting.

At this point the second step comes in. If it is doubtful whether the equal standing of these nonpersons for consequentialist reasons will hold the line, we will have to depend on other beliefs regarding the standing of these people to which members of society adhere, such as the belief that these people are owed equal respect simply because their lives have been part of the relationships that constitute our society. The problem is that the moral reasons derived from these other beliefs cannot be justified by reference to the narrow conception of public morality that is characteristic of liberal theory. That is, the inclusion of nonpersons can be justified on the basis of moral reasons that exceed the liberal framework of public justification. To solve this problem both Engelhardt and Rawls have to concede that liberal morality must rely on moral sources that it cannot recognize publicly. To be reasonably sure that such moral views obtain, both authors rely necessarily upon the fact that people in liberal society are committed to communal values other than those their liberal theories can support.[33]

This pattern of argumentation, it seems to me, is unavoidable for any theory that may be classified as liberal.[34] Presumably, some will want to respond by saying that liberal philosophy has sufficient instruments to repair the weakness to which I have been pointing, such as the doctrine of equality of opportunity. There need not be a problem for liberal theory in the fact that the mentally disabled cannot answer to patterns of normal functioning, at least not in the sense that this fact should exclude them from being treated equally. The varieties of liberal thought notwithstanding, many of them accept the principle of equality of opportunity.[35] On the basis of this principle liberal theorists may want to argue that people with special needs should be treated equally. Their argument would be that if we have moral reasons for treating people equally with regard to their opportunities in life, we also have moral reasons for taking into account inequalities preventing them from the benefits of equal opportunity. If these inequalities originate from scanty provisions of nature, as is the case with people affected by genetic disorders, the doctrine of equal opportunity requires that natural misfortune be compensated.[36]

If this doctrine can be justified within the conventions of liberal thinking, where does that leave my criticisms? The answer is that this response fails to address the issue at stake. The issue is not what equality should imply once we have accepted that the mentally disabled are also eligible for equal treatment. The issue is how to justify the basis for their being thus eligible in the first place. The doctrine of equal opportunity answers the question as to what equality should entail, but this already presupposes a decision on the range of creatures to whom equality applies. The doctrine as such, however, does not address the question of who should be included in that range. It is not easy to see how answering the latter question within the framework of liberal theory can avoid the pitfall that traps Engelhardt's and Rawls's theories.[37]

Is liberal moral and political philosophy to be blamed for its failure to answer the question of the moral standing of nonpersons satisfactorily? Yes and no. It is to be blamed to the extent that it accepts the burden of answering that question but then fails to provide a satisfactory answer. Presumably, the reason for accepting this burden is that, intuitively, many people in our society will be inclined to regard the mentally disabled as recipients of justice who should be included in our community. At least Engelhardt and Rawls seem to presuppose this intuition, which explains why they take the trouble of showing how to justify the inclusion of nonpersons in the first place.[38]

As the analysis of their arguments suggests, however, one can also say that liberal theory is not to be blamed in this respect because it only provides a moral framework for guiding interactions between free and equal human beings who are rational or reasonable creatures. Naturally, for such a theory, nonrational or nonreasonable creatures are not included. They are not included, this is to say, in the sense that their inclusion cannot be *publicly* justified in any direct way, without resorting to convictions and beliefs that exceed the public sphere as liberals understand it. This does not mean, of course, that people do not have valid reasons for accepting social responsibility for the mentally disabled and for caring for them and accepting them as fellow human beings. It only means that these reasons cannot be public reasons, given the presuppositions of liberal justification.

If this is true, as I claim, it suggests what I have called the parasitic nature of public morality in liberal society. This society takes pride in treating all of its citizens as equals, but its public morality is, as a matter of fact, incapable of providing adequate grounds for including the various categories of human beings whom we nonetheless do consider as citizens. Apparently, public morality in our society is actually richer in moral content than what liberal theory is capable of justifying in its own terms. This conclusion suggests that liberal morality is nourished, at least in part, by sources that liberal society fails to recognize publicly for their contribution.[39]

What follows from these observations with regard to a more satisfactory account of the moral standing of the mentally disabled in this society? If the pattern of argumentation that has been analyzed in the foregoing sections has been correctly identified, then liberal philosophy is at this point stuck with the choice between accepting inadequacy or accepting serious limitation. My own choice—and probably Rawls's and Engelhardt's as well—would be to accept the second alternative. Public morality as liberals understand it simply lacks the moral resources to make sense of why we care for mentally disabled persons and accept responsibility for them in our actual social practices. If we follow Engelhardt's suggestion of the 'social sense of person', it is clear where our theoretical reflections should go from here. The question that remains to be answered is, What sustains the social practices in which the mentally disabled appear as persons in the social sense if it is not liberal theory? What are the moral resources from which these practices derive their vitality and strength?

EIGHT

Imperatives of the Self

The fundamental problem of ethics has been expressed as the question: What ought I to do? The weakness of this formulation is in separating doing from the sheer being of the "I", as if the ethical problem were a special and added aspect of a person's existence. However, the moral issue is deeper and more intimately related to the self than doing. The very question: What ought I to do? is a moral act. It is not a problem added to the self; it is the self as a problem

Abraham Heschel

How could a bad person see that a true moral theory were in fact true, if he does not believe he is bad? If the theory conflicts with the considered judgment of a very good man, are we to believe the theory or the man? If the theory conflicts with strong feelings of conscience, is it possible that the theory is nonetheless true? And if the answer to the last question is "yes", as it seems it must be, in what sense do adherents to a moral theory maintain moral autonomy if they must override their sense of moral obligation with their loyalty to a theory?

Cheryl N. Noble

8.1 Two Claims

Public morality in liberal society incorporates a 'social sense' of the person which exceeds the conception of personhood that its philosophy can justify. It sustains social practices of accepting moral responsibility for people whose capacity for human agency is diminished for one reason or another. Since such people cannot possibly be included in contractual or procedural accounts of liberal morality, the question to be answered is therefore which moral resources our society has available for sustaining these practices. The main burden of this chapter and the next is to defend two separate but related claims with regard to this question.

The first claim regards the primacy of critical method that is characteristic for modern moral philosophy. Although conceived in various ways, the method follows a pattern. It invites us to step back from whatever particular moral convictions we may happen to have and to engage in the construction of critical principles that can be deployed for testing our convictions. The term 'critical principles' is reminiscent of utilitarian authors such as Richard Hare and Richard Brandt, of course, but it is not difficult to find similar approaches in contemporary bioethics.[1] Authors such as Peter Singer, Helga Kuhse, and John Harris are well known for their attack on tradional moral views as are entailed in the doctrine of the sanctity of life, for example, which they take to reflect a traditional view on the value of human life that is no longer tenable.[2] These philosophers claim that even though the traditional views they attack are deeply rooted in our moral consciousness, it is nevertheless perfectly all right to ignore this fact.[3] The point of critical principles is precisely to go beyond what our traditional morality tells us to believe.

Kantian thinkers such as Rawls and Engelhardt follow different avenues. Their concern is less with critical than with public rationality, but their resultant theories are not unlike theories presented by utilitarians with regard to how they treat traditional morality. They do not deny that our public morality is supported by background views derived from contentful moralities or comprehensive doctrines, but they do deny that these views should enter into our scheme of public justification. Even if these background views reflect our strongest convictions, the logic of 'public reason' requires that we ignore them. However, regardless of whether our convictions are scrutinized by 'critical' or 'public' philosophy, the implication in both cases is by and large the same: should our convictions happen to be at odds with philosophical reason, so much the worse for our convictions.[4] Against this primacy of critical method I will argue in this chapter that to ignore facts about our moral conscience is to ignore facts about the integrity of the moral self that can only be denied at the cost of impairing that self.

The second claim takes up a theme from the last chapter. It is based on the conclusion that neither Rawls's nor Engelhardt's Kantianism is capable of giving an adequate account of why our society accepts moral responsibility for dependent others such as the mentally disabled. Both authors defer substantial moral convictions that can support this responsibility to the private realm, where we are allowed to act upon whatever convictions we want to maintain as long as we do not violate moral requirements supported by public reason. But at the same time they presuppose the efficacy of such convictions in our society so that their theories will not stand accused as being morally bankrupt. My second claim, then, considers one of the views that resist the theorizing of Kantian and utilitarian philosophy, namely the view that it is our responsibility to care for the lives of dependent people who do not fit the description of rational persons, not because of what they are but because of who they are. This inclusion is based on the fact that they are part of the social relationships that constitute the moral fabric of our society. This is a moral conviction that the defenders of a liberal conception of the human person do not want to abandon, notwithstanding the fact that their respective theories do not provide them with strong grounds for maintaining it.

Before I explain the task to be accomplished in this chapter, let me comment briefly on how both of the claims introduced here are related. The first claim is intended to make a formal point: to question whether we have good reason to abandon whatever moral views we have merely because they turn out to be incompatible with the results of moral theorizing. For if the theories of critical or public morality do not provide us with adequate reasons for sustaining the lives of dependent people and we nevertheless are convinced that these lives ought to be sustained, what are we to do? This question is not about rational consistency but about moral integrity. As the quote from Cheryl Noble at the beginning of this chapter indicates, moral convictions can be abandoned only at the peril of undermining one's identity as a moral person.[5] They are deep moral convictions in the sense of being imperatives of the self. The second claim makes a material point. It says that the inclusion of dependent others such as the mentally disabled is not grounded in anything like their psychological and mental characteristics but in their participation in the social relations that constitute the moral fabric of our society. In accepting responsibility for these people we express how we understand ourselves in relation to them. Both claims are related in this way, then, that our views on social responsibility for dependent others is a reflection of our moral identity. Their moral standing does not depend on their individual capacities but reflects a particular way of how we understand the relationships we share with them. To give an account of this self-understanding I will turn in the next chapter to a particular description of the moral life. Its leading idea is that moral responsibility is grounded in the fact that the life of the 'other' is given to us, which requires that we respond appropriately.

To elaborate the first of these two claims in the present chapter I will switch to another mode of discourse and turn to a novel that makes the point about moral integrity with admirable literary genius. The novel is called *A Personal Matter* and is written by the Japanese Nobel Prize-winning author Kenzaburo Oë, who is himself the father of a mentally disabled son.[6] The story concerns a man who must come to terms with the birth of a severely handicapped child during the first few days. Having decided that he wants to get rid of 'the monster'—as he calls the baby—he then has to live with this decision which turns out to be impossible for him.

Although there is no explicit reference in this novel to moral theorizing, the crisis of Oë's main character is induced by the fact that he is tempted by the kind of questioning that moral theorizing generates with respect to the issue of handicapped newborn infants: If the baby is not capable of experiencing anything, if it is just like a vegetable, what good is keeping it alive? Or, Do human vegetables suffer from being born? Or, Can I consistently will to decline being the father of such a child? In pursuing the psychology of being tempted by these and other questions, Oë shows what abandoning deep convictions can do to people's integrity as moral persons.

My aim in retelling his story is to suggest that accepting responsibility for the social relationships in which we find ourselves is constitutive of the moral self, rather than being the object of our choice and decision. Trying to deny these responsibilities may very well be destructive to the self. To explain why, I will draw on an analysis of the connection between identity and accountability by Alasdair MacIntyre.[7]

Since the task of retelling the story of Oë's novel will take up most of the present chapter I will postpone the discussion of the second claim to the next one.

8.2 Kenzaburo Oë: A Personal Matter

Why would someone maintain that it is appropriate to care for severely disabled human beings who lack the powers of reason and free will and who are hardly consciously aware of the fact of their existence? Oë's novel tells the story of a young man who faces this question very directly when his first child turns out to be seriously deformed.

The novel begins when the main character, called 'Bird' because of his birdlike appearance, wanders through the city. He is restless because his wife is in the hospital. She is about to give birth to their first child. The reason for his restlessness is not concern about his wife but anxiety about his future. He spends some time in a warehouse looking for maps of Africa, which in Oë's novel is a metaphor for Bird's vain hopes of being saved from dreaded, ordinary life. These hopes seem to fall apart when he receives a phone call from the hospital. He must come immediately: "The baby is abnormal, the doctor will explain." It is the opening sequence of a drama that takes its main character on a journey into the dark alleys of the self in a desperate attempt to escape.

On his first visit to the hospital Bird introduces himself as the father and is painfully aware of the fact that the medical staff avoids looking at him. "The child is considered a monster and I am the monster's father," he says to himself.

The director explains the condition of the child: brain hernia. Part of the brain is protruding from a defect in the skull. "Even if we are lucky and succeed in getting the defect fixed, the result will be some kind of a vegetable human being," the doctor says. When Bird asks whether the child will die soon, the doctor replies that he does not expect the infant to die immediately, because it appears extremely vigorous. When asked what he intends to do, Bird is bewildered. What can he do? He inquires anxiously whether there is any 'alternative', without daring to make explicit what kind of alternative he has in mind. It is the first expression of the resistance that is mounting in the unfortunate father. The hospital director, however, refuses to respond and denies that there is any alternative, whereupon it is agreed that the child will be moved to the university clinic for further clinical investigation.

During the ride to the university clinic Bird asks the attending physician whether the baby is suffering. "Is it your opinion that a vegetable suffers?" the physician asks. Bird has never thought about it: "is a cabbage in pain when eaten by a goat?" He then looks at his son and sees its skull bandaged with bloody cotton, showing "something large and abnormal." The sight of it makes him infinitely sad: "My son has bandages on his head and so did Apollinaire when he was wounded on the field of battle. On a dark and lonely battlefield I have never seen, my son was wounded like Apollinaire and now he is screaming soundlessly" (24). Bird starts to cry at the thought that the image of Apollinaire evokes in him. Like the French poet, his son was wounded on a dark and lonely battlefield where the father will have to bury him like a soldier who died at war. Oë brilliantly catches the wretchedness of the father and allows it to develop into self-pity. The image opens up Bird's sorrow and even makes him feel redeemed: "He even discovered a sweetness in his tears."

Having left the baby at the clinic, Bird notices that after a few minutes he has already lost his clear image of the child. He takes it as an ominous sign that his son soon will be forgotten: a life that appeared out of darkness, "hovered for nine months in a fetal state" in order to live through a few hours of cruel discomfort and then descend again into "darkness, final and infinite." Wandering through the labyrinth of hospital corridors, Bird is caught by the shattering truth that he will never be able to escape the question "where is your son?" The birth of his deformed son is an undeniable fact about the world that will be there until the end of time.

After a while Bird receives a phone call from his mother-in-law. She is aware of the child's severe condition and questions the point of further medical examination. Bird responds quite aggressively that the point of further examination is that the baby happens to be alive. He promises to hide the fact of the child's brain defect from his wife but realizes the falsehood of his response. He will not only hide the truth about their newborn son from his wife but also the truth about his own desire to get rid of the child if he can.

8.3 An Inward Voyage

On his own again, the tortured young father discovers cruelly that from now on every innocent little thought and memory will be tainted by deceit. For example, having left his house in a hurry that morning, he decides to get a shave before visiting his father-in-law. Upon entering the barbershop he remembers a scene at a barber's years ago when he still was a boy. The remembrance brings a smile to his face. But when he sees his own smile in a large mirror in front of the shop, he is horrified: "Bird shuddered, shattering the smile, and began thinking about the baby. In the smile on his face, he had discovered proof of his own guilt. The death of a vegetable baby—Bird examined his son's calamity from the angle that stabbed deepest. The death of a vegetable baby with only vegetable functions was not accompanied by suffering" (30). So, the truth is out. The baby, being a vegetable, does not suffer, which means that there can be but one reason for wanting his son's death: his father does not accept him. Bird is horrified precisely because he has already decided that he does not want the baby to live, even if he is still very far from openly acknowledging it.

Oë now develops the theme of how Bird, by withdrawing into his inner self, holds himself accountable for his intentions in a way that takes on cosmological dimensions. Still in the same barbershop, Bird contemplates the life of his son. What would life mean to such a child? What would its death mean? Here is what the novelist has his character ponder about these questions:

> The bud of existence appeared on a plain of nothingness that stretched for zillions of years and there it grew out of nine months. Of course, there was no consciousness in a fetus, it simply curled in a ball and existed, filling utterly a warm, dark, mucuous world. Then, perilously, into the external world. It was cold there, and hard, scratchy, dry and fiercely bright. The outside world was not so confined that the baby could fill it by himself: he must live with countless strangers. But, for a baby like a vegetable, that stay in the external world would be nothing more than a few hours of occult suffering he couldn't account for. Then the suffocating instant, and once again, on that plain of nothingness zillions of years long, the fine sand of nothingness itself. (*A Personal Matter*, 30)

The child is doomed to return to that same eternal plane of nothingness for no other reason than being rejected by his father. Contemplating this possibility,

Bird faces what appears to him to be the ultimate question: what if all this will not remain unnoticed?

> What if there *was* a last judgment! Under what category of the Dead could you subpoena, prosecute, and sentence a baby with only vegetable functions who died no sooner than he was born? Only a few hours on this earth, and spent in crying, tongue fluttering in his stretched, pearly-red mouth, wouldn't any judge consider that insufficient evidence? Insufficient fucking evidence! Bird gasped in fear that had deepened until now it was profound. I might be called as a witness and I wouldn't be able to identify my own son unless I got a clue from the lump on his head. (31)

The death of the son will incur judgment upon the father, evidently, because who else is going to speak for his son on judgment day, if there is such thing? On that day the insincerity of the father will be exposed at last, for he will not be able to recognize his own son except in the state in which he left him to die.

From this point on the theme of guilt becomes central to the development of the story. It seems as if everything Bird says and does is intended to provide evidence of his base character. After he has visited his father-in-law-who against his own better judgment offers him a bottle of whiskey to drown his sorrow—Bird visits Himiko, a former girlfriend with whom he had a brief affair before his marriage. Bird gets very drunk and has intercourse with her in a way that, to put it mildly, is no tribute to their friendship. Himiko endures him, however, and does not even throw him out when he throws up in her bathroom the next morning. Later that day Bird, who is a teacher of modern literature at a college of higher education, feels sick in his English literature class and vomits again, this time in front of his class. The incident seriously offends some of his students who threaten to report him to the dean. Bird fails to be upset by any of these events, however, because they only prove what he already knows. It is as if he deliberately seeks to be degraded and punished.

Further proof of his guilt he finds later that day when he arrives at the clinic. Upon entering the building, he has to choose between two possible corridors. One takes him to the pediatrician's office to receive the message of his son's death; the other takes him to the intensive care unit where his son is still alive. He starts walking and finds himself approaching the pediatrician's office, which assures him that his desire for the baby's death dominates his consciousness. "Now he was the baby's true enemy, the first enemy in its life, the worst. If life was eternal and if there was a god who judged, Bird thought, then he would be found guilty. But his guilt now, like the grief that had assailed him in the ambulance when he compared the baby to Apollinaire with his head in bandages, tasted primarily of honey" (67). Inwardly convinced of his crime and comforted by the admission of guilt, Bird approaches the office. Anticipating the hopeful news of his son's death, he has mentally arranged the child's burial already. But unfortunately for Bird, things are not going his way. The nurse at the office congratulates him merrily on his strong son. "Does that mean that he is still alive?" Bird asks, hardly able to disguise his disappointment. "Of course he is alive!" the nurse says. When Bird sees his baby again, it appears to have become stronger and stronger, well prepared to enter life as a living vegetable.

The doctor who has examined the child wants to speak with him. Within a few days the child will be transferred to another hospital for brain surgery. "There will be an operation then?" Bird asks. The doctor is very stern about it: "Sure there will be an operation if it gets strong enough." Bird now understands that he not only has become the first enemy of his own son but that he will also have to act as his executioner. Nonetheless, however disgraceful, he wants to get rid of this child. What will become of his life if it lives? What of his trip to Africa? Seeing his life under attack, Bird prepares for battle. But for the moment he has to face the fact that he utterly lacks the courage to act upon his resolution.

> He blushed and began to sweat, ashamed of the tapeworm of egotism that had attached itself to him. One ear was deafened by the roar of blood hurtling through it and his eyes gradually reddened as though walloped by a massive, invisible fist. The sensation of shame fanned the red fire in his face and tears seeped into his eyes—ah, Bird longed, if only I could spare myself the burden of a monstrous vegetable baby. But voice his thoughts in an appeal to the doctor he could not do, the burden of his shame was too heavy. (75)

Apparently aware of the father's anxiety, the doctor then explicitly asks if he does not want his child to recover. Bird shivers, feeling that his ugliest thoughts are completely exposed by the docter's question, but he manages a feeble attempt: "Even with surgery, if the chances are very slight . . . that he'll grow up a normal baby . . ." Bird watches himself racing down the slope of contemptibility when the doctor comes to his rescue. After a pause of silence he answers that he, as a doctor, cannot take any direct steps to end the baby's life. Bird hurries to agree—"Of course not!"—but the doctor then continues and suggests regulating the baby's milk and giving him a sugar-water substitute. Only if the child still does not appear to weaken will they have to operate. Burning with shame but very much relieved, Bird leaves the hospital. He is told not to come back for a couple of days. The tension that Bird experiences is almost unbearable. The strong desire to save his own life—including his dream of going to Africa—collides with the undeniable fact that he is the father of this child. Thus the birth of his disabled son appears as a cosmic event that confronts him with a judgment from which there is no escape, because his own conscience will not let him. The self that ties Bird to the actual world, which he so desperately wants to escape, will bring him to the brink of self-destruction.

8.4 Himiko's Theory

An absolutely masterful key to this plot is the conversation that Bird has with Himiko, whose presence and importance in Oë's novel is far greater than I have space to show. Himiko is the only person to whom Bird dares reveal his secret desire, because she understands his sense of guilt. She has been through it herself, due to the fact that her husband committed suicide not long before Bird reappeared in her life. In a moving attempt to comfort him, Himiko explains her theory of the pluralistic universe.

When she was still a child she almost died of typhoid fever, an event that she experienced as standing at a crossroads: one way descending to death, the other ascending the slope to recovery. Since the Himiko who is telling this experience chose the road to recovery, another Himiko chose death!

> Do you see, Bird? Every time one stands at a crossroads of life and death, you have two universes in front of yourself; one loses all relation to you because you die, the other maintains its relation to you because you survive in it. Just as you would take off your clothes, you abandon the universe in which you are only a corpse and move on to the universe in which you are still alive. In other words, various universes emerge around each of us the way a tree's limbs and leaves branch away from the trunk. (45)

What is called the 'real world' is only one among countless other universes in which one may exist. Himiko herself was abandoned by her husband when he committed suicide in this universe, but in another universe, where he does not commit suicide, another Himiko is with him—or so she believes.

Himiko wants to share this piece of philosophical imagination with Bird so that he will not feel so sad about his baby and his desire to get rid of it. There is another universe in which the child is healthy and strong and in that universe Bird exists as a happy father. Himiko celebrates with him while they are having a drink together. Ignoring Himiko's intentions to comfort him, Bird denounces the idea as a "philosophical swindle" because, as he puts it: "one cannot tamper with the absoluteness of death by psychological tricks." So, he refuses to accept the cosmological escape that Himiko offers him and chooses to face what he experiences as inescapable reality. But he must then also face the actual world in which his intentions and motives are probed. In this world he is obsessed with one single fact, namely the expected phone call announcing the child's death. As long as it lives, his life is doomed. Bird clings almost pathetically to a state of self-pity that will end only with the affirmation of death. But this self-pity is not justified by the notion that he is the victim of natural disaster. For one thing, it is his son who is the main victim and, for another, Bird cannot wait to see the baby die. This hypocrisy is mercilessly exposed. One of Himiko's friends asks Bird if waiting for his child to die from malnutrition is not the worst of all possible alternatives. Fully aware of his deception, Bird knows that this is true and is heart-stricken when Himiko's friend suggests that what he probably dreads most is the possibility that his baby will not die. He does not know how to respond.

While he spends the night with Himiko, now his mistress, the phone rings at last. Bird is summoned to the university clinic next morning and this message makes him feel confident. But unfortunately, upon arrival he discovers that he has been deceived by his own false hopes: the baby has not died but is sufficiently strong to undergo brain surgery. The director of the clinic wants his approval. Feeling betrayed, Bird rises in anger and refuses, whereupon the doctor asks him bluntly if he will take the child home. Bird answers that he will.

Thus the last stage of the drama is set, because now the ultimate decision cannot be evaded: will he indeed become the executioner of his own son? Himiko suggests a possible way out. She knows someone at an illegal abortion clinic who might help him. Bird approves. But when he returns to the hospital to take the child home, a registration officer congratulates him with his baby and tells him that the clinic needs the name of the child for the hospital files.

> A name! thought Bird. Now, as in his wife's hospital room, the idea was profoundly disturbing. Provide the monster with a name and from that instant it would seem more human, probably it would begin asserting itself in a human way. The difference between death while the monster was nameless and death after Bird had given it a name would mean a difference to Bird in the nature of the creature's very existence. (146)

Giving him a name would indeed change the nature of the creature: ceasing to be a monster, it would now enter into the narrative of Bird's life, which is exactly what he has been so desperate to resist. Himiko implores him to hurry and just give the child a name. Bird hesitates: "I'll call him . . . Kikuhiko," he says abruptly, remembering the ominous name of an abandoned friend long ago. Then they leave the hospital with the baby.

Now that he is determined to go through with it, Bird manages to swallow what now appears to him as one repulsive decision after another. After a horrifying trip through the outskirts of the city, Bird and Himiko succeed in getting his son to the abortionist. Afterwards they go to a lonely bar owned by a former friend of theirs. Far from being at peace with himself, however, Bird is now confronted with the fact of his victory. He has saved his life from his abnormal son, but this victory soon loses its attraction: what was it about himself that he needed to defend so desperately? The answer is deafening in its emptiness: there is not one single thing left about which he can be proud, self-confident, or even moderately content.

This is the point where Bird's journey into his innermost being has come to an end, because there is nothing more to be discovered. That very minute he decides to go back to the abortionist and get his son. Himiko, for once, is furious because she immediately sees that their plans to visit Africa together will never be fulfilled. This is indeed so, Birds admits, because he is finally able to say what he has known all along: of all the possible worlds that he could have chosen to be happy without his abnormal son, it is only the actual world, for better or worse, that he can accept. In this world he is the father of this child.

8.5 Constancy and Truthfulness

Kenzoburo Oë's novel is a serious attempt to come to terms with the crisis in moral identity caused by the birth of a profoundly disabled child, a not uncommon phenomenon among people who go through a similar ordeal.[8] However, this crisis is not so much shaped by the consciousness of a moral dilemma as found in textbooks on bioethics. Rather, the crisis is one of constancy and truthfulness. The question is whether Bird will be faithful to his responsibilities as a husband and a father.

To warrant this reading, let me focus on a theme that I have neglected thus far: the relationship between Bird and his wife. Throughout the story his wife appears as a meek and timid woman to whom no husband would reveal his secret dreams and desires. Apparently, Bird's relationship with his wife is part of the cage from which he would escape if only he had the courage to do so. In Oë's novel both Bird's mother-in-law and Himiko are the strong women. His mother-in-law acts as a buffer between Bird and his wife. It is with her that Bird discusses what is to be done about their child even before he has seen his wife. It is not until the second day after the birth of their son, when the doctor tells him that the child will live at least for a couple of days, that he comes to visit her. With his mother-in-law still present, no word, no sign of tenderness or intimacy, passes between them. They even manage to quarrel over a bag with grapefruits that he bought forgetting that she does not care for grapefruit. Later on, his mother-in-law leaves the room and they are alone. "He sat down on the edge of the bed. 'You're all worn down,' his wife said, extending abruptly an affectionate hand and touching Bird's cheek. 'I am.' 'You've begun to look like a sewer rat that wants to scurry into a hole.' The slap caught him unawares. 'Is that so?' he said with a bitterness on his tongue, 'like a sewer rat?'" (97). At this stage Bird is clearly no longer capable of talking to his wife without presuming that she is suspicious of him. She tells him that her mother is afraid he will start drinking again. Remembering yesterday's scene of the hangover at Himiko's place, Bird answers that he will not. He feels that his wife has doubts about his inclinations. She mentions Africa and tells him that she has never been sure whether he would not leave her and the baby:

"When mother told me two days ago and then again last night that you were staying at the other hospital, I suspected you'd gotten drunk or run away somewhere. I really had my doubts, Bird." "I was much too upset to think about anything like that." "Look how you're blushing!" "Because I'm mad," Bird said rudely. "Why should I run away? With the baby just born and everything—" "But, when I told you I was pregnant, didn't the ants of paranoia swarm all over you? Did you really want a child, Bird?" (98)

Burning with shame because of his lie, he evades the question and tells his wife not to worry about him because it is the baby's condition that is the important thing now. Indeed, but that is exactly the reason for her doubt, because all will now depend upon him. "'I was trying to decide whether I could rely on you to take care of the baby and I began to think I didn't know you all that well. Bird, are you the kind of person who'll take the responsibility for the baby even at a sacrifice to yourself?' his wife asked" (98). What can he say? His wife does seem to know him quite well after all. Irritated by his silence, she withdraws her hand from his knee and then continues: "'Bird, I wonder if you're not the type of person who abandons someone weak when that person needs you most, the way you abandoned that friend of yours,'—Bird's wife opened her timid eyes wide as if to study Bird's reaction—'. . . Kikuhiko?'" (99).

Bird remembers this incident which occurred long a time ago. One night a lunatic escaped from a mental hospital in their village and Bird and his friend Kikuhiko together with other boys were summoned to chase him. When Kikuhiko became afraid and wanted to quit, Bird became very angry and humiliated his friend. He told him that he knew all about Kikuhiko's affair with a homosexual American officer and implied that he would tell others. Then he ran off, leaving his friend trembling with fear. The fact that his wife recalls this incident in connection with Bird's commitment to his son is further proof of his wife's doubts about him. "'What makes you feel like attacking me with past history like Kikuhiko? I'd forgotten I'd ever told you that story.' 'If we had a boy, I was thinking of naming him Kikuhiko,' his wife said. Naming him! If that grotesque baby ever got hold of a thing like a name! Bird winced" (100).

Connecting their son with the abandoned friend through a name was undoubtedly the most devastating blow Bird's wife could give him, even if she was completely unaware of it. As we already saw, the next day at the registration office, when Bird is summoned to name his son, he indeed betrays his intention to abandon his son by calling him Kikuhiko. Trying to escape from the actual world and his connections with it, he discovers that there is no way to do that *and* at the same time maintain his integrity. In other words, he can only remain truthful to himself when he accepts that his future life is with his wife and their child and not in an imaginary universe called 'Africa'. The crossroads at which Bird finds himself is the choice between losing or finding peace with himself.

Oë's story does not say that Bird is acting from a deep conviction about the inviolability of human life but rather that there is no way of continuing his own life by attempting to get away from it. Denying that he is attached to his wife and his son turns out to be the same as declaring himself morally bankrupt. The deep conflict is not about anything like the question: Am I allowed to make the decision to end the life of a profoundly disabled infant? Instead, the question for Bird is: Will I be able to abandon my wife and my son and at the same time be faithful to myself?[9] The prime question is who he wants himself to be. Throughout the story his main concern is to save his own life—whatever is worth saving—but at the same time the attempt to do so at the cost of his child evokes in him a sense of abhorrence that threatens his identity as a moral person. There is no satisfaction in escaping to a different world where his disabled son does not threaten his own prospects. In the end he can do nothing else except trust that the actual world in which he is the father of a disabled child will be merciful and, eventually, allow him the possibility of happiness with his family.

That this is not mere conjecture on my part, as far as Oë's vision is concerned, is shown by the way in which he ends his story.[10] Bird is able to retrieve his son in time from the abortion clinic and bring him back to the hospital, where the child is operated upon immediately. The operation is successful and the child recovers quickly, not least because of the many blood transfusions that Bird himself donates. On his return home, Bird reveals to his father-in-law the true nature of the events as they have evolved since the birth of the child. Then, for a moment, Bird's thoughts wander back to Himiko, who has resolved to go to Africa with another of her friends.

Through half-closed eyes Bird saw again the freighter bound for Zanzibar that had sailed a few days before with Himiko on board. He pictured himself, having killed the baby, standing at her side in place of that boyish man—a sufficiently enticing prospect to Hell. And perhaps just such a reality was being played out in one of Himiko's universes. Bird opened his eyes, turning back to the problems in the universe in which he had chosen to remain. "There is a possibility that the baby's development will be normal," he said, "but there's an equal danger that he'll grow up with an extremely low I.Q. That means I am going to have to put away as much as I can for his future as well as our own." (164–65)

Bird's redemption is found in the fact that he puts his trust in whatever possibilities life together with his wife and their son will generate. It does not only enable him to save his son but also to discover himself anew. The way in which Oë describes this in the last paragraph of his novel is, again, unsurpassable in literary imagination. The scene is the moment that he leaves the hospital with his family to return home:

> Bird waited for the others to catch up and peered down at his son in the cradle of his wife's arms. He wanted to try reflecting his face in the baby's pupils. The mirror of the baby's eyes was a deep, lucid gray and it did begin to reflect an image, but one so excessively fine that Bird couldn't confirm his new face. As soon as he got home he would take a look in the mirror. (165)

Oë's novel conveys a much richer perspective on what is involved in responding to the birth of a handicapped child than ethical theorizing about 'the value of life' can possibly provide. This is not merely due to the difference between narrative and theory, as might be objected, because there is clearly also a difference in moral vision. Oë's vision is shaped by accepting social bonds between human beings as constituents of their moral identity. Because such bonds exist prior to one's appreciation of their existence, they cannot be severed without endangering one's self-understanding as a moral person. This, I take it, is what Oë's narrative teaches us.[11]

8.6 Accountability as Self-Narration

In a recent paper Alasdair MacIntyre argues for a narrative conception of personal identity over against the Lockean tradition. That tradition interprets identity, as is well known, in terms of the continuity of mental states that are linked through time. It is MacIntyre's view that identity depends on the correspondence between first-person descriptions and other-person descriptions of the self (connecting my identification of myself with others' identification of me). On this view, he argues, it is possible to show how personal identity and accountability are interrelated. "Both identity and accountability have the place that they have among our concepts and in our lives," he writes, "in part because of the relationship between what we say of ourselves and what others say of us."[12] In this final section I will draw briefly on MacIntyre's views because of their explanatory force with regard to some of the elements in Oë's novel, particularly with regard to the crisis of identity that threatens the novel's main character. The father experiences a growing tension between his inner self and the expectations of his significant others. On the one hand, he tries to hide his inner self from these others: he does not want them to know what he knows to be true about himself. On the other hand, however, he does not want to accept what others say and think to be true of him. He does not want to identify with his role as a husband and as a father because he does not want the responsibility. Consequently, given this tension between how he appears to himself and how he appears to others, Bird is unable to account for his intentions concerning his son without being crushed by shame and guilt. It is precisely when his wife expresses her doubts about his intentions that he is exposed to himself as a liar and a traitor.

MacIntyre's explanation of accountability helps us understand especially the inevitability of this state of affairs, given the particulars of the story as Oë tells it. Put succinctly, what Bird lacks in order to be credible and truthful *to himself* is "the identity of the narrator with the subject of her or his narrative."[13] Refusing responsibility for the particulars of his life as they are apprehended both by himself and others, Bird effectively eliminates his self-esteem. The explanation is, precisely, that self-esteem is grounded in the kind of coincidence of self- and other-ascriptions that MacIntyre has explained. Like personal identity, self-esteem is not of individual but of social origin.

Among the characteristics of accountability, MacIntyre claims, is that in giving an account of ourselves we seek to establish or maintain our credibility. Such accounts invite the evaluation of *both* the truth of the account and the truthfulness of the narrator at the same time. In case the result of this evaluation is uncertain, others are uncertain as to whether the person presented in the account is identical with the person who is presenting it. In Bird's case, he disengages himself from his own narrated self but in doing so, he has to present an account of his *own* actions as the actions of someone that he does not want to identify with. His true self is hidden behind a veil of appearances. Hence in the novel we find that, on virtually every occasion, Bird is afraid that he will appear to be untruthful in the eyes of others or that these others will be suspicious of his motives.

Furthermore, MacIntyre explains, to be accountable is to be accountable in terms of a shared understanding of certain standards. The evaluation by others of the account I give of myself depends on the kind of relationship I have with them and on which particular activities or practices we are involved in. Thus the fact that Bird is a husband and a father implies that certain things may be expected from him. He will be held accountable by his wife for his participation in their marriage and for his contribution to the recovery of his son. This part of his identity is constituted by prior commitments, so that his wife holds him accountable for how he takes care of their son by questioning how his actions fit into their story as a married couple. Their marriage cannot continue unless each of them acknowledges his or her commitments to what they may expect from each other.

So here we see how the ascription of identity by oneself and others is closely connected with accountability. To account for himself Bird cannot but accept the identity that is constituted by the life that he shares with his family. Unless he is prepared to say that he is not the same person that he was before he cannot deny a commitment to the standards that are involved in the story of their marital relationship. Apparently, this is exactly what he secretly wants to deny, but now the question arises: Who then is he? Who is the other Bird? As we have seen, it is largely through his affair with his mistress Himiko that he finds the answer: the other Bird does not really exist. The truth about imagined selves is, indeed, that they are imaginary. The convictions that haunt Bird in his inward voyage are deep moral convictions because they are intricately connected to his own being. These convictions can no more be seen as options that can be chosen than his own identity can be seen as optional. Precisely because of his strong desire to create his own life, his attempts to evade responsibility for what he himself created must fail. As helpless as the child is, it exerts inescapable power over him.[14]

This observation is reinforced by the way in which his desire to let the baby die haunts his conscience. The very idea of considering the existence of the child as 'optional' is offensive to his conscience. His conscience does not allow him the option of being no longer the father of this child, for the only thing he can see is that he cannot escape the question Where is your son? There is no possible world in which he will not be this child's father: he can be held accountable for what he did to his child until the end of time. Although he desparately seeks to escape from it, this connectedness to his son is irradicably part of himself. In longing for his imagined universe called 'Africa', his imaginary world of secret hopes and dreams, Bird seems to be caught by the idea that many modern people have, namely the idea that they can choose who they want to be by way of a *creatio ex nihilo,* that is, by changing the relationships of which they find themselves to be part and start all over again.[15] Oë's main character fails in his attempt to do so because he tries to forget who he is. We are who we are and we are not someone else.

To conclude, let me return to the observations at the beginning of this chapter with respect to modern ethical theories. The method deployed by these theories,

I said, implies a strategy of disengagement. Assuming the contingent nature of our moral selves, we are invited to step back from the relationships and practices that shape our selves, including the standards they involve, and to engage in scrutinizing our convictions in the light of disengaged reason, that is, in the light of what 'the facts' and 'rationality' tell us. Should our convictions be at odds with the available facts and the canons of rationality we are supposed to abandon them. To abandon one's convictions in this connection is not seen as an assault upon the integrity of the moral self but rather as a commendable form of 'cognitive psychotherapy'.[16] We are supposed to become 'healthier' people from following the prescriptions of disengaged reason. But since disengaged reason—be it in its critical or public variety—is itself dependent on the presence of particular moral convictions, as we have seen in the previous chapter, moral philosophers do not provide us with good reasons to abandon the moral views we have only because they turn out to be incompatible with or lack support from the results of their own theorizing. In any case moral rationality—disengaged or not—is guided by a moral vision. The only way of scrutinizing the views we are committed to—as the main character of Oë's novel learns—is to find out what kind of life our moral vision implies and whether we can manage to live such lives with integrity. Given MacIntyre's explanation of our moral selves as constituted by the narratives that we find ourselves to be part of, the appropriate way to do so is by trying to understand the rationality of these narratives, that is, by finding out why we are who we are. With regard to our main subject we have to ask what kind of convictions and beliefs are underscored by the narratives that shape the lives of disabled and of people who are engaged in caring for them. In the last part of this inquiry we will turn to this type of question, but first we will consider the other claim introduced in this chapter concerning responsibility for dependent others.

NINE

Responsibility for Dependent Others

Man's relationship with the other is *better* as difference than as unity: sociality is better than fusion. The very value of love is the impossibility of reducing the other to myself, of coinciding into sameness. From an ethical perspective, two have a better time than one *(on s'amuse mieux a deux!)*

Emmanuel Levinas

Modern society aimed at the creation of a public space where there was to be *no moral proximity*. Proximity is the realm of intimacy and morality; distance is the realm of estrangement and the Law. Between the self and the other, there was to be distance structured solely by legal rules—no distorting influence of anything spontaneous and unpredictable, no room for powers as unreliable and resistant to universal legislation as those of the wayward moral impulse.

Zygmunt Bauman

9.1 On Accepting Responsibility

People who abandon moral views that cannot be justified by ethical theorizing run the risk of losing their integrity as moral persons. That was the claim in view of which our discussion of Oë's novel in the previous chapter evolved. As indicated in the introduction to that chapter, this claim is linked to another, stating that moral responsibility for dependent people is not grounded in their individual capacities or faculties. Whether they are persons in the Rawlsian sense of being agents endowed with a sense of justice and capable of carrying out a rational plan of life is not decisive for why we include them in our moral community. Nor is their inclusion dependent on whether they are capable of consenting to how they are treated by others. People with mental disabilities are part of the moral fabric of our society because they exist among us in the web of relationships that bind people together. To be aware of this fact is a sufficient reason to accept responsibility to care for these people.[1] Our moral lives are social lives and our moral selves develop within the social relationships in which we are involved. There is no philosophical grounding of our moral lives from the point of view of 'rational beings' who exist prior to these relationships to which we could refer in order to justify responsibility. Sociability constitutes morality, not the other way around.

This claim provides the subject of our discussion in this chapter. I will turn to the phenomenology of the moral life that the Danish theologian and philosopher of religion Knud E. Løgstrup presented in his book *The Ethical Demand*.[2] Løgstrup's thought has recently been reintroduced into the world of Anglo-Saxon moral philosophy through the work of the sociologist Zygmunt Bauman but was already well-known among theologians and philosophers of religion on the European continent. Particularly well-known is his theory of *Spontane Daseinsäusserungen*, i.e., spontaneous expressions of life, which Løgstrup developed in his later work as the primordial sources of morality. Bauman's reading of *The Ethical Demand* is guided by a critique of modern moral philosophy for its attempt to ground morality in reason. In Bauman's view this philosophy understands morality as an edifice of principles and rules functioning like laws that had to secure and improve social order and stability. In the modern era philosophers set out to construct their theories of morality side by side with legislators whose main concern—given the declining force of religion—was to control moral impulse and emotion. Hence the project of binding impulse and emotion to the rules of reason.[3] Theories of the rational self were constructed in order to show why rational agents should follow the moral precepts justified by critical thinking. In taking the rational self as the starting point of ethics, however, moral philosophers put the individuality of human persons before their togetherness. Thus they lost sight of the primordial source of moral responsibility, which—according to Bauman—is the 'moral party of two'. In order to retrieve the theoretical importance of this source he uses Løgstrup's phenomenology in a way similar to my intention in this chapter. Løgstrup's account of the moral life is particularly interesting because he does not start with the distinction between public and private or that between strangers and friends, which is the move characteristically made by modern moral philosophy. At the same time, however, he does not obliterate the distinction between the personal and the institutional but tries to show how they are connected.

Before we start, however, I should make the question to be addressed in this chapter more explicit, that is the question of accepting responsibility for dependent others such as the mentally disabled. This question can be understood in various ways. We can ask what reasons society has for accepting such responsibility, given its public morality, but we can also ask what reasons we think that our society has, given our own moral convictions. Ethical theories such as those presented by Kantians and utilitarians attempt to answer the first question by adopting a conception of disengaged reason, either in a critical or public sense, but they fail to provide adequate reasons for including dependent others as recipients of responsibility in the public domain. For example, Rawls's theory could not show why the principles of justice apply to nonpersons without relying on particular moral convictions that were presupposed to exist outside the domain of public reason. The conclusion was that Rawls' conception of public reason failed to account for all that it is supposed to account for.[4] If the question of why society should include nonpersons cannot be answered in terms of a 'freestanding' view of public morality, then the answer must be derived from particular convictions and beliefs held by particular people.

Something similar holds for utilitarian theories, as was suggested by our analysis of one of Engelhardt's theoretical moves. Given the claim that nonpersons are included for utilitarian reasons plus the fact that utilitarianism must allow for trade-offs to secure the maximization of preference satisfaction, there can be little doubt that the well-being of nonpersons is not going to carry much weight when it comes to a utilitarian calculus. If this is rejected as too crude a view because more sophisticated versions of 'indirect' utilitarianism accept a legitimate role for moral intuitions, then the conclusion must be, again, that whether 'non-persons' are included does not depend on the maximization of preference satisfaction but on certain intuitions that people in this society may or may not share to a sufficient degree.[5] In this sense the question What reasons does liberal society have to accept responsibility for disabled people? is inseparable from the question of why *we* think that liberal society should accept responsibility for these people, given our convictions and beliefs. Since both the critical and the public versions of disengaged reason fail to provide us with sufficient grounds to include the mentally disabled, it is not public morality in either of these versions, but our own convictions and beliefs that will be decisive.

This is only the first point to be clarified, however, because the question of accepting responsibility can be understood in yet another way. We can ask ourselves whether our society and its institutions should accept it, or, whether we as individual members should accept it. We have to consider the distinction between institutional and individual responsibility in this connection. I can hold that democratic society ought to include responsibility of the disabled in its institutional arrangements without implying that this view commits me to accepting a similar responsibility in my own life. Or can I? The importance of Løgstrup's—and Bauman's—view is that they criticize the separation between these domains of responsibility, because this separation is based on the assumption that they are grounded in a different kind of moral 'logic' instead of being interdependent. Not only do people who share their lives with disabled persons need the support as well as the security these institutions can provide, the reverse is also true: in order to sustain caring practices our institutional arrangements need to be informed by the convictions and beliefs that motivate people in sharing their lives with disabled persons. Without being so informed, our institutions deteriorate into bureaucracies that are no longer capable of discharging their responsibility in an appropriate way. Good institutions do not work well without good people.

It does not follow that anybody who claims that our social institutions should include the disabled in their arrangements should accept responsibility for them in their own life. But it does follow that unless there are those people who do accept this responsibility, and who have the character and the skills to discharge it well, our society will not be a caring society. This is a strong reason, it seems to me, for distinguishing between institutional and individual responsibility without separating them. The question before us is, then, what kind of moral convictions can support people who do accept this responsibility and guide them in their commitment to do so. To answer that question I will now turn to Løgstrup's account of the moral life.

9.2 'The Ethical Demand'

Decisive for Løgstrup's account in *The Ethical Demand* is that he begins with an affirmation of the pivotal role of trust in human existence. Human beings would not be able to exist in the world without trust. This is particularly true of our encounter with other people. The phenomenon of trust as Løgstrup describes it, however, is not an aspect of interaction between independent subjects. In addressing someone with a question or a concern, we place ourselves into the other person's hands.[6] In my encounter with the other person, I am giving myself partly in to her power, namely in respect of what makes me address her: a concern, a wish, a question, or a need. To express this expectation is a form of surrendering oneself to the other person. In that sense human interaction manifests a form of dependence.

Løgstrup focuses on the phenomenon of conversation in order to explain what this claim means. In the act of addressing someone we step out of ourselves and engage in a relationship of speech with the other. To address others is to give them some degree of control over oneself because the address must at least be interpreted, which can or cannot be done in accordance with one's intention. Therefore, the necessity of trust is closely connected with dependency. In the background of this analysis, Løgstrup presupposes that the denial of dependency explains the preoccupation with 'power' in contemporary social thought. That preoccupation is explained by the modern notion of the person as a self-governing being that seeks to realize its own ends independently from others:

> We have the curious idea that a person constitutes his own world, and that the rest of us have no part in it but only touch upon it now and then. If the encounter between persons therefore means, as it normally does, nothing more than that respective worlds touch upon each other and then continue unaffected on their separate courses, the encounter can hardly be very important. According to this reasoning, it is only when a person accidently breaks into another person's world with good or bad intentions that anything important is at stake. This is a very curious idea, an idea no less curious because we take it for granted. The fact is, however, that it is completely wrong because we do indeed constitute one another's world and destiny. (*The Ethical Demand,* 16–17)

According to Løgstrup mutual dependency consitutes the very fabric of our moral world. To reject the ontology of atomism that is connected with the ideal of independency and assert the primacy of trust, however, is not to deny that power is part of human exchange and relationship.[7] To be a self-in-relation is to be constituted, at least in part, by those to whom one is related. This state of dependency is a precarious and potentially vulnerable condition, which explains why human encounters are couched in moral language. Being in a position of having our expectations denied, we seek insurance against disappointment through moral claims and judgments in order to protect ourselves against this vulnerability.

The question now is: How are these facts about the undeniable role of power in human encounter related to what Løgstrup calls 'the ethical demand'? If we invoke moral claims and judgments to be insured against the threats involved in being dependent upon others, our encounters with these others apparently fail to ground responsibility. Nonetheless Løgstrup seems to argue that the ethical demand arises from these encounters. How is this to be understood?

9.3 Social Norms and Moral Judgment

In order to understand how the ethical demand arises from encounters with others and, at the same time, operates to oppose the abuse of power in the responses to these encounters, three qualifications of the demand are needed.

First, the ethical demand as Løgstrup understands it should not to be confused with a moral rule. It does not specify types of actions designated by a rule to guide us in specific circumstances. Nor should it be understood as a basic moral principle. The demand is 'unspoken'. It is distinct from the existing social norms that 'speak' to us in daily life.[8] This does not mean that the demand lacks any content or that it is purely formal. It tells us to accept responsibility for the other but does nothing to inform us how this obligation is to be discharged.[9]

Secondly, to accept responsibility for others who present themselves to us is not the same as granting a wish or fulfilling a desire. As far as the voice of recipients is concerned, the demand is 'silent'.[10] We must act for the best of the other person, but our own judgment decides what it is that 'for the best of the other' requires.

Both these qualifications indicate why Løgstrup opposes making the notion of individual independence pivotal in our account of the moral life. It causes us to believe mistakenly that human individuals are a world unto themselves and that the main problem is how to include other selves in that world.[11] To construe moral relationships in this way is to eliminate the manifestation of trust and replace it with the reciprocation of enlightened self-interest.[12] But the unavoidability of trust should not make us overlook the problem of power, however. The fact that the demand is unspoken and silent requires that *we* decide how to respond to the other who has placed trust in us. That is, we cannot escape responsibility for deciding what we think is best for the other person.

This consideration implies a third qualification of the demand. It is a radical demand in that it is followed for the sake of the other.[13] To fulfill responsibility for the other person from the perspective of one's own views on human flourishing is to be constantly at risk of denying the *otherness* of the other. Therefore the ethical demand requires the motive of unselfishness. For Løgstrup this motive is the nub of the problem of ethics because the possibility of trust is constantly jeopardized by the fact that human beings are tempted by the self-seeking gratification of desire, either by denying responsibility for the other or by determining what is good for the other in a egocentric way.[14]

So we see how Løgstrup's argument is to be understood. There is no human interaction that can properly proceed without trust, not even the interaction between self-interested individuals. But these individuals are particularly prone to ignore this fact and succumb to the temptation of perverting relationship with other human beings. The manifestation of trust as the primordial source of responsibility is understood as a necessary condition, even if it is not a sufficient one. The ethical demand rises from the givenness of the other who has placed her- or himself in our hands, but it needs articulation.

How then is the ethical demand to be articulated? How can we make sure that the otherness of other people is acknowledged in our encounters with them? This question is answered in two stages. The first stage refers to the role of social norms. Løgstrup argues that the demand is mediated by the norms of social convention, morality, and law.[15] Such norms protect us against one another by imposing limits upon our involvement in the lives of other persons. At the same time they are less demanding in that they can be obeyed even without the explicit purpose of caring for other people.[16] So, on the one hand there is the guiding role of social norms:

> We must know something about what a person's expectations are and how they may be realized. Also we must know something about the dangers his life holds for him and how he may be shielded against them. . . . Just how his life in the given situation is best provided for we will therefore in a great many instances have to learn from the social norms, because it is precisely these norms which protect the various human relations and institutions whose spiritual content has determined the content of the other person's life, his expectations and problems. The social norms thus serve as a guide in helping us to decide what will best serve the other person. (*The Ethical Demand,* 61)

Social norms mediate the practical content of the demand in any given situation, because it is in terms of such norms that agents and recipients understand what is morally appropriate.[17] Social norms do have a protective role to play in guiding our deliberations about how to take care of these others.

On the other hand, however, the mediation of the ethical demand by social norms is bound to remain inadequate. This takes Løgstrup's answer to the second stage. In fulfilling the requirements of a norm we can never be sure about what in fact we are doing with respect to the ethical demand. We may be answering the call of the demand, but we also may be caught in the web of moral convention that threatens the other person. To avoid this danger, Løgstrup insists upon the necessity of judgment as to the appropriateness of applying particular norms in particular situations, which requires that we are guided by the proper motive.[18]

Consequently, there are two sides to the question of how the ethical demand and its concrete articulations in particular situations are related. Actions guided by social norms and accompanied by selfish motives may have similar effects with regard to the expectations of others as when the same actions are performed for unselfish motives. Social norms are requirements of institutional arrangements that can be fulfilled regardless of personal motives. For example, paying taxes for fear of fiscal sanctions does allow the government to work for the poor just as much as when taxes are paid out of moral concern for their plight. At the same time, however, the interpretation and application of social norms require the radical openness and responsiveness of the demand.[19] This is the case when the appropriateness of particular social norms is in dispute with respect to what is best for the other person. In that case our judgment is called for and the contradiction between action and motive is no longer possible. In those cases we will be determined by our willingness to take responsibility for how the institutional arrangements in question affect the lives of others.[20]

This explanation helps us to see how the levels of personal and institutional responsibility can—and should—be distinguished without being separated. In discharging responsibility for people who depend upon social support, our society operates by means of institutional arrangements. These arrangements function regardless of whether everyone is well-disposed to support these people. Whereas our individual motives are not directly relevant on this level, they become quite important as soon as issues arise regarding which responsibilities our institutions are supposed to discharge, as in, for example, the issue of whether disabled people should be supported by society. Once institutional arrangements are in place the disparity between motive and action is not necessarily problematic. But in questions of who ought to be included as the beneficiaries of these arrangements and who not, the disparity between motive and action is potentially threatening to particular people. Society may refuse to include particular groups in its schemes for health care and welfare and leave the burden of support to their families. In such cases, these people have to rely on the personal motives and dispositions of others to counteract the threat of exclusion. Once the operation of institutional arrangements is in dispute, our judgment is called for, and much will depend on the motives and the beliefs guiding our judgment.

9.4 'Life as a Gift'

Since there is no way of judging social norms, according to Løgstrup, other than through our own 'outlook on life', he considers the question of which particular outlook justifies accepting responsibility for people whose lives are placed in our hands.[21] He answers this question in terms of understanding one's own life as a gift. Stated negatively, the argument is that if human beings are necessarily part of one another's world, then to claim sovereignty over one's life is to deny the contribution others make to it. I cannot with justification assert the sovereignty over my life and at the same time acknowledge that others have cared for my presence in their lives and continue to do so. Even if it is often suggested that it is 'rational' to act on the principle *do ut des,* the constitution of human life is such that it is more appropriate to reverse this principle: we can give because—and to the extent that—we have been and continuously are given.[22] According to Løgstrup, "The demand which invalidates the mutuality viewpoint does not arise exclusively from the fact that the one person is delivered over to the other. This demand makes sense only on the presupposition that the person to whom the demand is addressed possesses nothing which he has not received as a gift. Given that presupposition, the demand is the only thing that makes sense," (*The Ethical Demand*, 123). The radicality and one-sidedness of the demand is justified precisely by the fact that I have received my life and therefore cannot claim sovereignty with regard to the demand as such.[23] Again, Løgstrup does not deny that people can—and in fact often do—act as if they are sovereign of their own lives. If they do, they will agree to respond to others on the basis of what they see as the mutual exchange of claims and counter-claims, which is essentially a contractualist posture. This posture can only be maintained, however, at the cost of denying that one has received one's life as a gift. The demand that we care for the other person's life is rooted in the fact of our indebtedness for all the things we have received: intelligence, speech, love, and much more. These are the things that both enable and oblige us to respond to the needs of others.[24]

It is important to see, in this connection, that the notion of life as a gift can be accepted cognitively without moving the agent toward the appropriate action.[25] It is not cognition but motivation that matters. Human agents need their moral resources to be nourished by the experience of love, sympathy, and friendship. Unselfish motives are typically developed in stable and affectionate personal relationships, such as between parents and their children or between friends. Within these relationships our lives are bound together to the effect that the well-being of the one cannot be separated from the well-being of the other.

> This is why every time one cares for another person in love, sympathy, or solidarity, one is rewarded through the maintenance of those relationships in which a person has his life and which constitute his existence. The more intensely and comprehensively a person binds himself to other people . . . the more he will see that a selfish life lived at the expense of others is empty and unsuccessful, and the more he will refrain from that kind of life. (*The Ethical Demand*, 133)

Mutuality in personal relationships is therefore different from that in contractual relationships, because the latter are conditioned by expected benefits, whereas the former are not. The benefits bestowed by love and friendship are consequential rather than conditional, which explains why human life that is constituted by these relationships is appropriately experienced as a gift.

Furthermore, it is important to see that Løgstrup's account does not limit the scope of the ethical demand to the sphere of personal relationships where 'natural love' can be reciprocated. The point of the demand is that the other person to be cared for is *not* the same as the person from whose hands I receive my own existence. It extends beyond the symmetrical relationships with those who are closest to us and reaches out to people who do not benefit from our intimate affections. Although the willingness to accept our own lives as a gift is nourished within the sphere of natural affections, it provides us with a motive for action that is not restricted to that sphere.

9.5 Convention and Commitment

As indicated in the introduction to this chapter, Zygmunt Bauman has repeatedly referred to Løgstrup's phenomenology of the moral life as a very important source for his own thinking on postmodern morality.[26] According to Bauman, the postmodern condition has rendered obsolete the project of modern moral philosophy, because its attempt to control and replace moral impulse and sentiment by 'disengaged reason' has been largely discredited. The strategy deployed by modernity has been to depict itself as a 'frontier civilization' that confronts the backwardness and barbarism of unenlightened cultures and stands out as a beacon of hope for humankind. Its basic endeavor was to elevate disengaged reason to the throne of 'Universal Reason.' In the era of Western colonization, the project of designing society according to the rules of universal reason provided the philosophical underpinnings of wielding economic and military power in ways that betrayed the parochialism and partiality of this universal reason.[27] From the start, modernity set out to liberate human beings everywhere from historical trappings and influences so as to bring 'the human individual' to the fore. Stripped of all particularistic features, this individual became subject to the only remaining legitimate power, that of the nation-state. Cultural spaces of intimacy and togetherness were replaced by the legal realm of distance and estrangement.

> Between the self and the other, there was to be distance structured solely by legal rules—no distorting influence of anything spontaneous and unpredictable, no room for powers as unreliable and resistant to universal legislation as those of the wayward moral impulse. It was hoped that legal rules would be obeyed in as far as they appealed to the *self*-interest of those called to obey, and promised to deliver the best service there is or could be: legal rules were to assist and encourage individuals to seek what suits their self-interest and promised to show how to do it. The legally defined individual was one who had interests which were not the interests of others. (*Postmodern Ethics*, 83)

On the social level, the strategy of abrogating convention and tradition in the name of critical and public rationality inaugurated the philosophical 'expert' whose critique of traditional morality was grounded in the solid foundations of moral philosophy. But moral philosophy as a search for rational foundations was unmasked as a tale about the emperor's clothes: the foundations simply did not exist. Modernity's derogatory view of ordinary judgment, according to Bauman, left us with nothing to replace it. It is not without irony, as he points out, that people could do without 'foundations' as long as they stuck to the habitual and traditional and that it was precisely the elevation of philosophical expertise that prepared the way for the demise of foundationalism.[28] In the meantime, the collapse of this project indicates that "chaos and contingency" can no longer be expelled beyond the borders of rational order.

> The chaos and contingency which modernity spent two centuries to occlude out of the business of life is not just back in the field of vision, but appears there (perhaps for the first time so blatantly, and for so many viewers) naked, without cover or adornment, and without shame that would prompt it to seek clothing. Groundlessness is no more the guilty, shameful secret of being, for which society tried its best to repent and atone. It is hailed instead as the beauty and joy of being, as the sole ground of freedom. Postmodernity means dismantling, splitting up and deregulating the agencies charged in the modern era with the task of pulling humans, jointly and individually, to their ideal state-that of rationality and perfection. (*Life in Fragments*, 27)

The observation that postmodernity has no patience for philosophical attempts to reconstruct reason and accepts contingency and diversity does not imply the relativism of morality. That is only what the lingering fear of modernity wants us to believe, namely, that a world without ethics must be a world without morality. As Bauman repeatedly argues, postmodernism reveals the parochial relativism of ethical codes, and, in that sense, the crisis of ethics, which is not necessarily a crisis of morality.[29]

To support this claim, Bauman wants to retrieve the theoretical importance of the primordial 'moral impulse' that modern moral philosophy declared suspect. Ethically unfounded morality allows a true understanding of moral responsibility as the responsibility of the moral self. It is at this point that he turns to the notion of the unspoken demand that he finds in Løgstrup's thought. According to Bauman, the distinction between the demand as unspoken or spoken points to the difference between the unconditionality of commitment and responsibility on the one hand, and the conventionality of moral rules and precepts on the other. As can be inferred from my account of Løgstrup, however, this reading of his work is not correct because Løgstrup carefully avoids the separation between commitment and convention. Bauman reads Løgstrup's account of social norms as conventional norms only in a negative light.[30] Social conventions take away the 'ambivalence' of the ethical demand and delude us with the illusionary certainty of rule-following conduct. But moral responsibility cannot be discharged by way of conformity to social rules, according to Bauman, because of the radicality of the demand:

> The 'demand', unlike the comfortable precise order, is abominably vague, confused and confusing, indeed barely audible. It forces the moral self to be her own interpreter, and—as with all interpreters—remain forever unsure of the correctness of interpretation. However radical the interpretation, one can never be fully convinced that it matched the radicality of the demand. I have done this, but could I not do more? There is no convention, no rule to draw the boundary of my duty, to offer peace of mind in exchange for my consent never to trespass. (*Postmodern Ethics*, 80)

As we have seen already, Løgstrup points to the necessity of personal judgment to avoid the danger of conforming to rules regardless of moral motivation, but he does so only after having explained the nature of social norms as protections for the recipients of our actions. Since the expectations of these others will be determined within particular social relationships that we share with them, we will learn how to take responsibility through the guidance of conventional morality. As Løgstrup states, "The social norms thus serve as a guide in helping us to decide what will best serve the other person." But being only a guide they cannot replace judgment.

The difference between these readings of social norms is not merely a difference on the relative importance and priority of either commitment or convention. There is a more incisive difference lurking in the background. This is clear from Bauman's comments upon Løgstrup's attempt to justify the ethical demand by referring to 'the gift of life'. Bauman argues that Løgstrup's is an attempt to decenter modern moral philosophy by claiming the 'unconditionality' of moral responsibility, not unlike the attempt of Emmanuel Levinas who, according to Bauman, is engaged in a similar project. But he criticizes Løgstrup's attempt because he regards it as being caught in the framework it seeks to escape. It still accepts as valid the question of whether morality can be grounded in something which itself is not morality, i.e. the fact that life has been received as a gift.[31]

It occurs to me, however, that at this point Bauman mistakenly ignores the Christian background of Løgstrup's thought. Even though the latter insists on describing the moral life as a *human* rather than a Christian possibility, it is nonetheless clear that the gap between commitment and convention that Bauman postulates cannot exist in Løgstrup's view. At any rate, he does not only believe in the brokenness of human existence, he also believes in creation. The ethical demand is constituted by an encounter that is not responded to by the agent's mere *emotionality*, as is the case in Bauman's account, but by a particular kind of *sympathetic* response to the fact of life as a gift.[32] This response reflects the createdness of our moral lives in the sense that the notion of creation implies the belief that, somehow, our world is ordered toward the good. By the same token, social convention is not merely the deflection of individual responsibility, as it is for Bauman, but it also reflects the createdness of our lives in that it embodies the social reality of commitment. The notion of 'life as a gift' is intended by Løgstrup precisely to explain the meaning of createdness.[33] The ethical demand is a human possibility because we have been endowed with the gifts that make us the kind of beings who can fulfill it.

But the brokenness that is also part of our existence as human beings confronts us in our self-centeredness and complacency. The expression of moral impulse can be blocked or withdrawn by indifference or egotism. If it is, morality still calls upon us to treat others at least as we would have ourselves treated by them. But this recourse to a minimalist notion of reciprocity as a requirement of enlightened self-interest is what one might call a 'fall-back position'.[34] It reflects the modern notion of the individual who has to decide whether or not to become involved. This notion explains the central role of separate individuals in modern ethical theories. Such theories describe our relationships as reciprocal and construe morality as the mutual exchange of claims and counterclaims. The ethical demand conflicts with this minimalist notion of reciprocal relationships in that it is one-sided. We experience ourselves as being called upon by the demand; we do neither *choose* nor *decide* to experience its calling. In this sense, the experience of the demand precedes the will. It is a calling and a gift at the same time. The gift is that we are moral beings capable of fulfilling the calling because our lives have been shaped by what we have received from the hands of others. The task implied in the calling is to share these gifts with others who are dependent upon us.

The language of 'createdness' and 'gift' invokes the question as to what extent Løgstrup's account of the moral life depends upon religious views in order to be sustainable. Do we need religious views in order for this account to be rationally compelling? This is a question about the epistemological status of the arguments presented here that cannot be dealt with effectively, of course, within the space of a single section—let alone paragraph. I will address it here only by way of giving a few hints as to how an appropriate answer might go. First of all, the phenomenology of the moral life provided by Løgstrup is meant to describe the moral life in a way that, at the very least, can be recognized as valid by people who broadly share the moral culture brought about by Western Christianity. This is not to exclude people from other cultures—as a matter of fact I believe that the account is probably more accessible for these people insofar as their cultures accept religious traditions as the practical embodiment of received moral wisdom in their societies—but it is to include people within our own culture regardless of their explicit views on Christian convictions and beliefs. One need not be a Christian to understand what is meant by the moral life as a gift and to be motivated to respond to it accordingly. Secondly, things may become more intricate, however, as soon as substantial matters of moral controversy arise. In that connection Løgstrup invokes what he calls an 'outlook on life' which I take to be a vision of what our lives are ultimately about. Different visions may generate different responses to particular issues even in cases where there is general agreement as to what the issues are. To give an example in this context of this inquiry: in controversies about decisions whether or not to accept a disabled child, people may share the understanding of life as a gift, but it may make quite a difference whether or not they believe salvation to be greatest gift in their lives. To accept a mentally disabled child as a gift may appear to some as accepting the kind of gift that one rather would not have received. But things may appear differently if one knows that one's failures and weaknesses are forgiven and redeemed in a way that creates both the courage and the freedom to face whatever it is that life confronts us with. In other words the 'quality' of the gift is not necessarily the same as its meaning. Thirdly, even when we move toward broader issues that invoke these kinds of visions, such as, for example, issues about suffering and meaning, there can be many insights that are accessible when described in terms of human existence. Take for example the fact that human bodies are destined to wither away, oftentimes long before their actual death occurs. This fact inevitably raises questions about the meaning of human suffering and death that cannot be evaded by the endeavor to avoid and combat suffering and death whenever it occurs. Even if what we make of these experiences and how we think we can live with them is inspired by particular religious beliefs, this does not exclude the possibility of trying to give an account of these experiences and our responses to them that is accessible to other people. What cannot be assured, however, is that these people will be convinced about the truth of our views, even if they are 'fully rational'.

With regard to the epistemological status of the arguments that are presented in the last part of this inquiry, I take these remarks to suggest the importance of giving an account of what parents of disabled children think and believe about themselves and their children that helps us make sense of what they are saying and doing. Whether or not this account appears as revealing truth about human life depends on views that exceed the limits of the account as such. The extent to which these views need to be articulated in their own particular terms depends largely on what the issues are and whom one takes one's audience to be. In other words, the claim is not that the particular views sustaining the argument are optional insofar as they are taken to reveal (aspects of) truth about human life, but that they are optional with regard to where and when they need to be articulated in terms of particular, i.e., religious, views.

9.6 Appropriate Motivations

The final step in this chapter is to connect the insights it provides with those gained from the previous one. Løgstrup's account of the moral life confirms some of the insights gained from Kenzaburo Oë's novel. The main character of that story very much aspires to be the sovereign author of his own life, which tempts him to think about the relationships in which he finds himself as being the objects of decision and choice. He is unable to accept life as it presents itself to him in the real world and seeks refuge in an imaginary one. He desperately wants his life to be his own creation but finally comes to understand that this will lead him to destroy his own self. The suggestion is not that we have to take life as it comes and accept whatever occurs in it.[35] The suggestion is rather that conducting our lives responsibly starts within the fabric of actual relationships—personal and institutional—that constitutes our moral world, including our own selves. To accept responsibility is to accept responsibility for that world, which requires the willingness to account for ourselves in terms of these relationships, accept the responsibilities they involve, trust the potentialities they entail, treasure them as a gift and proceed from there.[36]

In this chapter we have considered the question of what moral reasons our society has to care for dependent others such as the mentally disabled. The answer depends, first, on whether we accept that the question of why our society should care for these people is inseparable from the question of why we should care for them. Secondly, the answer does not depend on whether or not they can reciprocate our actions. Nor does it depend on the extent to which they share the characteristics of a moral agent being endowed with the powers of reason and free will. Neither Kantian contractualism nor utilitarian universalism can provide our society with the motive to accept responsibility for dependent others such as the mentally disabled. In the case of the former, it is because the disabled do not fit its description of the kind of beings to whom we owe obligations of justice. Consequently, the proper motive for including them into our moral lives depends on sources that fall outside its conception of public morality. In the case of the latter, the failure is caused by its strategy of maximizing the satisfaction of preferences. This strategy requires that we detach ourselves from responsibility for particular others in order to be capable of trading off their happiness against that of other people.[37]

Following the lead of Løgstrup's account of the moral life, I have argued that dependent others are accepted because their lives are placed in our hands. We can reject their existence and consider their lives not worth living. We can leave them to be taken care of by their families and grant them the rights to be sovereign of their own lives. But we can also accept responsibility for the fact that they are part of the web of social relationships that constitutes our moral world.

The argument hinges on the connection between responsible action mediated by institutional arrangements on the one hand, and personal motives and dispositions on the other. The morality underlying our institutional practices of caring for the disabled is not that of universal maximization of happiness nor is it that of reciprocal respect for human beings as free, rational agents. We have these practices, and our society will continue to support them, as long as its members understand that it is appropriate for them to give to and support dependent others because of what they themselves have received.

The minimal condition for this possibility, I said, is that there are people who understand themselves and their moral lives in the light of moral convictions such as are exhibited in Løgstrup's account of the moral life, and who have the character and the skills to accept the responsibility that it entails.[38] But of course people may fail to see things this way, or they may fail to be this kind of people. They may not have received the opportunity to become caring persons who accept responsibility for others in what they themselves do *and* what their society does, or fails to do.[39] If my life has been such that I have failed—either by my own fault or that of others—to develop the motives and dispositions that constitute a caring self, there is no rational argument that logically forces me to accept this responsibility.

Particularly with regard to mentally disabled people, reason is impotent to repair what our character fails to do—which is to provide us with the proper motive. There is no compelling rational ground why *we* ought to try to share our lives with them, should we be inclined not to do so. In case we consider society to be the space of exchange between moral stangers, we can leave it up to our institutions to care for whoever needs to be taken care of. However, to the extent that we regard ourselves in a different light and understand our lives as a gift, we will not be indifferent to these matters. This is to say that there may be a compelling rational ground to share our lives with the disabled, but it can hardly be a compelling ground from anybody's point of view, which is to say that it cannot be a compelling ground from the perspective of disengaged reason. The appropriate motive for caring responsibility can be explained by reference to certain convictions and beliefs about ourselves, but these convictions and beliefs being absent, we cannot be argued forcefully into it on grounds of reason alone.

These observations, I take it, answer the question raised in this chapter. The reason for maintaining social responsibility for mentally disabled persons is grounded in an understanding of ourselves as relational selves who receive our lives and its potentialities from one another's hands. Although this understanding grows out of and is nourished by interpersonal relationships, it can provide us with motives to exert our moral imagination for the sake of dependent others through social institutions and practices. Whether we have these motives will make a difference for how we respond to their needs if we are called upon to do so. Regardless of whether they enter into our personal lives or into our society's institutions, in both cases we accept responsibility for dependent others—if we do—because we consider their lives and well-being to be entrusted upon us.

As Løgstrup reminds us, however, all of these claims are accepted—if at all—only on the basis of what he calls a particular 'outlook on life': a set of convictions, beliefs, and attitudes that guide us in living our lives in pursuit of what we regard as the good life for human beings. It is important to be reminded of this condition, because it implies that we cannot develop a philosophical account of how to think about accepting responsibility for disabled human beings in terms of a freestanding view. That is, we cannot develop such an account independently of the moral lives of people who are actually engaged in sharing that responsibility. Philosophical rationality is explanatory, not foundational. This reminder will guide us through the last part of the present inquiry, in which we will discuss some of the convictions and beliefs that may help to sustain the lives of those who care.

Part Three

TEN

The Presumption of Suffering

The power of modern medicine resides in its almost magical possibility of offering us a relief from biological necessity, granting us new powers to manage our fate and our destiny, presenting an image of unlimited hope, genuine knowledge, and great progress. It assumes the possibility of dominating, manipulating, and redefining nature and its potencies. This is a powerful and compelling image to a self all too conscious of its fragility.

Daniel Callahan

The conviction that some kinds of suffering can serve a moral project, and the correlative denial that all suffering is pointless, strikes at the very heart of the Baconian project and breaks the grip of the latter on the practice of medicine. Underlying it is a conviction that the attempt to render our bodies free from suffering and wholly subject to our choices is morally impoverishing in both self-regarding and other-regarding ways—that the kind of vigilance over the body it entails produces subjects who are incapable of understanding the nature and meaning of embodiment, of recognizing and accepting the limits of medicine, of caring adequately for those who embody those limits and fall victim to efforts to deny them.

Gerald P. McKenny

10.1 A Remaining Question

Among the convictions and beliefs that are important for our appreciation of disabled lives are those that concern the issue of suffering. Disabled children are generally taken to be a source of negative experiences, if not for themselves then at any rate for their parents.[1] Presumably, some would argue that even though the lives of the disabled are woven into the web of relationships that constitutes our moral world, this should not make us forget that a disabled life is often burdened by suffering. One of the questions remaining from our previous discussion is, therefore, what there is to say about the connection between disability and suffering. Occasionally, parents of mentally disabled children tell us that, though the diagnosis of mental disability was a blow that shattered their hopes and dreams about the kind of family they hoped to have, they learned to experience a sense of fulfilment. What to many outsiders looks like a life full of bleak necessity turns out to be a possible source of enrichment as well. In this chapter and in the next we will reflect how and why parents of mentally disabled children manage to derive positive experiences from their lives. What is it that can make caring for such a child an enriching experience?

In raising this question we are engaging evaluations of disabled lives from the point of view of a conception of the good life. The desire to have healthy children of one's own is widely accepted as an important part of the good life.[2] It is not only the desire to have children that is part of the human good: the same has been argued for parental preferences with regard to what their children will be like. No less confident than Edwards, Engelhardt wrote that "the use of technology in the fashioning of children is integral to the goal of rendering the world congenial to persons."[3] Presumably, the notion of having a mentally disabled child is not 'congenial' to many persons. Perceptions of disabled lives in our society are determined by the prospect of diminishing expectations and disappointments, both for one's family and oneself. Given these perceptions, the presumption that disabled people and their families suffer from their hardships is very influential in our society. Consequently, once the results of prenatal testing indicate the presence of a genetic defect, nothing seems more obvious than to avoid the birth of a handicapped child. Who would not save herself from such an ordeal?

The question is, however, where this leaves parents who tell us that sharing one's life with a disabled child can be a rewarding experience. In this chapter we will look more closely at what I will call the 'presumption of suffering' and ask whether or not there are sound reasons for challenging it. The intention of raising this question is twofold. First, I want to challenge current attitudes toward disability in order to see whether they are as compelling and rational as they appear. The presumption of suffering renders the option of prevention the natural thing to do. By the same token it renders the decision of people to accept a disabled child irrational. I will argue that this view is mistaken and that we can see why when we look at people's motivations for caring for dependent others. Second, I want to challenge the way in which the literature deals with stories about parental experiences. These stories are often presented as reports about how living with a disabled child makes people *feel* about their own life.[4] Thus understood, such stories report emotional states of affairs that enable us to assess both the positive and negative experiences with the implication that the appropriate response is, indeed, to balance these experiences in order to arrive at an overall picture. The objection to this presentation is that it reduces people's stories about their lives to accounts about emotional states rather than about the attitudes and beliefs that motivated and sustained them to become the kind of people they are. To take their motivations seriously, we should not only ask how their lives feel but also which beliefs and attitudes entered into the formation of the kind of character that produced these feelings.[5]

Unfortunately, there is not much in the current ethical literature on which to build. We enter upon largely untrodden ground. Characteristic of that literature, as I suggested in chapter 1, is that it looks at disability only in a negative light and approaches it in terms of the defect model and then discusses the moral issues with regard to prevention within the liberal framework of individual rights and social responsibilities.[6] In response to this literature, there is no point in denying that parents of disabled children have many things to worry about and go through rough times of grief and despair. But the question is what these parents are saying when they tell us that having such a child has enriched their lives. The point of raising this question is to suggest that the presumption of suffering in this context may depend more on beliefs and attitudes that prevail in liberal society than on informed views about the lives of disabled people. If this is true, it is an important point to consider in the debate on genetic testing for reasons of prevention. It is quite possible that disabled people and their families do not only suffer from natural conditions but also from prevailing attitudes towards disability.

Before beginning with the discussion I should make explicit what type of conditions I have in mind when speaking of disabled lives in this chapter. Essentially they are the conditions delineated in chapter 3: mental and physical disabilities that (1) are identified as impairments caused by genetic diseases and (2) allow people to live reasonably healthy lives but (3) preclude 'normal' social functioning and hence require adaptive strategies or devices. Included are conditions such as Down syndrome and fragile X syndrome. Excluded are conditions that, in one way or another, link disease with illness, such as, for example, Huntington's chorea, cystic fybrosis, or Duchenne's muscular dystrophy. Although I certainly do not exclude the possiblity that what is argued in these chapters will hold as well for persons with the latter conditions, I will not rest my case against the presumption of suffering on that possibility.

Furthermore, I should make explicit that individual decisions to prevent lives affected by genetic disorders are viewed in these chapters exclusively from the parents' point of view. In order to isolate their own point of view in a plausible way, I will focus on the case in which the prospect of having a disabled child is frightening, without this fear being grounded in the expected suffering of the child itself. Children with the type of disorder that is relevant in this connection have their difficulties in life, but they are nonetheless capable of reasonably happy lives. One thing they will never be able to do, however, is to live a life of their own without special concern and support from other people, most of all their parents.

Singling out this type of case will allow us to focus on the presumption of suffering of parents where the cause of suffering lies in their prospect of *being the parents* of disabled children.[7] The focus is therefore on people's judgments about what a disabled child means to them. In inquiring into the assumptions on which their judgments are based, I am never implying that these people are motivated by self-interest. But even when they are not so motivated, their judgments are open to question.

10.2 Reasons Regarding Quality of Life

In considering the presumption of suffering we are back to the point of passing evaluative judgments on disabled lives. It will be recalled that I proposed a distinction between two types of reasons on the basis of which such judgments can be made: reasons based on beliefs about moral standing (MS reasons) and reasons based on expectations about quality of life (QL reasons). Having discussed mainly the former in connection with discrimination—chapter 5—I will now turn to the latter type of reason. Obviously, the presumption of suffering concerns the issue of what sharing one's life with a disabled person will do to its quality. In this chapter I will therefore discuss some aspects of QL reasons.

The problems presented by QL reasons can be, and quite often are, very complex. Judgments based on such reasons can easily go wrong due to their prospective nature. First of all, the possibility of mistakes in prospective judgments rests on the fact that not everything about the future is unknown. We may be mistaken in some of our expectations about the future, of course, without there being a possibility of knowing that we are mistaken. But there is also the possibility of a mistake about the future that can be recognized as such. This is the easier case. If the future of a child with Down syndrome is considered, for example, particular things about this future are objectively known. Parents who fear that a child with Down syndrome will suffer from having a hydrocephalus are objectively mistaken. That fear is unfounded because having a hydrocephalus is not among the symptoms of Down syndrome. The diagnosis of particular conditions includes certain symptoms as possible, but it also excludes certain other symptoms as impossible, hence the fact that expectations about future states of affairs can be objectively mistaken.

There is, however, a far more difficult problem regarding the possibility of mistaken expectations. For example, a child with the condition of spina bifida—a neural tube defect—may or may not develop a hydrocephalus, but one cannot always be sure about whether or not it will. Nor can one be sure of how such a complication may develop. Neural tube defects are subject to a range of possible complications, some of which are dependent on where the defect is located on the spine. Consequently, there is a range of uncertainty that cannot possibly be eliminated at the moment of a deciding about the child's future. This is why estimations of the quality of life for children with spina bifida remain a matter of controversy among neonatologists.[8]

In more general terms, expectations can go wrong when based on predictions of facts that do not occur or do not occur in the degree predicted. There is, of course, the possibility of so-called follow-up studies which show how children with a given disorder actually develop. These studies can be used to obtain indications as to what can be expected with a reasonable degree of certainty. But the information that can be obtained from these studies is statistical, which implies that with regard to individual cases one cannot be certain as to what to expect. There is thus an empirical underdetermination in these cases that affects the rationality of judgments about future states of affairs.

When confronted by the fact or the risk that one's child will be disabled, people will want to know what their future is going to be like if they decide to accept the child or the risk. In this they are dependent upon medical information of the kind described above: which symptoms attend which disorder? Given the fact of empirical underdetermination, however, medical experts are also faced with the problem of uncertainty. They can be quite uncertain about what to predict in the actual case. This creates the further possibility that the expectations of medical experts may be biased by their own views on the quality of life. There have been reports of court cases where expert testimonies about expectations regarding the quality of life for neonates with certain defects have been mutually contradictory.[9] The most probable explanation for this is that individual experts argue from what they take to be the paradigm case of a given condition, while different experts have different paradigm cases in mind. Leaving this complication aside, however, even a general agreement on the paradigm case of a given disorder does not eliminate the possibility of attaching different values to these cases in terms of the quality of life. Suppose there is something like the typical male fragile X person. How will the prospect of life for such a person be presented from a medical point of view? Apparently, much will depend on how the prospect is depicted. Consider the symptom of hyperactivity as being characteristic of many people with fragile X. What according to some is a lively character will appear to others as a nervous, uncontrolled person. Ways of describing and ways of evaluating are difficult, if not impossible to disentangle. If so, the least we can conclude is that factual information about what to expect in a particular case will be difficult to isolate from normative evaluation.[10] This difficulty of disentangling factual and normative aspects of medical information implies a dependence that, to a certain extent, affects the possibility of independent parental decision making. Given their dependence on the information that is presented to them by their medical counselors, parents can be misguided in making their decisions on information that is biased by values different from their own without their being aware of it. QL reasons have this irradicable aspect of uncertainty attached to them, which cannot but render parental decision making in this context a bewildering responsibility.[11]

10.3 Ways of Suffering

The more interesting problem with regard to QL reasons—philosophically speaking, that is—does not arise from the limited possibility of obtaining objective factual information about future states of affairs, but from the qualitative aspects of the decisions in question. Assuming these decisions regard children that are dearly wanted, they cannot but invoke deeply held convictions about the meaning of our lives and the place of having children in it. QL reasons, in other words, necessarily force people to reflect upon issues regarding their own conception of the good life.[12]

The question arises as to whether it is possible to assert views about our lives that enable us to look critically at reproductive choices made in the face of genetic disease. Can it be argued that, given certain facts about human existence, people may make decisions in this area that are probably mistaken? Can we argue with some confidence, for example, that people may make decisions that rest on a misjudgment of their own character? To explore this question, let me start with a distinction between 'ways of suffering' developed in this connection by Stanley Hauerwas.[13] In facing the prospect of parenting a disabled child, people may fear the distress and sorrow that lies ahead of them should they accept this responsibility. People may say, as they often seem to do: I am not capable of bearing this burden.[14] The prospect they fear is a prospect of a life burdened by suffering. But what is it exactly that makes them suffer?

In answering this question, Hauerwas distinguishes between the suffering that happens to us because of things we undergo and suffering that is conditioned by our purposes and goals. He writes:

> This distinction helps us to see the wider meaning of suffering. We not only suffer from diseases, accidents, tornadoes, earthquakes, droughts, floods—all those things over which we have little control—but we also suffer from other people,

from living here rather than there, from doing this kind of job—all matters that we can avoid—because in these instances we see what we suffer as part of a larger scheme. This latter sense of 'suffer', moreover, seems more subjective, since what may appear as a problem for the one may appear an opportunity for another. Not only is what we suffer relative to our projects, but how we suffer is relative to what we have or wish to be. (*Suffering Presence*, 166)

Hauerwas's distinction, it seems, opens up the possibility of pursuing the question of whether we may misjudge certain characteristics of our lives. For example, it allows us to see how some of our beliefs and attitudes toward suffering may enter into the experience of suffering itself. 'Natural' events that cause us to suffer by subjecting us to their force are often connected with pain and illness. They enforce upon us the condition of being a patient. The language we use in this connection reflects our passivity: we 'undergo,' we 'submit to', we are 'incapacitated'. All of these notions express that while being in pain and ill we experience powerlessness over ourselves and are placed into the hands of whoever is there to care for us. As Hauerwas puts it, the suffering of pain and illness is "fate rather than choice."[15]

But not all forms of suffering are characterized by passivity. Suffering can occur simply because we fail to achieve the goals we have set for ourselves. For example, should the goal of my life be to become a good singer, I will most likely suffer from my own frustration at not achieving that goal. Assuming that the instrument of my voice is too poorly equipped to be a good singer, I can give up the goal of becoming a singer and switch to a different instrument: I can choose to become a violinist. We have the option of changing our objectives in order to remove the cause of frustration and, by the same token, of suffering.

There is yet another and also more complicated kind of active suffering, however, which is more important for our purposes. We encounter it when we suffer in a way that blurs the line between fate and action. For example, cancer patients do not necessarily resign their capacity for action when developing the clinical symptoms of the illness, not even when their condition is terminal. In its initial stages the disease will most certainly be experienced as an alien force intruding upon their lives, which may induce the patient to try to understand her disease in order to able to come to terms with it.[16] Eventually it may come to be accepted and become part of the patient's identity, precisely because she accepts the fact of impending death and tries to face it in order to continue and prepare for life in its final stage.

Obviously, many genetic disorders cause suffering of the kind that is largely beyond our control: a matter of blind fate imposing itself upon people through the mechanism of the 'natural lottery'. Natural fate is without reason and therefore the most frightening kind of suffering. The distinctions introduced here, however, enable us to look more carefully and ask how and to what extent suf-fering from natural fate is linked to the goals we pursue in life. Without any doubt, we should not suffer because of nature's whims. But this does not neces-sarily imply that when it happens to us the only rational response is to resent it as a force that alienates us from the goals we expected to achieve in our lives.

10.4 Enrichment? In What Way?

To pursue this line of reasoning—which, it should be noted, does not argue for resignation—we have to ask what parents of disabled children can possibly mean when they say that sharing their lives with these children has been an en-riching experience.[17] What these parents do not mean, presumably, is that their disabled child has increased their happiness understood as the emotional state of pleasure. This notion of happiness does not possess much explanatory force in this context because it contradicts the experience of what it takes to learn how to live with and how to care for such a child. Particularly children with a mental handicap require much effort, which means that their parents get far more than the average share of things to worry about. 'Happiness' does not seem to be the clue for understanding the enrichment claim insofar as this notion evokes images of living in peace, undisturbed by natural misfortune. Certainly those images are not what one has in mind when thinking about what life with a handicapped child will be like.

Perhaps we should look in a different direction. Maybe the clue to the en-richment claim is to think about how the experience of being confronted with difficulty and disappointment is overcome. Supposedly, in conquering the diffi-culties in our lives we can achieve something that may be less easy to obtain when we choose not to confront these difficulties. This appears to be generally true for many of the things we pursue in our lives. Less demanding tasks create less rewarding lives. People do not only take interest in achieving the goals they set for themselves. What it takes to achieve these goals is often equally impor-tant, as any artist or athlete can tell. In these cases the reward is not only—and perhaps not even primarily—achieving the goal but also in the experience of making the effort.

The question of whether the experience of mastering a difficult task con-tributes to happiness does not seem to be the correct question, therefore. What we are looking for is better expressed by the notion of 'fulfillment'. I take it that the enrichment claim has to be understood in this sense. The effort of over-coming more than the average amount of difficulty brings a sense of fulfillment because one has to tap resources beyond what one initially trusts oneself to be capable of doing. If correct, this means that a life requiring more than average effort to succeed can be experienced as enriching because it allows for personal growth. To invoke the notion of happiness in this connection would seem to suggest, mistakenly, that because one has succeeded, the effort proves in the end not to have been an effort at all. Trying to overcome difficulties and obstacles in our lives is not an easy task, but it has a prize that can be gained only by accepting that task. The sense of fulfillment is a reward precisely because of the effort that had to be made. In the same sense it is true that adversity in life does not in retrospect change into fortune because one has succeeded in overcoming it.

This explanation of the enrichment claim presupposes a theory of the good that does not consider happiness to be the comprehensive good, at least not in the Benthamite sense of pleasurable experience. That is to say, inasmuch as happiness in that sense is at odds with the struggle for ends that cannot be obtained without adversity, it is not the comprehensive good. There are other goods, such as self-knowledge, that are obtained only through personal growth in difficult circumstances. Accordingly, the experience of being in pain or distress does not obliterate the possibility of experiencing goodness, but it must be goodness of a different kind from what is implied in the notion of happiness as pleasurable experience. The intuition guiding this view was famously stated by John Stuart Mill when he wrote that it is better "to be a human being dissatisfied than a pig satisfied; better to be Socrates dissatisfied than a fool satisfied."[18] The failure to achieve certain goals in life may be painful, but even then—Mill tells us—the attempt itself can be more rewarding than the pleasurable satisfaction of desire. Everything depends on the sources of satisfaction or dissatisfaction.

It is important to see, in this connection, that Mill did not mean to imply that the sources of satisfaction can be used in more or less prudent ways. He did not mean to say merely that instead of attending to the immediate and maximum gratification of our desires—as pigs and fools do—we should better practice some moderation in fulfilling them. What he meant was that the question of how and when to satisfy our appetites is significantly different from the question of what goals to set, and that satisfying our appetites is only one of these goals, and not the most commendable one for humans. In Mill's view there are other goals for human beings, goals of a different and nobler kind. Even if the fulfillment of this nobler kind of goal remains beyond our reach, it is nonetheless preferable to strive toward fulfillment because it becomes our nature to do so. Given the naturalist background of his utilitarian frame of reference, Mill notoriously failed in giving a convincing account of these 'higher pleasures', as he called them, a failure that can be explained, perhaps, by the fact that what he had in mind were not pleasures but achievements. In reflecting upon the good, Mill may have thought, we do not only reflect upon how our experiences make us *feel* about our lives but also upon what we make of ourselves in the pursuit of what we take the good to be.[19]

A more convincing account of this distinction is offered by Robert Nozick in an argument based upon his well-known thought experiment of the 'experience-machine.'[20] The experience-machine connects our brain to an artificial source of neurological stimuli that causes us to have any experiental sensation we want. The machine thus guarantees the maximum satisfaction of desires. The question is: Would one volunteer to be hooked up to it? Nozick constructed this imaginary device to see whether the good can be conceived in terms of how our lives feel 'from the inside'. In his view it cannot, because life holds other goods in store besides our states of experience: "The view that only happiness matters ignores the question of what we—the very ones to be happy—are like. How could the most important thing about our life be what it contains though? What makes the felt experiences of pleasure or happiness more important than what we ourselves are like?" (*The Examined Life,* 102). Even if Nozick's machine is capable of satisfying any of our desires in every possible dimension and context, we still have strong reasons for not choosing to be plugged into it. The first reason is that we want the things we deem important to be real rather than fake. I would personally be thrilled to see the Dutch national soccer team win the next World Cup. Having this wish fulfilled will give me the desired thrill, but what counts about this thrill is not the fact that I experience it but that the Dutch soccer team actually wins the championship. If states of experience were all that mattered, we would then be satisfied by the belief that certain events that please us happen, regardless of whether they actually do happen.

The second reason is closely related to the first. The machine allows us to feel good about having accomplished certain objectives through our own efforts regardless of whether we ever made those efforts. Feeling good is a state of experience that does not necessarily have other states of experience as its object. In many cases we feel good about ourselves rather than about our experiences. As Nozick argues, the doctrine that experience is all that counts for a good life—the doctrine of hedonism—fails to acknowledge that a life that feels good 'from the inside' could depend entirely upon self-deception.[21] What we make of ourselves matters to us because it is in shaping our own person that we respond to and act upon reality as it is given to us.[22]

The argument is a strong one. Of course one could say that—in Nozick's terms—the value of 'what we are like' is included in what makes us feel good, but this only reinforces the distinction between the two. What we are like is itself not an experiental state, but presupposes a judgment on how well we do in mastering the tasks posed before us by the world as it is. We can feel good without delusion only because we actually do face these tasks instead of avoiding them. Feeling good about tasks that one never begins may be a cause of happiness—people often manage to deceive themselves about their achievements—but this happiness rests on a mistake. It is simply irrational to feel good about having done something that one never did. In setting a personal record, the track and field athlete has reason to feel good because of the effort that she put into it. "It is worth the sacrifice and all the hard work," she will say. This is only true because she actually did make the sacrifice not because she merely believes she made it.

Nozick's question regarding what we are like is the question of how we shape our own character in responding to the limits that the world as it is sets before us. This is a point to consider carefully. When we fail to see the distinction between what we ourselves are like, on the one hand, and how we feel about our lives, on the other, we are likely to avoid the effort of shaping our character, which 'happiness' as such does not require. Being happy—understood as the emotional state of pleasure—tempts us not to confront the question regarding our character, that is, the question of who we really are.[23] If Nozick is right in this—as I think he is—the failure to heed this distinction may very well deprive us of important goods, i.e., the goods that can only be won by the activity of confronting the tasks reality sets before us. Happiness in the sense of feeling good cannot be the objective of this activity itself. In responding to the tasks that reality confronts us with, it is not feeling good that validates the response. Rather, the reverse is true. Responding adequately gives a sense of fulfillment that befalls us. The state of feeling good in this connection is essentially a by-product: unsolicited by desire but received anyway.[24]

Let us now try to understand what the argument developed so far tells us about the enrichment claim that is presented occasionally by parents of children with mental disabilities. It has been reported by some of these parents that the task of parenting a disabled child has taught them the truth of the saying "no pain, no gain."[25] This truth goes beyond the insight of suffering now for a greater joy later—which is what prudential hedonism would advise—because the gain is of a different kind. It has to do with becoming a different kind of person. A mother says: "I don't know what kind of person I might have been if I hadn't had N——. I don't often spend much time thinking about, well, what if N—— had been 'normal'. But I do spend time thinking about what would I have been like if I hadn't had N——" (*From Devastation to Transformation*, 110). The fact that parenting a child with 'special needs' forces these parents to face so many new and unanticipated tasks is a source of personal change in itself. Another parent says:

C—— has helped me find a side of myself I didn't know existed. I went from seeing myself as not having a lot to give the world to having a new world open up to me—a world of advocacy. Before I felt voiceless. But then I recognized my child is voiceless. I am the only voice he has. Advocacy for others is now an important part of my life. So I have come to discover new pieces of who I am through C——. (*From Devastation to Transformation,* 147)

According to these testimonies, there is reason for considering the task of parenting a disabled child in terms of a transformative experience, an experience that takes on a central role in self-narration and that constitutes changes in people's identity which they themselves regard as personal growth.[26]

To understand the enrichment claim, therefore, we have to take note of the difference between parental experiences that are characterized by a sense of regret and experiences characterized by a sense of fulfillment. Presumably parents of disabled children are never happy to receive such a child and it very often may cause them grief or frustration. But they nonetheless may move beyond the state of experiencing their lives as a lasting source of disappointment with which they have learned to cope. If they move beyond mere coping, these parents may come to experience a sense of fulfillment grounded in what they have shown themselves to be capable of doing. This neither obliterates the memories of pain and despair nor does it preclude the possibility of further hardship. But it does foster their confidence and trust that life can be good and worthwhile when the difficulties it poses are faced rather than resented.

Bringing these considerations to bear on the issue of difficult reproductive decisions, we can say that when people decide not to accept the burden of a disabled child, this may be a wise decision. But it is not necessarily so. There are different perceptions of what it means to share one's life with such a child, and they can be based on good reasons. We do not need to promote the idea of the enriching experience that such a life can bring, but neither should we ignore—let alone belittle—the fact that it often does. Not only parents of disabled children but many others whose lives have been affected by difficult conditions, medical or otherwise, know from their own experience that the quality of their lives cannot be reduced to a question of happiness.

Prospective parents facing difficult reproductive choices may be mistaken not so much in what their future lives will bring—the kinds of mistakes our discussion started with—as in what to expect about themselves. They may be misguided about the strengths and weaknesses of their own moral character and skills. Obviously, this mistake can go either way. People can underestimate the burden that raising a disabled child will bring or they may overestimate the burden they are capable of bearing. There is no way of knowing in advance how well they will do. But there is the possibility of trying to find out and it is a possibility that deserves serious consideration.[27] The importance of finding out what kind of people we are and what our lives are like is, in fact, the importance of not being deluded by self-deception. The good life, in any case, is a life lived in truth. People can deceive themselves with respect to what they think they cannot do as well as with respect to what they think they can do. Thinking correctly in these matters requires self-knowledge, more than anything else. But self-knowledge is obtained in facing whatever it is that life has in store for us and in finding out what we can make of ourselves in facing it.

10.5 Identification, Not Resignation

One of the ways in which people can face the reality of life and find out what they are capable of doing is by using science and technology to confront the hardships they face. Consequently, the hardships caused by genetic disorders can be confronted by trying to eradicate them by means of preventive medicine. Moreover, the development of preventive medicine is not only just another way of making an effort to overcome adversity; it is arguably the most effective way. It is certainly not obvious that accepting disability or disease is the more appropriate way of facing the reality with which life confronts us. On the contrary: human suffering ought not to be, so there is no reason to face it with equanimity. This consideration suggests that there is yet one other idea lurking in the background of the enrichment claim, namely the idea that the acceptance of suffering is a virtue. Even if Nozick's point against happiness as the ultimate good is well taken, it does not follow that the appropriate way to respond to what reality confronts us with is acceptance. Why should one think that accepting a disabled child and making the best of it is the virtuous thing to do?

To begin modestly, the conclusion thus far is not that to accept and make the best of it is *the* virtuous thing to do. As I have indicated, this will prove to be a mistake for people with a misguided conception of their own character and skills. The claim was that there is a strong argument for seeing it as a possible response, given one's self-knowledge and the belief in a nonhedonist conception of the good. Even if acceptance is not necessarily a virtue, it is certainly a possibility that cannot be discarded as irrational. Having said this, however, let us consider the notion of acceptance somewhat further and see what it may entail.

Undoubtedly, there is strong resistance in our present culture to the idea of the acceptance of suffering.[28] It smacks of passivity and patience, of subjection and submission. It seems to imply a view of natural reality as fate. Given all these connotations, the notion of acceptance contradicts some of the core values of modern culture, i.e., the value of self-determination and of living a life of one's own. In McKenny's words:

Technological control over the body is not merely an accidental feature of modern medicine but one with enormous implications for the way medical care is given and received and even for the constitution of modern persons as subjects.

We become subjects in part by monitoring, acting on, and exercising vigilance over our bodies, and medicine, especially when it has the role and capacities it has in contemporary society, is a vitally important way in which we carry out these attitudes and performances on our bodies. From this perspective, it is possible to understand how the moral commitments to expanding choice and eliminating suffering depend in a twofold way on the formation of a subject who exercises control over the body. Most obviously, control over the body, as Bacon and Descartes saw so clearly, is necessary in order to realize the aims of expanding choice and eliminating suffering. But beyond this, those commitments require that one abstract one's moral identity from the body, which in turn becomes (through technology it is hoped) simply the object of one's choices and desires. (*To Relieve the Human Condition*, 216)

It follows that whatever appears to be contrary to human self-determination is perceived as an alienating force. Natural hazards such as illness and disease are an impediment to living the lives we choose to live. In its attempt to control forces that set limits on our freedom, modern culture exhibits the belief that the only acceptable natural conditions of our existence are those that would have been chosen voluntarily.[29] Since illness and disease are incompatible with 'free will', they ought to be eradicated from the natural conditions of human existence.

In this light acceptance of disease and disability seems to contradict everything for which modern culture stands, as is particularly clear from its achievements in science and technology. This critical rejection of the notion of acceptance betrays too narrow a view, however. It is only when we think of our natural conditions in terms of the power nature holds over our lives, that 'acceptance' will be understood as resignation and defeat. Only within a paradigm that takes power to be the ruling principle of the universe, the experience of being confronted by nature's powers calls for the organization of countervailing powers. Outside that paradigm things may appear different.

The notion of acceptance can be taken in a different way as soon as we escape the dichotomy between passivity and activity that constitutes the paradigm of power. To explain this, let me return to the earlier example of cancer patients who come to accept the terminal disease in order to learn how to live with it.[30] Following Hauerwas's phrasing, this example was presented as a case that blurs the line between fate and action. In the case of terminal illness, as cancer often is, people arrive at the stage where they accept the fact that they are going to die as a fact about themselves. In identifying themselves with their own impending death they may find a way which, paradoxically, opens a possibility for continuing their lives that otherwise remained closed. They learn how to face the last task they need to fulfill, which is the task of dying.[31] Accepting the fact of impending death as being part of themselves is not an act of resignation but an act of facing reality that allows them to respond to it.[32] This response is possible only because they accept that their physical condition is beyond control.[33]

This example indicates that even when we do suffer from the pain and distress nature imposes, it may still depend on our own beliefs and attitudes as to whether or not we are capable of responding adequately. Therein lies the possible cause of a secondary form of suffering. This secondary form of suffering can be mitigated by the beliefs and attitudes that we have regarding the limitations of our own existence. These limitations can be rejected as frustrating the goal of living an independent life, but they can also be accepted as being part of the human condition.

To return to our case, that of parents facing the risk of children with genetic disorders, the point is that being confronted by a genetic disorder can be—and often is—experienced as the end of one's hopes of living a happy life in accordance with one's own dreams and expectations. However, this experience need not be a lasting one. People can—and often do—learn to see that there are other ways of living a good life. In this respect the argument in the present chapter was designed for a particular type of case—namely the case of deciding about a child that will be disabled, possibly seriously disabled, but that is otherwise capable of living a reasonably happy life. The argument suggests that particularly in this type of case there is reason to believe that the presumption of suffering may be mistaken. In many instances it is not true that people suffer from being disabled, nor is it true that people necessarily suffer from being the parent of a disabled child in such a way that makes their life unbearable. If so, the conclusion stands that the decision to accept such a child is certainly not an irrational thing to do. This is especially true if the child itself will not necessarily live an unbearable life. In that case the cause of suffering does not so much reside in what nature does to these people but in how they themselves, their relatives, as well as the community in which they live are capable of responding.

Let me conclude with one final observation. Seemingly, the project of gaining control over nature hardly needs more justification than the fact that disease and disability are the cause of great suffering. What more justification could there be? Nonetheless, one should note that the success of modern medicine makes us more and more aware of the illusionary nature of the project of gaining control over nature's powers. The more successful modern medicine is in keeping us alive, the longer our lifespan will be. The longer our lifespan will be, the more inevitable is the fact that we are going to witness the decay of our bodies. The more we are going to witness the decay of our bodies, the less confident we can be with regard to the project of gaining control over disease and disability.[34] The belief that medicine will continue to conquer the natural limits of our bodily existence is obsolete, because the success of medicine itself shows that it cannot succeed in this. If so, the rational thing to do is to adjust our expectations to meet this reality. The 'reality principle' invoked here is not the Freudian one saying that prudence is the rational way of succeeding in the satisfaction of desire. It is different in that it suggests that accepting the frailness of our bodily existence as part of the reality of human existence is a sign of wisdom.[35] Moreover, it may liberate us from the contemporary ideal for bodily perfection that is not only deceptive but also threatening to those who in the light of that ideal must necessarily appear as imperfect. Instead of trying to live *despite* the hardships that human life holds in store and trying desparately to escape them, we might as well try to learn to live our lives *with* them. To continue to believe that the quality of our lives is determined by control over nature's powers does not help us develop the skills necessary for facing the fragility and mortality of our own bodily existence.[36] In any case, the argument in this chapter has shown that the acceptance of natural limitations is certainly not irrational. In the case of children with genetic disorders who are nonetheless capable of reasonably happy lives it is not at all clear why the decision to share one's life with such a child should eliminate the possibility of a rewarding life.

ELEVEN

The Transformation Experience

The transformations described by parents with disabled children are not simply adjustments or accommodations. Adjustments and accommodations may occur gradually or in phases as the child with special needs is incorporated into an existing social and psychological framework. Transformations tend to be abrupt, significant areas of an existing social and psychological framework must be torn away and new ones constructed to incorporate new feelings and ideas. Changes are enduring, substantial, and generally perceived as desirable by the people who experience them.

Dick Sobsey

Transformer man
You run the show
Remote control
Direct the action with a push of a button
You're a transformer man
Power in your hand
Transformer man

Still in command
your eyes are shining on a beam
Through the galaxy of love
Transformer man
Unlock the secrets
Let us throw off the chains that hold you down

Neil Young

11.1 Incoherent Views?

What is it that makes parents of disabled children move beyond coping with their lives as a lasting source of disappointment? What enables them to experience their lives with these children as a source of fulfillment? As I suggested in the previous chapters, these questions require us to look at the beliefs and attitudes that guide these parents and shape their perceptions. How does the task of caring for such a child affect how these people think about themselves, that is, about the strengths and weaknesses of their own character and skills? This is the main issue to be discussed in this chapter.

It is almost a universal experience that the birth of a disabled child throws families into a crisis that generates deep emotional problems. This is often only the initial stage of their experience, however. Parents may change their views over time and come to love and honor their child, often very deeply. The question is, What marks the change? With regard to this question, it has been reported that parents of disabled children sometimes describe the success of parenting these children in terms of a 'transformation experience'.[1] Only when they were ready to let this child change their lives, including their views of themselves, were they able to enter into a process of learning and sharing. In this chapter I will explore this notion of a transformation experience. The reason for doing so is that it may teach us something extremely important; it suggests that it takes a particular kind of people to care for disabled persons and to enable them to flourish. If so, this adds to the suggestion developed earlier in this study that the future of disabled people in our society will in large part depend on whether or not there will be such people. Given the conclusion from earlier chapters that the public philosophy of liberal society provides little basis for any kind of special pleading for mentally disabled people, the crucial question then becomes how liberal society can produce the kind of people who are willing to have themselves transformed by what their society portrays and evaluates as defective children.

Before we come to the main topic for our discussion, however, I will begin with the experience of ambivalence. Parents who consider their lives to be rewarding sometimes express what appears as a paradoxical attitude towards their disabled child. On the one hand they assert that they would not want to have missed this child—despite all the difficulties that they have been going through. But on the other hand they express doubt as to whether they would choose to have this kind of life were they confronted with that choice. A father writes:

> There is one other essential observation regarding the human side of the suffering that comes with genetic disease. I hate what this disease has done to our sons and our family through their suffering (and ours, with them). So if the genetic disorder could be dealt with for future generations through genetic therapy, I

would rejoice. Had I known ahead of time the agony that genetic illness would bring us, I would have preferred to avoid it. So I understand why people who approach this issue on a purely human level using secular values and reasoning may choose to kill unborn, genetically different children in an effort to avoid the kind of pain I have just described. But there is more than a purely human dimension to life. Spiritually speaking, when I ask myself would I rather that Jonathan and Christopher had never been born, the anwer is: absolutely not. Though it broke my heart twice to share their sufferings, through them I know a lot more about love and faithfulness, kindness, gentleness, and humility than I could possibly otherwise have known.[2]

Leaving aside the author's curious distinction between 'purely human' and 'spiritual', this quote expresses an experience that is widely shared among parents of disabled children. Sometimes these parents feel guilty about their ambivalence, however. It seems as if the love and dedication for their child is tainted by some sort of *reservatio mentalis*. Supposedly, there is a lingering sense of betrayal haunting them: "How can I say I love her when at the same time I think I might have tried to prevent her from coming into existence?" The first task in this chapter is to try and understand these conflicting feelings, not in the sense of whether we can sympathize with them but in the sense of whether we can explain their cognitive basis. For this purpose I will explore Thomas Nagel's distinction between the objective and the subjective point of view. The assessments people make of their lives all have in common that they exhibit a first-person point of view. In expressing what my life means to me, I give an account of it 'from the inside'. At the same time, however, I can imagine that my life could have been very different, or that I would not have existed at all. 'From the outside', that is, my current life does not have the same impact. I feel curiously detached from it even though it is very much me. I will explore this distinction to explain the sense of ambivalence mentioned above. In assessing their lives with their disabled child, parents adopt these different and often conflicting points of view. Subjectively, they honor their child as a source of fulfillment for which they are grateful. Objectively, they are aware that their lives could have been very different, that the grief and disappointment need not have been, if only the genetic disorder that caused the disability of their child would not have occurred.

11.2 Two Different Perspectives

There is a well-known argument in contemporary debate that living with a disability is not necessarily a loss or a disadvantage. The case for the argument is presented with regard to the deaf community.[3] Deaf people are a linguistic rather than a disabled minority. They have their own way of life, mediated by its own language and culture, that is as rewarding as any other. Faced with the development of genetic testing aimed at the prevention of their condition, these people argue that they would consider it a loss if the condition of deafness could be repaired.[4] Since being deaf is important to deaf people—at least to a number of deaf people, if not all—they would not want to change places with hearing people.

The case presented with regard to the deaf community does not easily translate to other conditions, however. The classification of deafness as an impairment can be disputed because of the distinct culture that the deaf community represents, but a similar argument cannot easily be made with regard to mental disability.[5] It presents us with a different and more difficult case. Presumably this is why people who share their lives with mentally disabled children often remain ambivalent about the development of genetic testing. They value their present lives as meaningful, which represents an evaluation from an internal point of view. At the same time, however, they concede that if they were to contemplate their kind of life as an object of choice they might decide against it, thus making an evaluation from an external point of view.

There is a significant difference between the two cases which resides in the fact that they are based upon different comparisons. When making their case, deaf people consider their present life and compare it with another life—that of a hearing person—and then decide for the former as being preferable. In the second case, however, parents of mentally disabled children evaluate the same life positively from an internal point of view, but negatively from an external point of view. On the positive side they say: "I experience my present life as rewarding." On the negative side, however, they say: "Were I to choose between two kinds of life, one of which includes living with a child like ours, I might choose the other."[6]

Characteristic for each of these responses, then, is the fact that in looking at their present lives from the inside, none of the respondents is interested in changing places. But while (some of) the people from the deaf community leave it at that, parents who remain ambivalent about genetic testing do not. It is important to be clear about the predicament in which these parents feel themselves to be caught. It is not that, as a matter of hindsight, they now think that had they been given a choice in the past, they would have decided against their present life. Nor is it the case that, even though they believe this decision might have been theirs at that time, they now know better, given their appreciation for their present life. Both these possibilities frame the problem diachronically: they reflect different attitudes conflicting between the present and some point in the past. The parental response we are considering here is more complex. In fact, what the parents in question are saying is that even though they would not change places now, looking at their lives from the point of view of their personal involvement, they nevertheless would not value their lives positively from a more detached point of view that allows them to consider what it might have been, for example with a healthy child. It appears that these parents are of two minds. The tension they experience is not fixed by two points in time: it is synchronic. They have to reconcile a positive and a negative judgment within their own soul. Parents who find themselves disturbed by the conflict between both judgments face a problem—the problem of looking simultaneously at one's life from two radically different perspectives. Thomas Nagel puts this problem very generally in the following way:

> The uneasy relation between inner and outer perspectives, neither of which we can escape, makes it hard to maintain a coherent attitude toward the fact that we exist at all, toward our deaths, and towards the meaning or point of our lives, *because a detached view of our own existence, once achieved, is not easily made part of the standpoint from which it is lived.* From far enough outside my birth seems accidental, my life pointless, and my death insignificant, but from the inside my never having been born seems nearly unimaginable, my life monstrously important, and my death catastrophic. Though the two viewpoints clearly belong to one person—these problems wouldn't arise if they didn't—they function independently enough so that each can come as something of a surprise to the other, like an identity that has been temporarily forgotten. (*The View from Nowhere*, 209; italics added)

The relation between both perspectives on our personal lives is necessarily uneasy because of the different and divergent attitudes that they exhibit. A detached view of our own existence, as Nagel puts it, is not easily integrated into the point of view from which it is actually lived. The person who is subjectively committed to her life finds herself at the same time detached from that life, a situation that threatens to undermine her commitment.[7] The awareness of this situation cannot but be unnerving. My life could have been very different from what it is now and there is a part of me that identifies with what my life could have been rather than with who I now am.

In Nagel's view my 'objective self' is as much a part of me as my 'subjective self' but in a distinctively different key. The objective self is the self that describes itself but from a non-subjective point of view: its self-description excludes the 'I'. It may talk about 'me' in a very general way: as a man sitting behind a desk, writing a philosophical text, working at a university, and so on. Regardless of the degree of generality or specificity, the life of 'me' can be described in a non-subjective way, such that from an external perspective it may look very different from how it looks subjectively to me. There is a perspective constituted by observation of facts and data about the individual sitting behind his desk—indicating 'what-ness'—that is radically different, in Nagel's account, from the perspective constituted by my identification of that individual as 'me'—indicating 'who-ness'.

The potential tension between the two perspectives is made concrete in Kenzaburo Oë's novel in the way its main character, Bird, is caught between his objective and subjective selves. On the subjective side Bird realizes that there is no escape from admitting "I am the father of a severely disabled child." On the objective side, however, he fantasizes about what his life would be like, if he left his wife and his son and went to Africa with Himiko.

11.3 A Capacity for Alienation

Nagel's account of the objective and subjective selves as the embodiment of two different perspectives that shape us as human beings helps to explain the ambivalence that parents of mentally disabled children may experience. From an objective point of view there are facts about their children that make these parents regard their lives as burdensome rather than attractive.[8] Presumably, some of these facts are that these children are incapable of living an independent life, they will never be self-supporting, pursue a career of their own, build a family, and so on. From this point of view, the state of their lives is such that the resulting picture does not unambiguously appear attractive. But at the same time these parents have memories of the happy moments they shared with their children, of the progress made in learning how to live. They are devoted to their children and love them dearly. There is an apparent conflict between these perceptions.[9] When they look from the inside they feel differently from when they look from the outside, despite the fact that in both cases the persons who are looking are identical.

The capacity for adopting an objective perspective on ourselves is often valued positively, because without being able to look at our lives from the outside we would not be capable of change. When we leave our subjective point of view behind, our actual existence appears in a different light. The philosophical expression for this phenomenon is that human beings are capable of transcending themselves. The notion that neither my life nor the world in which I live is necessarily what it appears to be at present, depends upon this capacity. According to Nagel, however, this capacity for transcendence is ambiguous, because it is the same as the capacity for alienation.[10] In looking at my life from the outside I can arrive at the point where the concerns I currently have start to crumble.

Each of us finds himself with a life to lead. While we have a certain amount of control over it, the basic conditions of success and failure, our basic motives and needs, and the social circumstances that define our possibilities are simply given. Shortly after birth we have to start running just to keep from falling down, and there is only limited choice as to what will matter to us. . . . We lead highly specific lives within the parameters of our place, time, species, and culture. What could be more natural? Yet there is a point of view from which none of it seems to matter. When you look at your struggles as if from great height, in abstraction from the engagement you have with this life because it is yours, you feel a certain sympathy for the poor beggar, a pale pleasure in his triumphs and a mild concern for his disappointments. (*The View from Nowhere*, 215–16)

The hardships we endure, the emotions we invest, the passions that absorb us in making an effort—all of which make our commitments look important to us—appear as simply a waste of energy. From the outside the struggle often seems pointless. Parents of severely disabled children are particularly prone to this kind of experience. A mother of a son with a severe hearing impairment says: "Even though I say I have accepted everything that has happened to G———, yes, I have accepted it—but there are always times when I will be listening to a song and all of a sudden it will hit me, he's never going to hear that exactly like I do. And I will go through all of this again. I will go through the grieving process and I will cry. And then away I go and I'm okay" (*From Devastation to Transformation*, 107). Parents of disabled children do have strong ties of affection and the occasional triumphs of their children fill their lives with joy and pride, but there is always 'the big picture' that does not look promising.[11] Given this potential tension, the truth about sharing one's life with a disabled child appears to be that the meaning that is found in that life alternates with the meaning that is lost. If one can discover the causes that explain why things happen the way they do, this may give hope and strength. Yet the why question may never be silenced. This is not only true of the experience of parenting a disabled child, however, it is true of the lives of each of us. The experience of alienation, according to Nagel, is part of each of our lives, even though both the frequency and intensity of this experience may vary.

In view of this threat of alienation to which the objective point of view—'the big picture'—exposes us, Nagel considers the objection that the problem it causes is unreal. Why should the question of how my life looks from the outside matter to me more than how it looks from the inside? Why identify with the objective self if this implies forgetting who I actually am? According to Nagel, this way of dismissing the problem cannot succeed because the objective point of view is not forced upon us from outside—it is our own. "Objectivity is not content to remain a servant of the individual perspective and its values. . . . The objective self is a vital part of us, and to ignore its quasi-independent operation is to be cut off from oneself as much as if one were to abandon one's subjective individuality. There is no escape from alienation or conflict of one kind or another" (*The View from Nowhere*, 221). Assuming that the 'objective' self has a life of its own, the problem resulting from the inner division of the self cannot simply be evaded. Our capacity for self-transcendence cannot be tamed, as Nagel points out, in the name of reaffirming who we 'really' are. Consequently, the experience of detachment from our actual lives poses the problem of integrating those aspects that describe us—or part of us—objectively but which we may find hard to accept subjectively.

Nagel's account of the divided self explains a great deal of the tension that people with disabled children experience. This tension looms large in languages that express the inner division of the self, such as the language of 'coping'. Coping is what humans do in facing the fact that they cannot live in harmony with themselves. On Nagel's view, human existence is irredeemably characterized by this tension, which leads him to conclude that the experience of absurdity is irradicably part of human existence. But this conclusion does not follow. As Nagel himself concedes we are occasionally engaged in ways that makes the distinction among points of view irrelevant.[12] People can sometimes be engaged by a given object or activity—Nagel seems to have in mind artists and poets—in such a way that even the awareness of the big picture does not detract them from it. But he remains skeptical about this possibility:

> It is hard to know whether one could sustain such an attitude consistently toward the elements of everyday life. It would require an immediacy of feeling and attention to what is present that doesn't blend well with the complex, forward-looking pursuits of a civilized creature. Perhaps it would require a radical change in what one did, and that would raise the question whether the simplification was worth it. (*The View from Nowhere*, 223)

Interestingly, this description of overcoming the inner division of the self is not unlike how some parents describe the way they learn to live with their disabled children. Indeed, to get on with their lives they must *radically* change. They have to accept what nobody wants to accept; they need to live with uncertainty. Not knowing what to expect next, they have to learn to live here and now and make the best of it. They need to learn to celebrate achievement where many others fail to see that there is any. All in all, there is a radical change in their lives that amounts indeed to a simplification of what matters and what does not, which leads them to believe that their lives are worth the effort. To understand this, let us look at what is meant by the transformation experience.

11.4 *"From Devastation to Transformation"*

In reviewing the recent literature on how people respond to the task of parenting disabled children, the American psychologist Kate Scorgie reports a tendency toward a seemingly negative approach with regard to counseling parents of disabled children. Sharing one's life with a disabled child is often described in terms of coping with stress. The general approach seems to be informed by the notion that the lives of families with such children are characterized by a deficit and that the professional task is to assist people in coping with its consequences.[13] In her own study Dr. Scorgie investigates the idea that to understand how parents of disabled children manage their lives, one has to include the potential benefits of being involved in such a task.[14] Interestingly she reports that the parents who agreed to participate in her study gave her reason to take this idea seriously.[15] They were much more motivated to talk about how they succeeded in managing their lives than about how they succeeded in coping. One parent in Scorgie's study said: "When I use the word 'coping', those are the days I'm barely holding on."[16] The explanation may be, following Scorgie, that 'coping' is what you do in response to a crisis that exceeds your ability to meet its demands. Parents of disabled children, however, not only manage to get beyond this point by learning how to live their daily lives but also experience positive transformations. Not only do they manage—rather than cope—they also change. They are personally transformed and become different people. Scorgie reports how the contribution of parents shaped her study:

> In fact, parents seemed to be describing their experiences as a journey—a journey from the devastation which accompanied the initial diagnosis to a place where they were beginning to discover, and often to their surprise, not only that they were able to manage life effectively, but that they were also being enriched along the way. Thus, the focus of the study broadened to include, not just life management strategies, but transformational outcomes. ("From Devastation to Transformation," 7)

Scorgie's study is designed to answer three questions. The first is what kind of strategies are used by parents who manage their lives with a disabled child effectively. The second is whether there are personal attributes and abilities that characterize such parents. The third is whether there are common themes in how parents talk about themselves as being transformed in parenting a disabled child. The answers to these questions enable us, one might say, to see what makes "the journey" a rewarding one. In interpreting these answers in terms of transformation, Scorgie distinguishes between personal, relational, and perspectival transformations.[17] Parents report personal transformations in an enhanced capacity to speak up for their children and reach out to others in need. They considered themselves to be more compassionate and confident. Interestingly, they also report an enhanced sense of humor. Some of the relational transformations include the ways they relate to others by taking people's perspectives on their own life seriously. In general, the task of advocacy has a strong impact on these parents' ways of relating to others. Perspectival transformations affect their attitude towards life. Parents report that they have learned to celebrate life, have changed in their conceptions of success and reward and, generally, have acquired a different view on what is important in life.

Scorgie's metaphor of life as a journey, however, evokes the notion of learning processes and of gradual development. Undoubtedly, there is this aspect and it is a very important one. But a preliminary question is: What makes the journey possible in the first place?[18] What kind of understanding, or insight, is required to make sense of the idea of a journey at all? To explore this preliminary question I will draw on Scorgie's material and focus on three key notions that she uses to describe 'successful' parenting of a disabled child. They are accepting the disability, a positive reframing of one's own beliefs and attitudes, and the ability of living with uncertainty.

The diagnosis of disability in one's child is a traumatic event for parents that creates feelings of profound devastation. Not seldom disbelief and denial of the permanency or extent of the disabling condition is the result. A mother in Scorgie's study says:

> When the doctor tells you that your child is behind and mentally handicapped, that is not something you want to hear—so you're going to prove him wrong. So you get out there and you do whatever you have to in order to make that a reality. Eventually it comes to the point where your life goes on and you realize that it doesn't matter what you do, you're not going to change what's happened. This is who your child is. ("From Devastation to Transformation," 104)

The realization of the fact that the disability will not go away does not by itself induce the redeeming response of acceptance. Resignation is also a possibility. Like other people, parents of disabled children can also be trapped in 'negative coping'. But there are those for whom acceptance marks the change of being able to concentrate upon what is rather than upon what could have been. Only then are they capable of learning to love their child as it is. Another parent recalls:

> You know, I bargained with God. I could handle all this for the next year if he just smiled or if he learned how to walk or talk. A year later he hadn't changed at all. And I remember being hit on this birthday thinking I made this deal and he

hasn't changed. . . . And I looked back at that point and realized that nothing had changed, except that I'd learned to love him for what he is. ("From Devastation to Transformation," 104–5)

Scorgie reports that several parents in her study spoke of a distinct moment in time "when reality clicked in." It was at that moment that they realized the need to give up the dream about the child they could have had and get down to the business of raising the child they had.[19] Acceptance is thus a key notion in getting started on the journey. However, some of Scorgie's parents rejected the notion of acceptance as too superficial to describe that change. 'Acceptance' leaves room for the suggestion of resignation and defeat which is not what they experienced. From what they say, 'embracement' would seem be the more accurate description. The experience of change through embracement does not obliterate the moments of grief that occasionally return. It rather sets people free to express their emotions without being captivated by them. Embracement marks a change, a painful change that consists in abandoning one's expectations but also a change that opens up the possibility of seeing one's child not as disabled but as lovable and endearing as it is.

What induces this change? This question takes us to the second notion. In Scorgie's interpretation it is the fact that the initial sense of devastation is reframed by a shift in perspective. Her parents report that:

It was only as they began to modify the way in which they perceived or appraised their circumstances, that they were able to view their own lives and their corporate family lives as potentially 'manageable'. That is, the parents engaged in the process of reframing (reformulating) their original thoughts and attitudes about their circumstances, which now included parenting a child with special needs. ("From Devastation to Transformation," 103)

Reframing one's beliefs and attitudes includes, among other things, that parents become more focused on their child rather than on their own feeling of disappointment: not only in the sense of being responsive to the child's needs but in the much more radical sense of being open to what this child, even when severely disabled, has to give. Furthermore, it includes allowing the possibility that the arrival of a disabled child in one's life may have a meaning and that the challenge of parenting that child is to discover what it could be. One parent remarks: "You can choose to be a victim of your circumstances. There's no doubt about that. You can also choose to make the most out of what you've been given in life. Ultimately we have a responsibility to our lives. There's a difference between 'putting in time' and 'making the most of it'. And it's primarily a choice" ("From Devastation to Transformation," 106).

Supposedly, the remarkable thing about these parents is that they are capable of accepting their child as a gift. As this parent indicates, there is more to this than that each of us has his or her responsibilities in life. We have a responsibility *to* our lives, as she puts it, for the very reason that our lives are given—not in the sense in which data are given but in the sense of its being a gift. What this means is suggested by another parent who talks about her child as her teacher:

> C—— is my teacher, my mentor, my inspiration. I just see his willingness to go out into the world every day and face every challenge with joy and acceptance. He doesn't let things get him down. . . . He's taught me about unconditional love. No matter how people act toward him, he's always there with hugs and smiles. ("From Devastation to Transformation," 106)

To engage in a reframing of one's perspective requires a strong determination to succeed. As indicated, it involves personal choice. The language of choice is an important part of the vocabulary of Scorgie's parents. The same is true for the language of control. But these languages have an interesting twist in meaning, because these parents are very much aware of how little choice they have and of how little they control. Many parents report irregularities in their children's functioning and behavior to the effect that they face the need to change their plans and schedules very often. This brings us to the third key notion, the notion of living with uncertainty.[20]

Living with uncertainty—not knowing what to expect next—does not mean that one cannot make any plans nor that one does not have any control. But it does mean that plans and schedules are tentative and that one must be very flexible. One has to learn to live "one day at a time." While the parents of the study admit that there are many things they do not control in their lives, they do claim to be in control over how much they permit the future to dominate the present. Scorgie interprets this claim by saying that while control is important for her parents, it is even more important to control one's affective response to events that one is unable to control.[21] A mother says, for example, that she is surely worried about "what's down the road," but she does not let that control her present life. The notion of control and choice as these parents use it, therefore, does not refer to causality. It is not about the extent to which they can make things happen or prevent them from happening. Rather, it is about intentionality. A parent of a child with an unknown prognosis comments:

> I guess it's caused me to look at what's real, what's important, and to live one day at a time, because I don't know how things are going to be from one day to the next. I think I appreciate life probably more than I ever used to. Every day I have

with L—— is a new day and it's an important day, and I have to make the most of that day. ("From Devastation to Transformation," 151)

These parents emphasize the importance of celebrating achievements regardless of how minimal they are, given that they experience failure so often. Celebrating achievements taught these parents how little things can bring a sense of fulfillment to one's life. Thus we learn that for these parents 'control' and 'choice' exist, paradoxically, in their capacity for receptivity and responsiveness. Another parent of a child with a degenerative condition remarks similarly: "So maybe later on he'll have to have a gastronomy. But that's okay. We'll just deal with it, but there is not a darn thing they can do that will stop the deterioration. I mean, if it's going to happen it's just going to happen," ("From Devastation to Transformation," 115). Far from believing that they are in control of what is going to happen to their children, let alone think that they have a choice in it, parents do know where they can choose and what they can control in *themselves*. What will be, will be. But how they respond is up to them.

With regard to this issue of parental response, Scorgie refers to literature that focuses on the narrative structure of experience, which implies that people do not respond to events but to their own reading of these events.[22] Thoughts, feelings, and perceptions do not determine what we experience but how we experience. For example, individuals who experience negative outcomes of critical events explain these events in narratives that underscore themes such as victimization, blame, and meaninglessness. In contrast, individuals who experience positive outcomes explain events in narratives dramatizing positive meaning, self-esteem, and beneficial effects.

These insights suggest the importance of maintaining a sense of coherence between how we experience what happens in our own lives on the one hand, and our view of the world at large on the other. If we only experience discontinuity between the two, we are either trapped in our lives or lost in the universe. Either way alienation and disengagement are what remains. This was, of course, the point of Thomas Nagel's distinction between the 'subjective' and the 'objective' selves. But while Nagel believes that the experience of alienation and disengagement—the absurd—cannot be suppressed, I have used Scorgie's study to describe how, after the experience of initial devastation, parents with disabled children come to experience the world again as a meaningful place by opening up to their children and accepting them as a fountain of joy and love.[23] As their testominies show, this has very little to do with heroic attitudes in facing adversity; it has rather to do with being prepared to be radically changed by these children. Their transformation experience corroborates a human possibility, the possibility of love, that Nagel only reluctantly concedes.

11.5 Transformation and the Power to Respond

Many of the themes and observations in Scorgie's study can be found in a book on transformation written a few decades ago by Rosemary Haughton. Haughton's prime interest is theological but her method is not: she discusses fictional narratives to discover general insights and ideas about the human condition.[24] One of these narratives is about a man who goes through a crisis that "separates him from the safety of life as he knows it, from the soothing framework of customs and routine and accepted behaviour."[25] The symptoms Haughton describes are similar to those produced by the kind of crisis we have been considering:

> This kind of condition can be produced by illness or catastrophic loss of fortune, or by moral collapse, or a mixture of these. The essential is that something happens that makes the normal structure of security, the life of the world, seem no longer safe or even very real. There is a loss of self-respect, a loss of feeling of belonging to anything. . . . This condition of estrangement from normality is not in itself transformative. It has no particular value at all, indeed it is dangerous, it can lead to panicky efforts to find *any* kind of sense or refuge, or to withdrawal into a semi-animal life of minimum response. (*The Transformation of Man*, 107)

Haughton interprets this critical condition as the disintegration of 'formative' forces, that is, the disintegration of the self that is shaped by prevailing rules, conventions, and practices that guide us through life and direct us toward the good.[26] The crisis is a crisis of the self, which makes the 'natural' response of this beleaguered self defensive and protective. Let us recall the mother who said that "when the doctor tells you that your child is behind and mentally handicapped, that is not something you want to hear—so you're going to prove him wrong." In holding on to expectations that her formative forces had installed in her, she was determined to do everything to turn these initial expectations into a reality. But in doing so, she prevented herself from opening up to that other reality, which is the reality of love that creates hope and joy. Professionals who talk about denial tend to conflate the two and fail to distinguish between denying the reality of the handicap on the one hand, and accepting the loss of the old self on the other. Parents who deny the reality of the handicap refuse to accept their child as it is, because they cling to the self as it has been produced by the formative forces that shaped their views and expectations about their future as parents. That is, they cling to their old selves. Parents who manage to abandon these expectations and manage to accept their child as it is, have somehow learned to see another possibility. In accepting the child as perfect in its own right, they abandon lingering thoughts about what could have been, including thoughts about what life with a different child could have been. In other words, they have changed and discovered themselves as a 'new' self. The reason that professionals are prone to miss the distinction lies, supposedly, in the fact that they are committed to the conventional framework of 'normal expectations'. Professionalism that is necessarily shaped by formative forces, especially when understood as a form of expertise, will lead them to regard the parents described by Scorgie's study as deluding themselves with false hope when they demonstrate optimism about their parental tasks.[27]

In this connection it is important to emphasize that the transformation experience has little to do with the self-seeking motive of feeling good about yourself because of what you do for others.[28] What Scorgie's parents report does not reflect a sense of gaining strength from other people's weakness. The experience that the life with their child has brought them is just too painful to be self-gratifying. But the abandonment of the old self that their life involves, though very painful, can nonetheless be rewarding.

However, according to Haughton it is not the loss of self as such that is transformative, for in itself it is primarily destructive. But it is the key to transformation. There is a truth to be faced and it is a very painful one. In facing it, one has to open oneself to the possibility of changing in the sense of 'letting go'. This possibility is the possibility of *self-giving* that is not driven by a sense of achievement, because—as Haughton puts it—there is "nothing to achieve against."[29] In the case of the mother referred to above, for example, there is no one left to be proven in the wrong about the condition of her child. In this respect, the main character in the narrative from which Haughton derives these insights is like the parents in Scorgie's study. Having accepted that the life that he used to live is in shambles, he has no reason left to reassure himself that all is well. Even though there are many difficulties lying ahead, he also has that kind of quiet conviction that made Scorgie's parents say: "what must happen is going to happen, but we'll make the best of it." This confidence is neither boastful nor self-gratifying because it is grounded in surrender. The transformation experience is one of accepting the loss of one's old self in the face of a future that does not look bright. In this experience a new self can be found, which releases the power to respond. But it is not the power of "look how strong I am." In a remarkable book called *Uncommon Fathers*, Rabbi Henry J. Karp[30] writes:

> Even in the darkness of our despair, a new light was beginning to dawn. All of a sudden, Joshua had been transformed. No longer was he that incorrigible little imp. No longer was he the fount of my frustration. No. There was something heroic about him. He had become a little warrior, waging a tireless battle against a relentless adversary. His was the struggle to live his life best he could. That he was battling forces beyond him—beyond us all—forces he could never come to

comprehend, mattered little to him. He would continue to explore and expand, albeit at a slower pace than others, and albeit down a twisted trail, but continue he would. It was at that moment that we bonded; the bonding so long delayed, but so well worth the waiting. Yet in truth, Joshua did not change at all. He was the same little boy who insisted upon scaling the shelves of the preschool. Rather, it was I who had changed. It was I who had opened up. The little hero was always there, always the hero. It was I who was late in perceiving it. (*Uncommon Fathers*, 107)

As the bellicose metaphors that Karp uses to characterize his son bring out so nicely, nothing has changed in the life of the little boy other than that his father finally understands that there is nothing he can do about this child but to love him. Only then does he discover that this love makes the boy appear in a completely different and radiant light, a little hero in his own right. This phenomenon, which appears as a kind of rebirth of the disabled child, is not uncommon in the literature.[31]

What is perhaps most striking in reading stories by parents of special children is how the air of paradox that surrounds many of these stories evaporates once we understand that the power of these people to respond is the power of love. Many of these stories speak of the experience of losing oneself to find oneself and of deep despair turning to hope. To close with a final, quite humorous example from these stories, told by Dick Sobsey, an American psychologist and himself the father of a severely disabled son: an Australian friend confessed believing that the only way God could remove his arrogance for being a smart guy was by presenting him with his mentally disabled son. Though grateful for this gift the friend commented: "I have also wished at times God had used sandpaper and not a chain-saw!"[32] Accordingly, Rosemary Haughton brings out this paradoxical nature of the transformation experience as follows:

The transformation occurs in the moment of self-surrender to love. Each is responding to an invitation that comes to him or her through the other, and could not do so otherwise. The response of each is a total gift of the whole person as it then exists, it is unconditional and unreflective. It is of their own deeper self, yet it is not possessed but only exists in its givenness. (*The Transformation of Man*, 80)

Allow me in the conclusion to this chapter to return to Nagel's account of the divided self and to his claim that there is no escape from alienation and conflict between the objective and the subjective selves. Intuitively, this claim appears to me to be mistaken. I suggest that Scorgie's account of the transformation experience provides us with an argument for why it is mistaken. In Nagel's view the problem is that I cannot help but find myself to be part of a reality so immense—the expanding universe—that part of me, the objective self, can only shatter the meaning I find in my present life, that is, the life of the subjective self. Nagel overlooks the possibility attested by the experience of parents with disabled children, namely the possibility of abandoning the self that is impressed by the sense that life could have been very different from what it turns out to be. Nagel's self, I suspect, is a self that believes that somehow our lives should be the product of our own projection. Since life as it could have been is so very different from what it actually is, we can never be sure that this particular life is worth living at all. We could only be sure of that, if it were true that we chose it, which is not the case. Nagel's belief in the inevitability of estrangement is grounded in the scepticism that we can never be sure about our lives because we control so little, which seems to betray the further belief that to value our lives, we need to be in control of how they come to be what they actually are.

The example of parents who have gone through the transformation experience, however, indicates why this belief is false. The self that is shattered by the misfortune of fate is transformed into a self that knows how not to be distracted by projections about what might have been. The initial devastation of giving birth to a disabled child is an experience of the absurd, if anything is. It is the experience of being the victim of the blind force of nature, which clearly represents the crushing power of objective reality invading the realm of one's personal life. The alienation resulting from this initial experience is superseded, however, not by denying objective reality, but by giving up the idea that our lives are worth living to the extent that we can choose its conditions. If I commit myself to the particular life that I am currently living, why should it bother me that I could have chosen a different life? The absurdity that Nagel believes to be irredeemably part of human existence stems from the fact that we live lives that we did not choose and that for that reason might have been very different. But why should I believe that my ability to maintain coherence in my experience depends on my own controlling activity? As I understand the transformation experience that Scorgie describes, it is rather when people manage to abandon this view and open themselves to the possibility of love for the other that is entrusted upon them, that they overcome the experience of the absurd. This is precisely what happens to the main character in Oë's novel, Bird, who goes from regarding his disabled son as a monster that somehow evokes the absurd world of Apollinaire, to accepting him as his child that wants to be loved and cared for. This possibility is not chosen, but elicited by the presence of his son. The transition marks the abandonment of his old self—the self longing to go to Africa in order to escape its current life—and the finding of a new self that has accepted this child. Only once he comes to regard his son as "inviting him to love," as Haughton puts it, the experience of being a pinball in nature's gambling machine—the experience of the 'objective self'—loses its alienating force.

I began this chapter with the ambivalence that parents of disabled children sometimes feel with regard to the development of genetic testing. The ambivalence in question was explained by saying that these parents adopt two different perspectives on their lives simultaneously. These parents are of two minds, I said, one informed by an internal perspective generating a positive judgment, the other informed by an external perspective generating a negative judgment about living with their disabled child. What worries these people is the fact that they are still not sure whether they would accept that possibility for themselves were they to make the decision now. That is, they are still not sure about themselves. The account of the transformation experience indicates that parents who attest to this experience will not look at their lives in this way. They will probably readily admit that, looking at the person they once were—*that* person might have decided to prevent the birth of their child, had he or she been given the choice of genetic testing. But having been transformed in such a way as to experience their disabled child as a gift, these parents no longer identify with their 'old' self. The choice for prevention no longer is a possibility that they find relevant to contemplate for themselves.

TWELVE

The Meaning of Life in Liberal Society

It will not do to allow that a meaningful life is a life involved in projects that seem to have positive value from the perspective of the one who lives it. Allowing this would have the effect of erasing the distinctiveness of our interest in meaningfulness; it would blur the distinction between an interest in living a meaningful life and an interest in living a life that feels or seems meaningful. . . . When one wakes up to the recognition or the thought that one's life to date has been meaningless, one is not weaking up to the thought that one's life to date has seemed meaningless.

Susan Wolf

12.1 Discovered or Made?

In this last chapter I will relate the issue of sharing one's life with a handicapped child to the broader issue of the meaning of life in contemporary society. Many of our contemporaries seem to believe that the meaning of life is something of our own making: it is neither received nor discovered as somehow 'out there', i.e., it is not inherent to external reality but is produced by our own deliberate activity. This modern view of the quest for meaning is characterized by activist notions such as 'giving', 'constructing', and 'inventing', which indicate their displacement of previous notions such as 'receiving', 'finding', and 'discovering.' In the first part of this chapter I will try to explain this semantic shift in some detail, including some of the key notions it involves. The discussion will be largely theoretical, but it aims at showing the practical implications for our appreciation of mentally disabled persons who are incapable of giving meaning to their lives. Although they will not appear in my argument until the very last stage, I hope it will become clear by then that I had these persons in mind all along the way.

Particularly with regard to profoundly mentally disabled people, one is occasionally confronted by skeptical views about the meaning of their lives, as, for example, when it is said that the lives of such human beings are pointless because they exist merely as 'vegetables'. I will argue that this skeptical view stands in the way of our ability to share our lives with such people. It presupposes that the possibility of a meaningful life is grounded in an individual capacity, i.e., the capacity for reflective experience. My aim is to argue against this kind of skepticism. Its basic claim is that, given the absence of reflective experience, there is nothing that can make the lives of the profoundly disabled worthwhile for themselves. My strategy of argumentation will not be to try to refute this claim directly, i.e., by showing that the profoundly mentally disabled *can* have meaningful lives even if their lives cannot be meaningful to themselves. Instead, I will focus on the question of how the sceptical view may affect one's ability to share one's life with such people. My suggestion will be that people will have no idea of what it means to share one's life with a mentally disabled person and care for her unless they are actually engaged in doing it. In this connection I want to recall what the exploration of the transformation experience taught us about parents who manage to live rewarding lives with disabled children. At some point they came to understand that nothing would ever change in their lives unless they opened themselves to the possibility that their child has something to give. This suggests that there is an element of receptivity that is constitutive of the meaning they have found in parenting their disabled children. I will argue that, unless we see the importance of this element, we are most likely to misunderstand what these parents are saying. If there is anything threatening to the future of disabled people in our society, it is the individual subjectivism that dominates current conceptions of the meaning of life. But it will take us quite a while to reach this conclusion by means of philosophical analysis.

12.2 Some Conceptual Clarifications

Let me begin with a few sketchy remarks on the two opposing sets of notions that were introduced above: 'receiving,' 'finding' and 'discovering' versus 'giving', 'constructing', and 'inventing'. Clearly, we cannot make too strong a distinction between these two sets, otherwise it must logically collapse. Even if 'meaning' is a matter of receiving, someone who is 'doing' the receiving, is still needed. The reverse is also true: even if meaning is a product, something that is made, we still need something it can be made of. We could not invent meaning from scratch even if we tried. The philosophical issue does not seem to lie in an either/or.[1]

To identify the philosophical issue let me attempt a clarification of the key notion of the meaning of life. What does it entail? There are many ways in which things can have meaning, but we may start by distinguishing between objects and projects on the one hand and words and phrases on the other. There are some poems that mean a lot to me, but were I invited to explain what that meaning is, I would not start with talking about the meanings of separate words and phrases. So, the meaning that these poems have for me cannot be reduced to the level of semantics. According to Vincent Brümmer, to say that a given object is meaningful to us, whether it is a person, a thing, or an experience of something, is to ascribe prescriptive properties to that object.[2] This indicates that in this usage 'meaning' is a relational term. To find 'meaning' is to be involved in something that is external to oneself.[3] Furthermore, to find meaning also signifies that the object is valuable. To say that opera means a lot to me is to indicate a particular attitude, a sensibility that I have for this particular form of art. 'Meaning', in other words, is an axiological term. In ordinary life, many 'objects' are meaningful to us in this axiological and relational sense. Family dinner has a special meaning in many homes, because it is the only hour that the members of families meet together. To be absent one needs an excuse or at least an explanation. Our lives are filled with many such everyday experiences that are meaningful. But even if there are these many experiences we nevertheless can simultaneously experience a kind of emptiness, a void, a lack of direction. On the whole, the meaning of our lives escapes us at times.[4]

The explanation for this possibility is given with a further characteristic of meaning. Things have meaning because they are embedded in a larger whole. The family dinner has its specific meaning because of a complex structure of expectations, values, and institutional variables such as school and work, that inform the patterns of our family life. Meaning is not attached to isolated things but is conferred upon objects by the larger context within which they have their proper place or function.[5] Whether or not our daily experiences appear as meaningful depends on whether the larger contexts within which we have these daily experiences appear meaningful. These contexts operate as horizons against which our daily experiences fall into place. They create the possibility of experiencing meaning on lower 'levels'. For example, going to church is meaningful to me in the context of being a member of a religious community; being a member of such a community is meaningful to me in the context of what my religion teaches me about my place and task in the world. Similar things can be said about any of our daily activities. Teaching a course in philosophy is meaningful to me because training students to think critically about important questions is meaningful and this, in turn, is meaningful because I believe that the world will be a safer place if people use their intellectual capacities in a self-critical way. In this connection 'horizons', 'contexts', and 'levels' are designations that can refer to various things, not only intellectual frameworks but also social and cultural environments.[6]

This feature of contextuality explains why questions about meaning *in* our lives—the things we do, the people we meet—have a tendency to slide back to the question of the meaning *of* our lives. The big picture which holds everything together may itself become unclear. Fortunately, questions about the meaning 'of' are not constantly on our mind because questions about the meaning 'in' our lives do not constantly create problems. But occasionally they do come up. Occasionally the experience of embeddedness is missing, because the larger picture has been blurred or has collapsed. At such moments the meaning of life has turned into a problem. The question What is the point of my life? or What is it that makes my life worth living? makes us fall silent. We do not know for certain. Consequently, we find ourselves in doubt as to whether or not the things we value and to which we can relate in our daily lives are as important as we usually think they are.

To leave these conceptual remarks on the notion of the meaning of life at this point, 'meaning' as understood here is *axiological* in that it reflects the fact that the object in question evokes a positive attitude; it is *relational* in that it depends on the fact that we are moved by something external to ourselves, and it is *contextual* in that it is constituted by our experience of being embedded in, and part of, larger structures and frameworks.

These remarks help us understand more clearly the peculiar aspect of modern conceptions of giving meaning to our lives, which is the focus of this chapter. Characteristic of these conceptions, it seems, is that modern people consider themselves to be the author of their lives. The meaning of life is of their own making. Whatever meaning there is to be found, can only be found in the initiative of their own self-conscious and reflective activity. This belief renders the notion of 'discovering meaning' notoriously suspect in so far as it implies that meaning is part of the structure of reality, of how things really are. Many of our contemporaries do not accept that meaning is given with reality as such. That notion is what disturbs the modern mind more than anything else because it interferes with the modern belief in ontological freedom.[7] Human beings are self-projecting beings, it is believed, who have no fixed ends set before them. The ends that make our lives meaningful are chosen by ourselves. They are not given as inherent in some larger and ultimate, metaphysical structure, because such structures are also of our own making. This essentially constructivist view is characteristic of the modern view of humanity as being in control of its own destiny. Even when many of our contemporaries seem to have lost faith in the powers of humanity in this regard, that does not stop them from believing that at least individual human beings can choose who they want to be. Accordingly, on this view, my personal identity is a construct of which I myself am the constructor. Or, to switch to another metaphor, even if it is true that there are many actors on the stage of my life, I am nevertheless the director of the play. Thus the modern view denies that there is a reality 'out there' that somehow shows itself as 'meaningful.' It makes external reality appear a large screen on which our conceptions of meaning are projected and not a source where meaning can be discovered. Even when our contemporaries still use the language of 'finding', they understand this language in a constructivist way, i.e., as invention rather than discovery.

12.3 Bricoleurs Rather Than Engineers

The language of construction introduced above can be misleading, however. Construction is the business of engineers who build whatever it is they make—tools, machines, tunnels, bridges—literally from blueprints. But even engineers do not seem to have complete control over their constructive work, given the resistance of the material with which they work. Similarly, it is impossible for human beings to construct their own lives. What they can do, however, is to identify themselves with culturally given patterns of meanings, inscribe their lives into these patterns and live accordingly. In shaping our lives, we do not construct our own model. Instead we choose from a possible stock of meanings that our culture has attached to various ways of living one's life.

It seems more accurate, therefore, to switch to postmodernist language in order to understand how our identities are shaped. According to postmodernists, personal identity is not constructed like an engineering project but is assembled according to the model of the *bricoleur*, to use Claude Lévi-Strauss's famous expression. The *bricoleur* is not a constructor but a collector. He does not work from a blueprint, but sorts out whatever materials he is able to find and puts his objects together from bits and pieces.[8] In shaping our lives, according to postmodern thinking, we are engaged in *bricolage* in this way. We take apart, revise, weed out, and put together, using bits and pieces from the variety of cultural ideas that are available to us. Some of these materials are inherited from previous generations, some are reassembled and some are new.[9] On this view, developing one's identity is an ongoing process of restyling. People have their own languages, expressing their own histories and the histories of their cultures and subcultures, without there being a core of fixed meanings that is universally shared. The identity of postmodern individuals is characterized by a high degree of plasticity: it develops on the crossroads of constantly shifting interferences of various spheres and modes of thinking. Accordingly, our individual identity appears to be a mixed bag of many possible meanings from which we as agents are free to choose which is more central and more peripheral. Postmodern identity is the identity of 'nomadic subjects'.[10] This does not necessarily mean that the languages we use are our own invention, but it does mean that there is room for creative activity in putting together the bits and pieces of available languages in order to arrive at new metaphors that express our individuality. As Richard Rorty's 'poetic' criticism of traditional philosophy indicates, we express our own meanings on the plane of language by stamping our mark on the languages available.[11]

If we accept this postmodern account of how we can live meaningful lives, the conclusion appears to be this. The notion of giving meaning to one's life is not so much a matter of invention and construction as it is a matter of creative reassembling. A meaningful life is not a creation in the sense of a *creatio ex nihilo*, but a creation from available fragments of 'meaning' that our culture has on offer. Since our imagination is informed by current linguistic resources we cannot want just anything, but we can choose and use these resources creatively. As this account shows, however, there is a strong continuity between modernism and postmodernism in this respect. The continuity exists in their joint rejection of external reality as a source of meaning mediated by ideas representing how things really are.[12] In other words; meaning is an expression of the self rather than an impression that the world makes upon the self. Or, better, since on the postmodernist view the self is not something 'beyond' its own expressions, the meaning we find in our lives is the manifestation of what we came to see as possible and important.

12.4 Culture as a 'Context of Choice'

This account can find further support by looking at how our moral culture—both from the perspectives of modernity and postmodernity—appears as a *context of choice*. This characterization of culture forges a connection between modernity, postmodernity, and liberalism. Contemporary liberalism is often accused of lacking sufficient interest in the mediating functions of cultural traditions. However, many liberals deny this charge. As Will Kymlicka explains, liberals do not deny the value of being rooted in a particular cultural tradition, but they make the value of what is received from this tradition dependent on individual judgment and choice. Culture provides us with options and examples from which we can choose. Thus John Rawls, for example, argues that we do not decide our 'rational plan of life' *de novo* but we examine the models set before us by those who have preceded us.[13] Crucially important to liberals, however, is that the cultural narratives which our culture provides do not have authority above our own judgments of their value.[14] As Kymlicka puts it: "we decide how to lead our lives by situating ourselves in these narratives."[15] In shaping our lives we adopt beliefs and values available to the community into which we grow, but these values and beliefs are subject to possible revision or rejection.[16] If at one time we made choices about what is valuable given our commitment to a particular way of life, we can later come to question that commitment. According to Kymlicka: "Beliefs give meaning to our lives, they make sense of why we do what we do. But we may be wrong in these beliefs. We may come to question the value or worth of many of the things we do, from going to church to writing novels. These beliefs underlie the most important decisions we make in life, and we care whether these beliefs are true or false," (*Liberalism, Community and Culture*, 163–64).

The possibility of revising and rejecting our previous views and commitments is thus required by the fact that we want our beliefs and values to be grounded in truth. The important question, however, is how liberals think that the revision of our values and beliefs is brought about. The answer seems to be that in order to reexamine the values and beliefs transmitted to us through cultural narratives, we need to detach ourselves from these narratives. In other words, a worthwhile life is a reexamined life and a reexamined life requires a form of personal detachment. This explains why liberals insist on the so-called exit option for individuals to move freely in and out of whatever cultural environment is available to them. As free individuals we can decide with whom to socialize, which books to read, which places to visit, which group to leave, and which to join. Consequently we have a choice with regard to the patterns of meaning that enable us to associate or dissociate ourselves from cultural ideals. The right to exit manifests the predominantly critical stance of liberalism toward both tradition and culture. When Kymlicka insists on the revisability of our beliefs and values he insists not only on our freedom to make revisions but also on our *duty* to do so: "We can and *should* acquire our tasks through freely made personal judgments about the cultural structure, the matrix of understandings and alternatives passed down to us by previous generations, which offers us possibilities we can either affirm or reject" (*Liberalism, Community and Culture*, 50–51, italics added).

Truth can be found only by adopting a perspective from outside, from where the value of what tradition passes on is judged. The important thing to notice here is that in this view our cultural resources are understood as options. At any time we may put the models and ideals our culture has in store on display before us and then decide to reject or affirm them on the basis of personal judgments uncoerced by institutions or other people. It is against this conception of culture as a context of choice that I want to raise a philosophical objection.

12.5 The Redundancy of Choice

The objection is that the belief that the meaning of life is of our own choosing is incoherent. Both the experience of meaning and meaninglessness are largely beyond our own control. Whenever we find ourselves asking questions about the meaning of our lives, we cannot attempt to fill the void by our own self-conscious activity. Meaninglessness is, in a sense, like sleeplessness: the harder one tries to overcome it, the more manifest it becomes. The act of finding, in this connection, is an unreflective one.[17] It succeeds to the extent that the agent has already identified with certain meanings that she found attractive before she chose them.[18] To explain, let me focus once more upon the opposition between giving versus receiving meaning and related oppositions such as between creating and discovering. I have already indicated that the language of finding can be used in all these oppositions but in different ways. On the one hand, finding indicates receptivity, a sense of openness to the world that reveals itself. On the other hand, however, it indicates creative activity in which finding comes close to inventing. This distinction should not be taken as a radical gap but as a matter of perspective where the difference is between what comes first and what follows, or, better, between initiative and response.

Now the question is: Why would the view that finding is our own creative activity be mistaken? Why should my life be subject to receiving or discovering rather than giving or creating meaning? Why should it be mistaken to think, for example, that I give meaning to my life by devoting it to the art of music, supposing that this is what I care about the most? The answer must be that this way of putting the question makes the very act of giving meaning self-contradictory. If the art of music is what I care about mostly, this is not because I chose it for that purpose. I could never choose a life devoted to music or anything else as a way of giving meaning to my life. Meaning cannot be extracted from objects that our will deliberately presents to itself as options among which we can choose. If meaning is not found *in* what we do—singing, reading poetry, gambling, saying our prayers, playing football, whatever—we will not find it by deliberately choosing to do these things either. Music fascinates me, captures my imagination, kindles my passion—these are all experiences that happen to me rather than experiences that I *make* happen. Meaning is not something that we can make or produce. I cannot deliberately choose to find meaning in my life by devoting it to the art of music, because I cannot deliberately choose to be fascinated or excited or to become passionate about such a life. I cannot even choose to see the point of such a life, if there is one. To think that I can produce meaning by making music the cause of my life is to put the cart before the horse. Finding meaning as activity is a way of responding to what has already been found. Something 'discloses', 'presents', reveals', or 'shows' itself to us as meaningful. These terms suggest that the quest for meaning will fail if the objects examined are approached as the 'raw material' of a world that carries no meaning in itself. 'Meaning' demands that we open ourselves to being engaged by the world as it presents itself. This aspect of disclosure also explains why we are vulnerable in these kinds of engagements. In order to find meaning we have to open up and allow ourselves to be moved, to be excited, to be thrilled. The experience of meaning is therefore characterizied by vulnerability.[19] 'Meaning found' can wither away and disappear, thus becoming 'meaning lost'. That is why we cannot find meaning unless we are prepared to be hurt, to be disappointed and disillusioned. The vulnerability of meaning has as its counterpart that we cannot avoid exposing ourselves to the possibility of suffering. We cannot avoid, that is, facing our own vulnerability in the quest for meaning.

Where does this alternative account leave us with regard to the gap between what we can find or receive and what we can give or make? It seems to me that the answer is something like the following. In being attracted to a life devoted to music, I can choose to answer the call, but I can also refuse to answer it. In either case the call precedes the response, but it is only with the response that my activity comes into play. The possibility of 'finding' in this example is dependent on being involved in the practice of loving music. Such practices produce what MacIntyre has called 'internal goods'.[20] These are goods that cannot be obtained other than by engaging in a specific activity and submitting oneself to the standards of excellence that govern it. To love music and to do it well requires skills that must be learned. The better one learns them, the more rewarding one's engagement in a given practice becomes. Thus practice mediates the possibility of being attracted by whatever it is that attracts. In other words, being attracted, excited, captured, moved—all of these notions signify meaning found in the experience of being engaged in a specific practice. Acting upon the standards of this practice signifies the other side, that is, meaning found as a response. My desire to achieve a particular goal is already a response to the attraction by the internal object of that goal, which impresses me and in which I want to take part in one way or another. Reflective activity is preceded here by passive receptivity. Without a doubt, something like finding meaning as self-conscious, reflective activity occurs, but it occurs in the activity of responding.[21] This activity is secondary to the experience which is prior to it, namely the impression that a given object makes upon me.[22] The point is not to claim a strong discontinuity between activity and passivity but rather to suggest that in experiencing meaning the latter necessarily precedes the former.

On this view, we can now raise some questions regarding Will Kymlicka's account of culture as a context of choice. For example, Kymlicka claims that people decide how to lead their lives by "situating themselves in cultural narratives." But is it true that we situate ourselves in these narratives—as if it could be our choice which narrative we will be part of—or is it rather that we find ourselves embedded in particular narratives? Kymlicka also argues that we can re-examine our commitments and acquire different motivations from the ones we had before. Surely we can do such things, just as we can question the desirability of our desires. But the point of doing these things is precisely that we have already come to regard our desires and motivations in a different light, which gives us reason to reflect. In other words, the fact of changing motivations signifies that we are already attracted by and responding to an alternative narrative. If so, what does the notion of choice or decision add to that change?

Furthermore, Kymlicka states that different motivations present us with reasons for choosing an option that is more valuable to us.[23] But how does this claim make sense? As Kymlicka explains: "Central to the liberal view is . . . that we understand ourselves to be prior to our ends, in the sense that no end or goal is exempt from possible re-examination. For re-examination to be reasonably conducted I must be able to envisage my self encumbered with different motivations than I now have in order that I have some reason to choose one over another as more valuable for me," (*Liberalism, Community and Culture*, 52–53).

Surely the idea that people choose their motivations is a curious one. However, leaving aside the psychology of that claim, the idea leads easily to an infinite regress. For the question is what motivates us to imagine certain motivations rather than others. Rather, is not the correct explanation that different motivations indicate a change that has already occurred, so that the notion of choosing is rather redundant in this context? At some point in my life I discovered the thrill of classical opera which then became my favorite genre in music. What does it add to say that once I made that discovery I *chose* to become an opera fan? Is it the fact of affirming this discovery that makes being an opera fan meaningful to me or do I affirm that meaning has already been found? Of course, we can revise our judgments and adopt different motivations but not because we choose to do so. As human beings we experience our lives such that at times we come to see things in a different light. But the reason has as much or as little to do with choice as switching one's taste from peanut butter to marmalade. It is simply that the light by which we are guided can change. Presumably, one could say that we choose at least whether or not we are going to expose ourselves to this new 'light': visit a different church, try another therapy, or try marmalade instead of peanut butter. Presumably one could also say that the point of exposing oneself to these things is nothing else than trying something new. But again, even then our choices are induced by what appears attractive to us to try.

The concept of culture as a context of choice, says Kymlicka, does not require liberals to deny that there is something given in the meaning of our lives. They maintain only that this something given is valuable because of our own judgment. However, this claim is mistaken for the same reason that radical constructivism is mistaken. It is not because of our judgment that something appears to be valuable but because our judgment is grounded in the fact that it so appears. Likewise, in revising our judgment, we attest that we have found a different meaning and not that we chose a different meaning. We did not even choose to find a different meaning. We simply found it. To paraphrase Heidegger, we did not choose to find this new meaning, but it found us.

12.6 Caring for the Disabled in Liberal Society

Given the modern view of 'meaning' as the object of choice and decision it is not surprising that the lives of profoundly disabled people appear to be meaningless in the eyes of those who are committed to this view. Against this kind of skepticism I want to raise a few points, however, drawing upon the foregoing analysis. The first point is that to be capable of experiencing a life shared with a disabled person as meaningful one has to care about that person. Without being personally involved, very little meaning can be found. Being engaged in their lives is where it all begins. Whatever meaning can be found will only be found in the context of that relationship.

Suppose I am friends with Jerry who is a profoundly disabled young man with the 'mental age' of a toddler. To say that Jerry means a lot to me is to say that there is something that attracts me not only to Jerry but also to his well-being. I could not leave him unhappy and remain unperturbed about it. I would lose something. In caring about him, I experience something that presents itself to me as meaningful, but this experience is not at my disposal. I cannot manipulate it. Taking Jerry out to the park, for example, is a meaningful activity because I know that he loves the sound of birds. I cannot make the sound of birds attractive to him nor can I make taking him out to the park meaningful to me. Meaning escapes control in the sense that it is essentially a by-product.[24] To find it we have to be engaged in doing something else and then receive it as a gift. I already referred to the analogy of intending to fall asleep, but there are many other examples of meaningful experiencing that cannot be the object of willful, intentional activity. Reporters of soccer games occasionally observe that a particular player is not "in the game," or that a team is "playing against themselves." Being in the game means losing oneself in it. Playing against oneself means trying so hard to play well that one's intention gets in the way of doing what one wants to do. Experiencing meaning seems to have a similar structure. Only to the extent that one is capable of opening up and losing oneself in an activity does the experience of fulfillment come, precisely because one's attention is directed otherwise. The skeptical view, in contrast, is a view that betrays the perspective of the outsider. The outsider is not involved. Oftentimes she does not want to become involved because she considers being consumed by disappointment and disillusion to be a waste of energy. The skeptical outsider is motivated by the desire to avoid vulnerability.

Second, the conception of 'meaning' as a matter of choice and decision has implicatons for how people think about the meaning of having children. It encourages them in thinking that having children can also be part of their plan of choosing a meaningful life. I can decide to have children in order to make them part of the life that I planned. No doubt that is a possibility, but it is not very likely that I am going to succeed. Children, whether handicapped or not, are not a means to a meaningful life. Not only because it is morally questionable to regard one's children as instrumental to one's happiness, but also because it is rather shortsighted. Parenthood is a bad idea for people who want to be in control of their own lives. The more we tend to regard children as instrumental to fulfilling our expectations in life, the greater the chance that we will fail. The reason is that parenting is one of those activities that can confer meaning upon our lives only if we give ourselves to that activity in a noninstrumental way. The reports of the parents portrayed in Kathryn Scorgie's study prove the point. Parenting a disabled child changed their view of life. It taught them to value each day, to celebrate life; it changed their view of success and taught them the wisdom of what is truly important in life. But these transformations only occurred after the moment of surrender in which they had no choice but to accept that their lives would never be what they originally planned them to be. Obviously, if we regard our children as a means to our own fulfillment, the presence of a mentally handicapped child is going to cause a great deal of stress and frustration, not only because the presence of such a child reduces our capacity to control our lives but (if we regard our children as a means to our own fulfillment) also because we are committed to a conception of a meaningful life that is inevitably going to make our disabled child look like a failure. According to Scorgie's study, one of the things the parents had to learn is to define meaning in terms that were very different from what these notions mean in liberal culture. The quality of their lives was more a matter of personal growth in respect of their character than in respect of status and success. One parent characterized this shift as changing from a perspective that was goal oriented to one that has an "attributional emphasis."[25] Meaning and success are connected to how lives are lived rather than to the states of affairs they produce. Were meaning to depend on the extent to which parents succeeded in realizing their original plan of life, their days would have been filled with the task of negative coping, which is the task that remains once one cannot do what one really wants to do. However strong and self-confident these parents may appear, their strength and self-confidence have been gained only on the condition of accepting vulnerability and the loss of self.

Thirdly, to find meaning in sharing one's life with a disabled child has not much to do with the self-gratifying activism that characterizes the contemporary role model of the achiever. Nor has it much to do with the self-regarding feeling good about yourself because of what you do for others. From the point of view of these contemporary role models, the lives of people like my friend Jerry cannot appear as anything but a burden that frustrates their parents goals. Consequently, the lives of those who care for such people look anything but great or attractive. What can one possibly get out of one's life by caring for someone who does not even know he exists? From the point of view of the skeptical outsider the lives of parents of disabled children are captivated by natural necessity. Their difficult task of parenting these children nullifies their options to lead an interesting, eventful life. It is time and energy consuming without much return.

Clearly, the skeptical outsider in liberal society is not going to deny people like Jerry's parents the option of caring for their child if that is what they prefer, but that is as far as the spectator's appreciation for the lives of people like Jerry goes. To put this in terms of the phenomenon of by-products; as long as the question of what I can get out of caring for someone like Jerry is in my mind, I will hold back rather than open myself to the experience of whatever can be found in spending my time with him. Whatever meaning is found, it will not be found unless I am motivated by different intentions in engaging in the activity of caring. For anyone who adopts the perspective of the outside spectator, the most likely conclusion will be that there is nothing to discover—not because the meaning sought is thoroughly subjective, but because it is grounded in involvement.

The main issue in both this chapter and the previous one has not been the question of what the lives of profoundly disabled people mean to themselves. As a matter of fact, the question of what the lives of such people mean to themselves is a potentially threatening one. The prevalent idea in contemporary culture that creating meaning is an individual activity has serious implications for human beings to whom the notion of agency does not apply. It is this very ideal that makes their lives appear to be deficient. Where there is no agent, there must be a deficit of meaning. Where there is a deficit of meaning, it is difficult not to perceive human existence as the cause of grave suffering. If it is merely a cause of great suffering, the question of why these people are kept alive becomes hard to avoid indeed. Not only is it hard to avoid, it also appears to have a definite answer. The centrality of agency and all that it stands for—'choice', 'decision', 'freedom', 'self-determination', and so on—is the default position of liberal culture. It makes us blind to other dimensions of our existence, such as our lack of control, our vulnerability, and our dependence on other people. For this very reason, it also makes accepting disabled people as human beings in their own right, without expecting them to meet contemporary standards of success, a difficult task indeed. Within liberal culture the question of whether profoundly disabled lives have meaning in themselves creates a vexing, almost paralyzing problem. What I have been trying to do in these chapters is to dislodge this problem—not by trying to solve it but by opening a different perspective that makes it look less important. Once the conceptual framework that generates the problem is displaced, there is no reason to think that the problem must be solved before one can meaningfully share one's life with someone like Jerry.

12.7 Conclusion

In this chapter I have discussed issues concerning our attitudes and beliefs about disabled lives, and have tried to think through their practical consequences on the level of our personal projects and commitments. In this concluding section I will try to connect these issues with the issue of genetic testing. Even though our society is willing to maintain its commitment to care for disabled people, it is certainly possible that the proliferation of genetic testing will undermine the strength of this commitment. Given the framework of moral convictions that dominate public morality in our society, which I dubbed 'the liberal convention', I do not think that liberal democracy is in a very strong position to do much for the disabled and their families in that case. Individual freedom and equality of opportunity will be used to break down cultural and institutional barriers for these people to participate in society. But at the same time these liberal values will effectively support the proliferation of genetic testing for reasons of prevention as a matter of reproductive freedom. That this development may have negative side effects, including the possibility of genetic discrimination, is a price that liberal democracy will most likely be ready to pay for that freedom. Consequently, much will depend on whether or not there will be sufficient people around who are committed to sustaining the lives of dependent others. As I have tried to argue, it takes particular beliefs and attitudes to shape the character of such people.

Contemporary role models and ideals make the lives of those who lack the capacity to choose look burdensome. There is no point in denying that it often is a burden, but it can be denied that it is only a burden that one rather would have removed from one's back. To appreciate this alternative view, it helps to think about the meaning of life as essentially a by-product, a freely received and gladly accepted gift. From the point of view of the skeptical spectator who considers caring for disabled people from the outside, none of my arguments may appear convincing because, unless one believes that there is something to be found in that kind of life, there is no reason to become involved in the first place.

On the view I have proposed in this inquiry, the presence of people who are willing to engage themselves in the practice of caring is crucial for liberal society. When people no longer want to get involved in the lives of dependent people, because these lives appear to be burdened with a deficit of meaning, this signifies a cultural rather than a political problem. The reason is that no public policy can resolve this problem unless it can tap cultural resources that motivate citizens to value the commitment that it requires. The role model of personal achievers that pervades contemporary culture is certainly not going to help, particularly not those for whom we call profoundly disabled. The lame can be trained to use a wheelchair, the deaf can be taught how to use sign language, the blind can learn to read their own alphabet, but people with profound mental disabilities can at most be taught to do things that each of us is hardly aware of doing, such as picking up a spoon, or opening one's mouth to take a bite. To the extent that our culture advertises the ideal of getting as much as possible out of our lives, the profoundly disabled look quite miserable indeed. Therefore, whenever people face the decision to share their lives with a disabled child and ask themselves whether this will frustrate their future plans, the answer to *that* question will most likely be in the affirmative, assuming that they never planned having such a child. As I have tried to argue, however, the question itself is open to criticism. To perceive the birth of any child, disabled or not, as instrumental to a meaningful life is unsound. This is true regardless of the fact that its eventual contribution to a rewarding life can, indeed should, be gladly accepted as a gift. The main argument presented in favour of this view has been philosophical, not moral. Caring for a sick friend may give me a sense of fulfillment, but the reverse is not true: I will not achieve a sense of fulfillment by deciding to care for somebody. For one thing, I may lack the character and skills required for such a task. Actually, the mistake is twofold. The first mistake is that the acceptance of caring responsibilities cannot be instrumentalized as a means to the end of personal fulfillment. The second mistake is that a rewarding life is not a matter of belief about future states of affairs. The reward is not grounded in *what* kind of lives we think we should live but in *how* we live our lives. It is not belief about states of affairs that matters. What matters is to be engaged. The decisive context is not belief but practice.

This is the last point I want to emphasize. Whatever meaning can be found in sharing one's life with another person, it cannot be known outside that activity itself. The experience of joy and fulfillment, despite hardships and difficulties, will often come as a surprise. Likewise, the loss of meaning in times of anxiety and grief will come as a shock. Both experiences testify to the same thing: both the gift of meaning and the loss of it happens to us. The harder we look for it, the harder it will be to find. Even when we use the practice of caring in our own plans of life, it will not likely be found.

What I have *not* been arguing in this inquiry, however, is that if people only would try harder, or if they would be more prepared to take on the burden of caring for a mentally disabled person, they would find personal fulfilment in their lives. Some do but others do not. The only thing one can say with certainty is that there is no other way of finding out than to expose oneself to the vulnerability of meaning and to accept the other as a fellow creature with whom one can share one's life and do the best one can.

Notes

1. Quoted from the foreword to *Playing God?: Genetic Determinism and Human Freedom,* by Ted Peters (New York: Routledge, 1997), ix–xi.

2. Cf. Hugo W. Moser, "Prevention of Mental Retardation (Genetics)," in Louis Rowitz, ed., *Mental Retardation in the Year 2000* (New York: Springer Verlag, 1992), 140–48. In this connection it may be argued that genetic testing is also used to serve purposes other than prevention. To give one example, the possibility of diagnosing fragile X syndrome has been used to identify the cause of disabilities in people whose condition previously remained unexplained (see L. B. A. de Vries, "The Fragile X Syndrome: Clinical, Genetic, and Large-scale Diagnostic Studies among Mentally Retarded Individuals" (Diss.: Erasmus University Rotterdam, 1997). The identification of their condition as 'fragile X' makes better care possible, in both medical and psychological respects, which can significantly enhance the quality of their lives. Consequently, there can be important goals for gene technology besides that of prevention, even from the perspective of the disabled.

3. The classical texts on normalization are B. Nirje, "The Principle of Normalization and Its Human Management Implications," in R. Kugel and W. Wolfensberger, *Changing Patterns in Residential Services for the Mentally Retarded* (Washington, D.C.: President's Committee on Mental Retardation, 1969); W. Wolfensberger, *The Principle of Normalization in Human Services* (Toronto: National Institute on Mental Retardation, 1972); W. Wolfensberger, "Social Role Valorisation: A Proposed New Term for the Principle of Normalization," *Mental Retardation* 21 (1983): 234–39. For recent 'updates' see H. Brown and H. Smith, eds., *Normalization: A Reader for the Nineties* (London: Tavistock and Routledge, 1989) and B. Perrin, *Beyond Normalization: Its Continuing Relevance for the 1990s—and Beyond* (Helsinki: IASSID 10th World Congress, 1996).

4. Cf. Paul R. Dokecki, "Ethics and Mental Retardation: Steps towards the Ethics of Community," in Louis Rowitz, ed., *Mental Retardation in the Year 2000* (New York: Springer Verlag, 1992), 39–51.

5. See J. Mansell and K. Eriksson, eds., *Deinstitutionalization and Community Living* (London: Chapman & Hall, 1996).

6. See World Health Organization, *International Classification of Impairments, Disabilities and Handicaps* (Geneva: WHO, 1980). See also United Nations, "Decade of

Disabled Persons 1983–1992," *World Programme of Action Concerning Disabled Persons* (New York: United Nations, 1983). In chapter 3 I will return to the issue of defining disability.

7. See Alexander Rosenberg, "The Political Philosophy of Biological Endowments: Some Considerations," in Ellen F. Paul et al., eds., *Equality of Opportunity* (Oxford: Basil Blackwell, 1987), 1–31, 7–17. Rosenberg has the following example to assess the value or disvalue of biological endowments: "In a population of Polynesians with no interest in coconuts, an agile tree climber will have no capital advantage. And in one in which all crave coconuts and can climb equally well, he will have no advantage either, though in both cases his biological endowment remains unaltered. . . . But things might be quite different. Suppose the coconut trees are too high for any method but climbing, and there is nothing to eat but coconuts. And suppose that time preference is quite high because, lacking coconuts today, the population will starve to death tomorrow. And suppose, finally, that everyone has acrophobia and only a handful have a talent for climbing. Here, the present value of the talent becomes extremely high" (15). Rosenberg concludes that "biological endowments are difficult to identify even biologically, and differences among them are distributed in ways that are difficult to summarize in terms of normality and abnormality. The role of environmental factors in the fixing of biological endowments is so great that to call such endowments hereditary may be seriously misleading." (16 f.). Although in making this comment Rosenberg does not seem to have genetic disorders in mind, his point is well taken and applies to these disorders as well. That is, the disorder of Down syndrome, for example, may be hereditary, but the disability resulting from it depends as much on socio-cultural responses. The best evidence for this claim I found in watching a tennis game between two people with that syndrome a few years ago. Given a different institutional setting—in this case the Special Olympics Tennis Championship—the game was every bit as much a match as the games played at the U.S. Open and the winner was no less of a champion than the winner of any 'grand slam' tournament.

8. Cf. Anita Silvers, "(In)equality, (Ab)normality, and the Americans with Disabilities Act," *The Journal of Medicine and Philosophy* 21 (1996): 209–24: "In speaking of the 'medical model', I refer to assumptions embedded deeply in current health care practice. I do not intend to stereotype all health care practitioners as accepting these assumptions. Nor do I contend that the relationships governed by these conceptions are injurious in every instance. Rather, my argument is that individuals with disabilities are confined to these relationships by the medical model" (222, n. 1).

9. The British Nuffic Council on Bioethics notices a similar inconsistency in the fact that on the one hand there is great effort to care for and integrate disabled people in our society and on the other hand huge resources are spent on preventing the birth of (severely) disabled people. Nuffic Council on Bioethics, *Genetic Screening: Ethical Issues* (London: Nuffic Council on Bioethics, 1993), 77.

10. Cf. Hauerwas: "Our humanism entails that we care for them [the mentally disabled] once they are among us, once we are stuck with them; but the same humanism cannot help but think that, all things considered, it would be better if they did not exist. As modern people we think we are meant to be autonomous beings. In view of such an overpowering presumption, how do we make sense of those among us whose very existence can be nothing but dependence? We live in cultures for which rationality and consciousness are taken to be

the very essence of what makes us human. What are we to make of those who will never, even with the best efforts, be able to read or write? Should they be considered human?" Stanley Hauerwas, *Sanctify Them in the Truth: Holiness Exemplified* (Nashville: Abingdon Press, 1998), 145.

11. ILSPMH, *Just Technology? From Principles to Practice in Bioethical Issues* (North York, Ont.: L'Institut Roeher, 1994), 11.

12. See Susan Wendell, "Toward a Feminist Theory of Disability," in Helen B. Holmes and Laura M. Purdy, eds., *Feminist Perspectives in Medical Ethics* (Bloomington: Indiana University Press, 1992), 63–81, 63. Wendell did a search in *The Philosopher's Index* in 1989.

13. See, for example, Neil A. Holtzman, "Genetic Screening: For Better or for Worse?" reprinted in Samuel Gorovitz, et al., eds., *Moral Problems in Medicine,* 2d ed. (Englewood Cliffs, N.J.: Prentice Hall, 1983), 375–77; Victor A. McKusick, "The Human Genome Project: Plans, Status and Applications in Biology and Medicine," in Tom L. Beauchamp and LeRoy Walters, eds., *Contemporary Issues in Bioethics,* 4th ed. (Belmont, Calif.: Wadsworth, 1994), 622–29, 628.

14. See for example Joan Retsinas, "The Impact of Prenatal Technology upon Attitudes toward Disabled Infants," *Research in the Sociology of Health Care* 9 (1991): 75–102; Kenneth D. Alpern, ed., *The Ethics of Reproductive Technology* (New York: Oxford University Press, 1992), which has a section called "Why Have Children?"; Deborah Kaplan, "Prenatal Screening and Its Impact on Persons with Disabilities," *Clinical Obstetrics and Gynaecology* 36 (1993): 605–12; Paul R. Billings et al., "Discrimination as a Consequence of Genetic Testing," in Beauchamp and Walters, *Contemporary Issues,* 637–43; Dorothy C. Wertz and John C. Fletcher, "A Critique of Some Feminist Challenges to Prenatal Diagnosis," in Françoise Baylis et al., eds., *Health Care Ethics in Canada* (Toronto, Montreal: Harcourt Brace, 1995), 385–403; Philip Kitcher, *Lives to Come: The Genetic Revolution and Human Possibilities* (London: Penguin Books, 1996); Peters, *Playing God?;* Ted Peters, ed., *Genetics: Issues of Social Justice* (Cleveland: Pilgrim Press, 1998).

15. Editorial, *Nature* 380 (1996): 89.

16. Lee M. Silver, *Remaking Eden: Cloning and Beyond in a Brave New World* (New York: Avon Books, 1997), 15.

17. Ibid., 10. Cf. also Arthur L. Caplan, "If Gene Therapy Is the Cure, What Is the Disease?" in George J. Annas and Sherman Elias, eds., *Gene Mapping: Using Law and Ethics as Guides* (New York: Oxford University Press, 1992), 128–41. Caplan writes with regard to scientists: "Those who are actually engaged in mapping and sequencing the human genome, or the genomes of other organisms, often do not have any particular practical goal or application motivating their work. Despite all the hand wringing that has accompanied the evolution of the Genome Project, and the promises of therapeutic benefits that it will produce, many of those involved are simply interested in understanding the composition of the genome, its infrastructure or anatomy. . . . If uncertainty about what to do with the new knowledge in the realm of genetics is a cause for concern in some quarters, then those who want to proceed quickly with mapping the genome might find it prudent to simply deny that any application of new knowledge in genetics is imminent or to promise to abstain from any controversial applications of this knowledge" (129 f.).

18. Robert Pritchard, "Public Participation in the Scientific Adventure," in Barry Holland and Charalambos Kyriacou, eds., *Genetics and Society* (Wokingham: Addison-Wesley, 1993), 1–11.

19. The same judgment is expressed by James Watson, who discovered the double helix structure of DNA together with Francis Crick: "So what is worse: not finding the gene or worrying about whether it will be misused? I think that by far the worst thing is not to find the gene. We should first find the gene, and then ensure that it will not be misused at the public level." James Watson, "The Human Genome Initiative," in Holland and Kyriacou, *Genetics*, 13–26, 25.

20. Holland and Kyriacou, *Genetics*, 9 f.

21. Accordingly, Pritchard accounts for moral decisions about the proper uses of genetics in terms of what 'providers' and their 'clients' may freely chose to decide. What remains outside this justification is a critical analysis of the value judgments on which their decisions are based. Moreover, no attention is paid to the fact that these judgments are mediated by socio-cultural patterns of meaning. The feminist literature on human genetics and reproduction has emphasized the political importance of this fact. For this literature see, for example, Christine Overall, ed., *The Future of Human Reproduction* (Toronto: The Women's Press, 1989) and Holmes and Purdy, *Feminist Perspectives*. For a defense of the position held by Pritchard see also Max Charlesworth's 'Millian view' of liberal society as the normative background of bioethical discourse in *Bioethics in a Liberal Society* (Cambridge: Cambridge University Press, 1993), 10–27, 16 ff.

22. See chapters 5 and 6.

23. Cf. Stanley Hauerwas, "Suffering the Retarded: Should We Prevent Retardation?" *Suffering Presence: Theological Reflections on Medicine, the Mentally Retarded, and the Church* (Notre Dame: University of Notre Dame Press, 1986), 159–81, 160. The project of widening the scope of the moral debate on medical technology by relating moral questions in health care to the task of living a morally worthy life is the subject of Gerald McKenny's outstanding book *To Relieve the Human Condition: Bioethics, Technology, and the Body* (Albany: State University of New York Press, 1997).

24. In this respect the growing influence of medical concerns in our lives and the subsequent rise of 'health promotion' can be argued to result in the paradox of health: the more people pay attention to their health status the less confidence they have in the solidity of their health. See Marcel Verwey, "Preventive Medicine—Between Obligation and Aspiration" (Diss., Utrecht University, 1998), 83–86, who concludes that "probably the best indicator of good health is being unaware of it," (85, n. 29).

25. McKenny signals the overall tendency in contemporary bioethics to restrict itself to the "narrowness of modern moral theories" and focus on issues of rights and duties in health care (*To Relieve the Human Condition*, 8, 20). He discusses three explanations of this phenomenon. The first is provided by the self-understanding of 'standard bioethics', which says that unprecedented moral issues have arisen with medical technology for which traditional medical and religious moral views cannot provide adequate solutions (11 f.). McKenny gives a couple of examples to suggest that this explanation is incorrect, because the issues are neither unprecedented nor have religious ethical systems failed to provide adequate solutions. The second explanation is provided by an analysis of "the crisis of moral authority" (referring

again to the breakdown of traditional medical and religious ethical systems). The author argues that this explanation is closer to the mark, but that it fails to detect a deeper cause. The claim of 'standard bioethicists' that the parochialism of these traditional ethical systems is superceded by common moral rationality drawing on secular reason is implausible given "the embarrassing fact that bioethicists do not agree on either the method or the substance of their allegedly common morality" (15). 'Standard bioethics' suffers from the crisis of moral authority just as badly as traditional ethical systems. This argument leads McKenny to propose a third explanation that says that 'standard bioethics' is deeply committed to the 'Baconian project'. This project is based upon the imperative to eliminate human suffering and to expand the realm of human choice by submitting 'nature' to human control by means of science and technology (25–38). Its commitment to the Baconian project shows that 'standard bioethics' is about neither new and unprecedented issues nor new forms of moral reasoning but about a new set of values, namely the values attached to the submission of the human body to the will of autonomous individuals: "From this follows the expectation that the expansion of the reign of technology over the body should be accompanied by, and in fact should make possible, the expansion of the reign of human choice over the body, and that medicine should enable and enhance whatever pattern of life one chooses" (20).

26. This commitment is clearly present in one of the early classics of the field by Joseph Fletcher, *Morals and Medicine* (Princeton: Princeton University Press, 1954); on the history of medical ethics in the early period see Leroy Walters, "Religion and the Renaissance of Medical Ethics in the United States: 1965–1975," in Earl A. Shelp, ed., *Theology and Bioethics: Exploring the Foundations and Frontiers* (Dordrecht/Boston: Reidel, 1985), 3–16.

27. See Susan Sherwin, "Feminist and Medical Ethics: Two Different Approaches to Contextual Ethics," in Holmes and Purdy, *Feminist Perspectives,* 17–31. Sherwin writes: "The institution of medicine is usually accepted as given in discussions on medical ethics, and debate has focused on certain practices within that structure: for example, truth-telling, obtaining consent, preserving confidentiality, the limits of paternalism, allocation of resources, dealing with incurable illness, and matters of reproduction. The effect is to provide an ethical legitimization of the institution overall, with acceptance of its general structures and patterns" (22 f.). McKenny also acknowledges the contribution of feminist authors in showing how the discourse and practices of modern medicine form us as subjects partly by shaping the understanding of our bodies (*To Relieve the Human Condition,* 198).

28. Put in this way the issue is a familiar one in feminist ethics, for example, with regard to the question of abortion and 'free choice'. See Holmes and Purdy, *Feminist Perspectives;* Susan Sherwin, *No Longer Patient: Feminist Ethics and Health Care* (Philadelphia: Temple University Press, 1992); Susan Wolf (ed.), *Feminism and Bioethics* (New York: Oxford University Press, 1996). See also McKenny, *To Relieve the Human Condition,* 184–210.

29. Cf. Robert M. Veatch, "Models for Ethical Medicine in a Revolutionary Age," in Daniel Callahan, *Ethical Issues in Professional Life* (New York: Oxford University Press, 1988), who writes: "Authority about what constitutes harm and what constitues good . . . cannot be vested in any one particular group of people [the medical profession]. To do so would be to make the error of generalizing expertise" (90). In one of his earlier essays, H. T. Engelhardt went even so far as to define health as "a state of freedom from the compulsion of psychological and physiological forces," from which he concluded that "while there are many diseases,

there is only one health—a regulative ideal of autonomy directing the physician to the patient as person, the sufferer of illness, and the reason for all the concern and activity." H.T. Engelhardt, "The Concepts of Health and Disease," in Arthur L. Caplan et al., eds., *Concepts of Health and Disease: Interdisciplinary Perspectives* (Reading, Mass.: Addison-Wesley, 1981), 31–45, 43. A more explicit commitment to what McKenny calles 'the Baconian project' than this is hardly possible.

30. The distinction—if not the terminology—goes back to an essay by P. F. Strawson, "Social Morality and Individual Ideal," in G. Wallace and A. D. M. Walker, eds., *The Definition of Morality* (London: Methuen, 1970), 98–118 (original publication in *Philosophy* in 1961).

31. Influential accounts of this view have been presened by G. J. Warnock, *The Object of Morality* (London: Methuen, 1971) and J. L. Mackie, *Ethics—Inventing Right and Wrong* (Harmondsworth: Penguin Books, 1977).

32. This characteristic is brought out nicely by a distinction found in Henry Sidgwick's *The Method of Ethics,* 6th ed. (London: Macmillan, 1901), 112, where he distuinguishes a 'morality of constraint' from a 'morality of direction'.

33. McKenny anticipates this suspicion by expecting 'standard bioethicists' to argue that the project of relating moral problems in health care to the task of living a morally worthy life cannot be universally binding and that in establishing autonomy as a core value, bioethics enables individual conceptions of morally worthy lives to flourish (*To Relieve the Human Condition,* 31). McKenny denies the second part of this claim—'standard bioethics' is incapable of addressing the issue of how the Baconian project shapes our understanding of our bodies as being the object of technological control such that we are more and more incapable of incorporating its mortality and finitude in our lives—but he accepts the first part. That is, he accepts that ways of conceiving the meaning and value of our health as integral to the meaning and value of our lives will fail to win general support, given moral diversity in our culture. In my view, however, this means that insofar as bioethics locates itself in the public domain, it will refuse to reconsider and widen the scope of its agenda by severing itself from the Baconian project. Although I take the present inquiry to be very close to McKenny's, I focus much more strongly than he does on the failure of 'standard bioethics' to account for our practices of health care strictly in terms of its narrow conceptions of public morality. Maybe he is right in pointing to the Baconion project as the real cause of the narrowness of contemporary bioethics. But it seems to me that the space for widening its scope is going to be mediated by an argument about its conception of public morality. This marks the difference between our respective strategies even though our inquiries aim at the same goal.

34. Let me repeat once more that what I say regards people with *mental* disabilities, even though in many instances one could argue that specific claims and arguments may also hold for disabled people in general.

35. See John N. Gray, "On the Contestability of Social and Political Concepts," *Political Theory* 7 (1977): 331–48, 332; by the same author, "Political Power, Social Theory and Essential Contestability," *British Journal of Political Science,* 1978: 385–402.

36. Cf. Nicholas Wolterstorff, "Audi on Religion, Politics, and Liberal Democracy," in Robert Audi and Nicholas Wolterstorff, *Religion in the Public Square: The Place of Religious Convictions in Political Debate* (Lanham, Md.: Rowman & Littlefield, 1997), 145–65, who de-

fines liberal democracy as incorporating 'the libertarian principle', 'the equalitarian principle', and 'the neutrality principle' (149). Although I am concerned here with liberal *morality*, Wolterstorff's account of liberal democracy pertains to what he and Audi call 'the ethic of the citizen' (148), implying that these three principles constitute the normative framework for public debate in liberal society.

37. Readers familiar with the recent debate on 'liberalism' will recognize that my account of liberal morality fits theories by liberal philosophers such as John Rawls (*A Theory of Justice* [Oxford: Oxford University Press, 1971] and *Political Liberalism* [New York: Columbia University Press, 1993]); Ronald Dworkin (*Taking Rights Seriously* [London: Duckworth, 1977] and *A Matter of Principle* [Cambridge, Mass.: Harvard University Press, 1985]); and Will Kymlicka (*Liberalism, Community and Culture* [Oxford: Clarendon Press, 1991]). To a lesser extent the same holds for the libertarian theory in Robert Nozick's *Anarchy, State and Utopia* (New York: Basic Books, 1970), while 'communitarian' theories of liberalism such as presented in Michael Walzer's *Spheres of Justice: A Defence of Pluralism and Equality* (Oxford: Blackwell, 1983) and William Galston's *Liberal Purposes* (Cambridge: Cambridge University Press, 1992), are harder to squeeze in. This is probably even more true of the perfectionist liberalism in Joseph Raz's *The Morality of Freedom* (Oxford: Clarendon Press, 1986).

38. The issue of inclusion will be discussed in chapter 7.

39. Hauerwas has persistently argued that liberalism relies on moral practices—and on the convictions and beliefs underlying these practices—that its own presuppositions cannot account for, and that at the same time, it undermines these very convictions and practices. See for example *Dispatches from the Front: Theological Engagements with the Secular* (Durham: Duke University Press, 1994), 190 f.

T W O   *The 'Liberal Convention'*

1. I use the term 'narrow' here in the same sense as was introduced in the previous chapter by reference to Strawson's distinction. See above, page 11.

2. Unlike, for example, the latest editions of the 'classic' of contemporary bioethical literature, Tom L. Beauchamp and James F. Childress *Principles of Biomedical Ethics*, which are flawed by the fact that the authors tend to answer critical responses by incorporating their critics' views in newly added chapters and sections of their text. As a matter of fact it is very well possible—and quite instructive—to read the subsequent editions of Beauchamp and Childress's book as a history of the field in the last twenty-five years. It provides an illuminating insight into the question of what happened to ethical theory in the attempt to apply it to contemporary moral issues.

3. I use the term 'convention' in a sense similar to how David Hume uses it. A convention reflects the ways in which the members of a particular society deal with one another. A moral convention reflects the moral practices and convictions that people within a particular society hold as binding upon the members of that society. See David Hume, *A Treatise of Human Nature*, 2d ed., trans. and ed. P. H. Nidditch (Oxford: Clarendon Press, 1978), 484–501.

4. In the next chapter I will return to the use of quantifiers such as 'some', 'many', and 'most of us' with regard to particular moral views held by people in our society. In using such

terms I do not suggest an empirical basis, but simply assume that the views indicated are held by a sufficiently large number of people in our society to make them interesting enough to be considered in this inquiry.

5. Isaiah Berlin, "Two Concepts of Liberty," in *Four Essays on Liberty* (Oxford: Oxford University Press, 1969), 118–72, 122 f.

6. Cf. Will Kymlicka, *Multicultural Citizenship: A Liberal Theory of Minority Rights* (Oxford: Clarendon Press, 1995), characterizes the morality of liberalism as based on two preconditions for the fulfillment of our interest in leading a good life: "The first is that we lead our life from the inside, in accordance with our beliefs about what gives value to life. Individuals must therefore have the resources and liberties needed to lead their lives in accordance with their beliefs about value. . . . The second precondition is that we be free to question those beliefs, to examine them in the light of whatever information and examples and arguments our culture can provide. Individuals must therefore have the conditions necessary to acquire an awareness of different views about the good life, and an ability to examine these views intelligently" (81).

7. This view is quite forcefully defended by John Harris, *The Value of Life: An Introduction to Medical Ethics* (London: Routledge & Kegan Paul, 1985).

8. In recent times 'age' and '(dis)ability' have been added to the list of characteristics that are to be exempted from the justifiable grounds for treating people differently. This fact raises the question of how the antidiscriminatory stance of the liberal convention with regard to the disabled relates to the issue of genetic discrimination. This question will be dealt with extensively in later chapters.

9. I take this to imply that the state should not favor any particular conception of the good and, in that sense, remain neutral between them. The point is impartiality, not separation. There is no need to take the neutrality principle in the stronger sense that the state should refrain from either not advancing or hindering any such conception. See on the distinction Wolterstorff, "Audi on Religion," 145–65, 149.

10. Cf. Thomas Nagel "Moral Conflict and Political Legitimacy," *Philosophy and Public Affairs* 16 (1987): 215–40, where he argues that accepting the framework of liberal thinking about public morality often means a setback for people arguing from particular philosophical or religious views: "Liberals ask of everyone a certain restraint in calling for the use of state power to further specific, controversial moral or religious conceptions—but the results of that constraint appear with suspicious frequency to favor precisely the controversial moral conceptions that liberals usually hold" (216).

11. Alasdair MacIntyre, "The Privatization of the Good: An Inaugural Lecture," *Review of Politics* 52, 3 (1990): 344–61.

12. On this connection, see for example Ronald Beiner, "Liberalism in the Cross-Hairs of Theory," in Ronald Beiner, ed., *Philosophy in a Time of Lost Spirit* (Toronto: University of Toronto Press, 1997), 3–17.

13. H. T. Engelhardt, *The Foundations of Bioethics,* 2d ed. (New York: Oxford University Press, 1996).

14. Engelhardt, *Foundations,* 3.

15. There are two main principles in Engelhardt's theory (*Foundations,* 102–34). Apart from the principle of permission it also includes the principle of beneficence, but this second

principle has no independent standing in his theory. In Engelhardt's version, the principle of beneficence *permits* people to attend to the interests of others to the effect that violation of this principle does not occur when someone fails to attend to such interests, but only when he or she fails to respect someone else's right to do so. There is then a clear conceptual priority to the first principle. See the introduction to *Reading Engelhardt: Essays on the Thought of H. Tristam Engelhardt, Jr.,* edited by Brendan P. Minogue et al. (Dordrecht: Kluwer Academic Publishers, 1997), 1–14, 3.

16. Engelhardt, *Foundations,* 7.

17. Engelhardt adds several qualifications to these distinctions to the effect that they should not be taken as absolute. Many people, if not all, live in various capacities as moral friends and as moral strangers. Besides, there are ways in which moral strangers can understand one another, but there are also ways in which moral friends can be divided (see *Foundations,* 80 f.).

18. Here and elsewhere we see that Engelhardt is committed to the modern view of regarding 'method' as the criterion for rational inquiry. At one point he claims that answers to moral questions are found if one knows how to resolve moral controversies. He then continues, "The procedures for answering a question disclose both the meaning of the question and the significance of its answer" (*Foundations,* 35).

19. Engelhardt, *Foundations,* 7.

20. The superiority of the sources of moral friends is clearly implied by the ostentatiously negative characterizations that Engelhardt gives of the moral predicament of secular society after the failure of the project of modernity. For example: "this volume offers secular means for coming to terms with the chaos and diversity of postmodernity. The means are meager and offer no transcendent fulfillment. But they are all that is available in general secular terms" and "the author recognizes in the landscape of secular bioethics a diversity that is often perverse, but which the secular state cannot find warrant to set aside. This volume does not celebrate the chaos, or even much of the diversity, and surely not the moral perversity and vacuity of this landscape" (*Foundations,* 10). The content-full morality of particular communities, in contrast, is what allows us to have "full meaning in life and concrete moral direction. It is within particular communities that one possesses a content-full bioethics" (74).

21. The adjective 'general' in phrases referring to secular morality—for example 'general secular moral reason'—is meant to allow the distinction between a content-full religious morality and a content-full nonreligious morality. This distinction makes it possible to characterize the morality of, say, egalitarian socialists as an example of a moral vision within a particular community, which should be distinguished from a general secular morality governing the public square.

22. The author hints at a difference between ethics and political theory in the context of secular society but does not explain what it might be: "This book provides not simply a political theory, but an account of the morality that should guide individuals when they meet as moral strangers to fashion health care policy" (*Foundations,* 11). Consequently, Engelhardt conceives bioethics as a theory about moral issues in health care that is restricted to the perspective of political morality. Very generally, this appears to be one of the main characteristic of contemporary bioethics—if not the main characteristic—that accounts for its oftentimes narrow focus.

23. Engelhardt, *Foundations*, 11. Cf. Rawls, *Political Liberalism*, 42 f., where he argues that a democratic society is not a community governed by a shared comprehensive religious or philosophical doctrine. If we overlook this limitation we fall prey to "a zeal for the whole truth" that "tempts us to a broader and deeper unity that cannot be justified by public reason."

24. Engelhardt, *Foundations*, 13.

25. I concur with James L. Nelson's interpretation, and to some extent with Stanley Hauerwas's and Cynthia Brincat's, each of whom reads Engelhardt's theory in the light of the attempt to control brute force by reason, which results in the notion of peace as the absence of war. See James L. Nelson, "Everything Includes Itself in Power: Power and Coherence in Engelhardt's *Foundations of Bioethics*," in Minogue et al., *Reading Engelhardt*, 15–29; Stanley Hauerwas, "Not All Peace Is Peace: Why Christians Cannot Make Peace with Engelhardt's Peace," in *Reading Engelhardt*, 31–44; Cynthia A. Brincat, "The Foundations of the *Foundations of Bioethics:* Engelhardt's Kantian Underpinnings," in *Reading Engelhardt*, 189–203.

26. See Mackie, *Ethics*, 106.

27. Protagoras holds that human beings are capable of surviving the scanty provisions of stepmotherly nature only because they possess the art of politics (*politike techne*). (*Protagoras*, 322b1–322c4; see also Mackie, *Ethics*, 108 f.).

28. Terence Irwin notes that Plato does not raise the question as to whether the teaching of the virtues that is advantageous for the individual agent is also conducive to the public good. At this point of the dialogue both Socrates and Protagoras assume that this is so. T. Irwin, *Plato's Ethics* (New York: Oxford University Press, 1995), 79 f.

29. Mackie uses the same distinction that I borrowed from Strawson (Mackie, *Ethics*, 106).

30. Engelhardt, *Foundations*, viii, 74, 78. The author argues that without content-full moralities secular morality would have no content (78) and attributes greater importance to the former ("Just as important, indeed more important than the morality of moral stangers, is that which can bind moral friends. This morality gives content" [103]). As we will see, however, the truth of the matter is that his *justification* of secular morality depends on certain elements of a content-full morality, namely one that has peaceableness as its core value.

31. The editors of *Reading Engelhardt* seem to have both readings in mind when they write: "The Kantian Engelhardt thinks that secular bioethics should establish a transcendental account of how free persons can derive rational (i.e., universalizable and impartial) justifications for specific moral rules involving individual liberty and the common good. But the skeptical Engelhardt argues that secular bioethics can establish few of the moral rules that might bind men and women in a common effort," whereby the 'common effort' refers to the establishment of social peace and order (Minogue et al., *Reading Engelhardt*, 2). On the Kantian reading of Engelhardt's theory, see in the same volume Brendan Minogue, "Engelhardt, Historicism and the Minimalist Paradox" (205–19) and the essay by Cynthia Brincat referred to above (note 25). She establishes the similarities between Kant and Engelhardt but only to explain what she takes to be a crucial difference (189), namely the fact that Kant aims beyond a 'civil commonwealth' (governed by the principle of right) at an 'ethical commonwealth' (governed by 'laws of virtue' that aim at a content-full morality), 197 f.

32. The following discussion is based on an analysis of two consecutive sections in Engelhardt's book: "The Way Out of Nihilism: How to Save the Moral Legitimacy of

Secular Bioethics" and "Moral Authority in Postmodernity: Legitimating Health Care Policy" (*Foundations,* 67–74); both of these sections are in my view crucial to Engelhardt's entire project.

33. See the earlier quote from Engelhardt's text: "If individuals are interested in resolving issues peaceably (i.e., without a basic reliance on force itself as authority), and even if the individuals do not hear God in the same way, and despite the fact that secular sound rational argument cannot establish a particular content-full moral vision, what is offered will still function to secure a general secular bioethics" (12).

34. Cf. *Foundations,* 69: "The appeal to permission as the source of authority involves no particular moral vision or understanding. *It gives no value to permission.* It simply recognizes that secular moral authority is the authority of permission" (italics added). The same argument appears in another passage: "The morality that binds moral strangers is contentless in being committed to no particular ranking of values, thin theory of the good, or vision of proper action. Because the morality of moral strangers derives the only comon secular moral authority from the agreement of those who collaborate, it does have content-full moral implications (e.g., one may not use competent individuals as living organ donors without their permission). But these implications follow from the centrality of this practice that can with general moral authority bind moral strangers in common endeavors: persons are to be used only with and through their permission. *It is not that this practice is good, worthwhile, or to be valued. Even peaceable action is not to be valued.* At least, no such judgment can be justified in general secular moral terms" (*Foundations,* 120 f.; italics added).

35. The distinction between the instrumentalist and the formalist option in Engelhardt's argument is suggested in Minogue's essay ("Engelhardt" 210 f.).

36. At this stage of Engelhardt's exposition the most important points appear in the notes where he deals with Kant (see nos. 81–87, 94–97). According to Engelhardt the very act of engaging in moral behavior—giving justified praise and blame—'creates' the reality of our moral world (note 82, 94 f.).

37. Engelhardt, *Foundations,* 97 (note 86). The passage referred to here reads: "Following Kant, I underscore the presupposition of respect of freedom as the necessary condition for the possibility of justified blame and praise. Justified blame and praise (e.g., blame and praise that is due to another, not just useful to assign) as well as acting with *moral* authority, presuppose grounds for showing some actions to be right or wrong. The minimum foundation for this moral nexus is provided by using persons only with their permission" (italics added).

38. Cf. James Nelson, "Everything," 23. I concur with Nelson's criticism of Engelhardt's transcendental deduction (21 ff). Nelson presses the question of what *moral* reasons I have to consider my agreement as binding upon myself. His conclusion is that Engelhardt's theory does not provide such a reason. Engelhardt's response in the same volume is that Nelson conflates justification and motivation, moral reasons with reasons to be moral (Engelhardt, "The Foundations of Bioethics and Secular Humanism: Why Is There No Canonical Moral Content?" in Minogue et al., *Reading Engelhardt,* 259–85, 264). This response is too easy, however, because Nelson's question—What moral reasons do I have to consider the agreements that I have entered upon as binding upon myself?—does require an answer. Since I am not supposed to share the moral value of peaceableness with the strangers with whom I

have reached an agreement, I do not seem to have moral reasons prior to the agreements themselves. However, the brute fact of these agreements per se cannot be sufficient to ground a moral reason, because nothing stops me from cheating or from cancelling the agreement at any time that I think fit. Unless Engelhardt shows why this would be morally wrong—independent from any assumption derived from particular moral visions—his theory falls short of what it seeks to establish. Moreover, the distinction between moral reasons and reasons to be moral collapses in many of Engelhardt's formulations, for example where he argues that the principle of permission "derives from this being a necessary condition for the possibility of a major endeavor of persons: a secular moral fabric that *can be justified to, and that can bind,* moral strangers" (*Foundations,* 70; italics added).

39. Engelhardt, *Foundations,* 97 (note 97).

40. At a later stage in his book, Engelhardt says, "The concrete fabric of morality must then [when shared moral premises are absent] be based on a will to a moral viewpoint, not on the deliverances of rational argument. The secular moral point of view in its most generally definable sense will be that intellectual standpoint from which one understands that conflicts regarding the propriety or impropriety of a particular action can be resolved intersubjectively by mutual agreement" (*Foundations,* 103 f.). This assertion again shows that Engelhardt's argument works for those who accept the moral viewpoint that defines morality as constituted by mutual agreement. His theory does not offer a foundation; at best it explains what many people in liberal society think about the public morality they share. That is to say, it is based on the liberal convention, e.g. something of the nature of what I sketched in the second section of this chapter.

41. For a powerful critique of consensus and agreement as the aim of procedural conceptions of morality, see N. Rescher, *Pluralism: Against the Demand of Consensus* (Oxford: Clarendon Press, 1993), 16–20, 55 ff.

42. Hauerwas reaches a similar conclusion in his essay ("Not All Peace," 41). Surprisingly, Engelhardt seems to concede that his conception of public morality can be assumed to work to the extent that it is operated by good people, that is to say, by people who are themselves motivated by interest in the good of others prior to any agreement. Having explained secular morality as a morality of restraint, he adds with regard to the practice of health care, "If one were to understand bioethics only in terms of these restraints, one would have forgotten why one had decided to engage in health care to begin with, namely, to achieve a set of important goods for patients and potential patients" (*Foundations,* 118).

43. A major achievement in this connection in the United States is the *Americans with Disabilities Act* (ADA), adopted by Congress in 1990.

THREE *Genetics and Prevention in Public Morality*

1. Cf. Julius Kovesi, *Moral Notions* (London: Routledge and Kegan Paul, 1967), 119: "Moral notions do not evaluate the world of description but describe the world of evaluation."

2. For the view that there are clear cases in which there is a duty to prevent disabled lives see, Laura M. Purdy, "Can Having Children Be Immoral?," in Gorovitz et al., *Moral Problems,* 377–84. See also D. W. Brock, "The Non-Identity Problem and Genetic Harms—

the Case of Wrongful Handicaps," *Bioethics* 9 (1995): 269–75; R. M. Green, "Parental Autonomy and the Obligation Not to Harm One's Child Genetically," *Journal of Law, Medicine and Ethics* 25 (1997): 5–15.

3. The so-called wrongful life cases could not have been taken to court unless there is a legally recognized principle that parents should refrain from harming their children even before birth. In the same connection one can also think of the fact that all liberal abortion laws have limited legal abortion to a certain point of time in gestation, indicating that free choice is limited even for abortion on demand.

4. See Verwey, "Preventive Medicine," 13 f.

5. Verwey's distinction between 'primary' and 'secondary' prevention is relevant in this connection: in the first there are no patients (yet) and the preventive measures are intended to preclude that there will be; in the second there is at least an early stage of the disease process in particular individuals who are already identified as patients (13).

6. When Verwey suggests as one of the moral criteria for preventive medicine that "preventive measures should focus on a contribution to a disability-free life expectancy," (38) this can be taken to refer to two different things in the context of our subject. It can refer to abortion as a measure of preventive medicine in the strict sense in which an early pathogenic stage of disease has been detected. But it can also refer to preventive medicine in a wider sense, in which measures are intended to enhance positive health promotion, for example the promotion of taking folic acid by pregnant women. I return to this distinction in chapter 5.

7. This view was defended at an early stage in the abortion debate by Daniel Callahan, *Abortion: Law, Choice and Morality* (London: Collier Macmillan, 1971); see also, among many others, Lewis W. Sumner, *Abortion and Moral Theory* (Princeton: Princeton University Press, 1981); Bonny Steinbock, *Life before Birth: The Moral and Legal Status of Embryos and Fetuses* (Oxford: Oxford University Press, 1992); and Ronald Dworkin, *Life's Dominion: An Argument about Abortion and Euthanasia* (London: Harper/Collins, 1993).

8. See the volume edited by Joel Feinberg, ed., *The Problem of Abortion* (Belmont: Wadsworth Publishing Company, 1984). According to Elizabeth Mensch and Alan Freeman, *The Politics of Virtue: Is Abortion Debatable?* (Durham: Duke University Press, 1993), 126 ff. the question of whether or not the fetus is a person gained considerable weight in the abortion debate due to the Supreme Court's decision in *Roe v. Wade*.

9. For a defense of this view see Sumner, *Abortion*, 126 f.

10. World Health Organization, *International Classification of Impairments, Disabilities, and Handicaps* (Geneva: WHO, 1980). See also United Nations, "Decade of Disabled Persons 1983–1992," in *World Programme of Action Concerning Disabled Persons* (New York: UN, 1983).

11. See James Trent, *Inventing the Feeble Mind: A History of Mental Retardation in The United States* (Berkeley: University of California Press, 1994). See also Joanna Ryan and Frank Thomas, *The Politics of Mental Handicap* (Harmondsworth: Penguin Books, 1980); R. C. Scheerenberger, *A History of Mental Retardation* (Baltimore: Brookes Publishing Company, 1983).

12. Recent versions of influential classification schemes of the American Association of Mental Retardation (AAMR) and American Psychiatric Association (APA) indicate similar concerns in defining mental handicaps as "subaverage intellectual functioning" and "deficits

in adaptive functioning" whereby the latter deficit may result from social systems that demand particular levels of adaptive functioning without sufficient accommodation for people incapable of attaining those levels. See R. Luckasson et al., *Mental Retardation: Definition, Classification and Systems of Supports* (Washington, D.C.: AAMR, 1992); American Psychiatric Association, *Diagnostic and Statistical Manual of Mental Disorders,* DSM-4, 4th ed. (Washington, D.C.: APA, 1994).

13. For a similar criticism see Wendell, "Toward a Feminist Theory," 65–81, 66.

14. For the distinction between disease and handicap, I found helpful Heinz Krebs, "Social Medicine and Social Ethics on Health and Disease of Persons with a Mental Handicap" in *Workshop Bioethics and Mental Handicap: Report on the European Workshop 6–8 November 1989* (Utrecht: Bishop Beckers Foundation, 1990), who argues that disease is "an exceptional case" with respect to health while handicap is "a special case" with respect to health (31). I will return to this distinction in the next section.

15. This does not rule out, of course, that many mentally disabled persons suffer from psychiatric conditions as well. See Antal Dosen and F. J. Menolascino, eds., *Depression in Mentally Retarded Children and Adults* (Leiden: Logon Publications, 1990).

16. At any rate, this is the dominant view of liberal bioethics. See, for 'classical' versions of this view, Michael Tooley, *Abortion and Infanticide* (London: Clarendon Press, 1983); Harris, *Value of Life;* Peter Singer and Helga Kuhse, *Should the Baby Live?: The Problem of Handicapped Infants* (Oxford: Oxford University Press, 1985); and Helga Kuhse, *The Sanctity of Life Doctrine: A Critique* (London: Clarendon Press, 1987). The designation 'liberal bioethics' is appropriate in this connection in the sense that the conception of the person found in the work of these authors is equivalent to the conception of the person as it appears in theories of political liberalism, such as Rawls's, and in Engelhardt's theory of bioethics in liberal society. A characteristic of these theories is that they subordinate ethics to the political philosophy of liberalism. See in the present inquiry also chapters 2 and 8. For a general, sympathetic account see Charlesworth, *Bioethics,* 10–27. Bioethical discussions, according to Charlesworth, should be much more sensitive to the context of liberal society: "some of the stances adopted, especially in the field of the ethics of assisted procreation and reproductive technology, the ethics of death and dying, and the ethics of health resource allocation are so authoritarian and paternalistic that one wonders if their supporters realize that they are supposed to be living in a liberal democratic society. It is the contention of this book that those engaged in bioethical discussion must become aware of the fact that they are living in a liberal society and take account of its basic values" (27).

17. I follow here Steven D. Edwards in his criticism of Nordenfelt's theory of health, according to which the concept of disability is central to the concept of illness (L. Nordenfelt, *On the Nature of Health* [Dordrecht: Kluwer, 1995], 36). Against this view Edwards claims: "A serious difficulty with this view stems from the intuition that a person can have a disability but not be ill. Hence, whilst disability may be a necessary condition of illness, this intuition suggests that it is not a sufficient condition, and hence that disability and illness are separable" ("Nordenfelt's Theory of Disability," *Theoretical Medicine and Bioethics* 19 [1998]: 89–100, 94). Edwards continues to argue that Nordenfelt's view betrays the view that is known as 'the medicalization of disability'. The separability of 'disability' and 'illness' is crucial to the general strategy followed by the argument in the present inquiry.

18. Cf. Christopher Boorse, "On the Distinction between Disease and Illness," in Caplan et al., *Concepts of Health,* 545–60. Boorse links the notions of disease and illness to theoretical and practical senses of health. Disease is a theoretical concept that applies indifferently to organisms of all species, according to the author, while illness constitutes a subclass of disease that requires medical intervention because of its incapacitating effects. This distinction explains why plants can have diseases but they they are not said to be 'ill' (550). Albert Jonsen has a characterization of the famous British physician Thomas Sydenham, "the English Hippocrates," which he found in Henry Sigerest, *The Great Doctors* (New York: Dover Publications, 1933), that illustrates the distinction quite neatly. Sigerest points out the difference between the empiricist Sydenham and Hippocrates by noticing that "Hippocrates recognized only illness, not diseases. He knew only sick individuals, only cases of illness. The patient and his malady were for him inseparably connected as a unique happening, one which would never recur. But what Sydenham saw above all in the patient was the typical, pathological process which he had observed in others before and expected to see in others again" (Albert R. Jonsen, *The New Medicine and the Old Ethics* [Cambridge: Harvard University Press, 1990], 84 f.).

19. Klinefelter's syndrome produces boys with at least one extra 'female' chromosome that causes underdeveloped male attributes (sparse body hair and beard growth, small genitals, extremely low sperm production) and overdeveloped female attributes (developing breasts). Although there are mental problems such as insecurity and shyness, the intellectual performance of boys with this syndrome is 10–15 percent below that of their normal siblings, but they will develop quite normally when adequately treated with testosterone. They have jobs, marry, and, though exceptional, have families. See K. Sorensen, *Klinefelter's Syndrome in Childhood, Adolescence and Youth: A Genital, Clinical, Developmental, Psychiatric and Psychological Study* (Chippenham: Parthenon Publishing, 1987).

20. On the distinction between 'normativists' and 'non-normativists' with respect to the concept of disease, see Caplan, "Gene Therapy," 128–41, 132 ff. The issue between these positions is whether disease is necessarily a value-laden concept, as normativists argue. Their argument is that an exceptional or abnormal condition of the body is only classified as a disease because it is disvalued. Caplan argues sensibly for a middle ground between both positions by showing that 'abnormality' and 'disvalue' are not coextensive. Being a seven-footer and having exceptionally large feet is surely abnormal but it need not be disvalued, for example if one wants to be a professional basketball player. Analogously, every human being may at times suffer from headaches which makes headache a universal condition. But this does not mean that it is not disvalued even though is it quite normal that most people occasionally suffer from it.

21. The relevance of this distinction and how it might shape different moral perspectives on the prevention of disability is the subject of a lengthy discussion in chapter 10.

22. One of the recurring features that Engelhardt mentions in connection with his conception of secular morality is that it entails the possiblity of 'a right to do wrong'. This phrase combines the two respective judgments: from the point of view of public morality we can defend a right to perform certain acts, while we may be appalled from the point of view of our own 'content-full' morality when people actually perform such acts (see, for example, *Foundations of Bioethics,* 78, 84). See also Nagel, "Moral Conflict," 215–40.

23. This is the argument made by Wertz and Fletcher, "Critique of Some Feminist Challenges," 385–403.

24. See C. H. Krishef, "State Laws on Marriage and Sterilization," *Mental Retardation* 10 (1972): 36–38; R. P. Petchesky, "Reproduction, Ethics and Public Policy: The Federal Sterilization Regulation," *The Hastings Center Report* 9 (1979): 29–41; A. Grubb and D. Pearl, "Sterilization and the Courts," *Cambridge Law Journal* 46 (1987): 439–64; R. Gillon, "On Sterilizing Severely Mentally Handicapped People," *Journal of Medical Ethics* 13 (1987): 59–61; Philip J. Reilly, *The Surgical Solution: A History of Involuntary Sterilization in the United States* (Baltimore: John Hopkins University Press, 1991); J. Smith et al., "Institutionalization, Involuntary Sterilization, and Mental Retardation: Profiles from the History of the Practice," *Mental Retardation* 31 (1993): 208–14.

25. Cf. J. A. Robinson, "The Potential Impact of the Human Genome Project on Procreative Liberty," in Annas and Elias, *Gene Mapping*, 215–25: "While some restrictions based on age and marital status, and to a much lesser degree mental competence, exist, it is fair to say that married couples have a fundamental right to reproduce by coital means. That is, the state would have to demonstrate a compelling need and the absence of less restrictive alternatives to limit the number, the timing, or the fact of coital reproduction" (215).

FOUR *"The Condition, Not the Person"*

1. See for example Richard West, "Ethical Aspects of Genetic Disease and Genetic Counseling," *Journal of Medical Ethics* 14 (1988): 194–97: "The aim of genetic counseling is to inform the patient or patients of the risks of genetic disease occurring in their offspring or those of other family members, and to advise them of the options for reducing that risk. This should have the effect of reducing the number of individuals being born with severe handicapping conditions of genetic origin" (195).

2. See International League of Societes for Persons with Mental Handicaps (ILSPMH), *Just Technology?: From Principles to Practice in Bio-Ethical Issues* (North York, Ontario: L'Institut Roeher, 1994).

3. See for example Adrienne Asch, "Reproductive Technology and Disability," in S. Cohen and N. Taub, eds., *Reproductive Laws for the 1990s* (Clifton: Humana Press, 1989), 69–127.

4. ILSPMH, *Just Technology?*, 9–22.

5. For a justification of clinical genetics in terms of individual choice see, for example, Ruth Macklin, "Moral Issues in Human Genetics: Counseling or Control?" in Gorovitz et al., *Moral Problems*, 364–75; also Eike H. Kluge, "Genetic and Pre-Natal Screening," in *Biomedical Ethics in a Canadian Context* (Scarborough: Prentice Hall, 1992), 330–52. A survey of recent reports by standing committees on bioethical issues in Britain, Denmark, and the Netherlands indicates that there is a marked shift in the aims of genetic screening and counseling from preventing and alleviating disease to the aim of offering individual options (Roger Hoedemaekers et al., "Genetic Screening: A Comparative Analysis of Three Recent Reports," *Journal of Medical Ethics* 23 (1997): 135–41, 135).

6. Cf. Singer and Kuhse, *Should the Baby Live?*

7. The more recent literature is covered in a review essay by Wertz and Fletcher ("Critique of Some Feminist Challenges," 385–403, 396 f.). The authors argue in particular that feminist worries about women's choice are unfounded and that discouraging women from having prenatal diagnosis will not likely benefit disabled people. On the other hand, they recognize some 'legitimate fears' regarding the attitudes towards disabilities in connection with rationing of health care budgets.

8. See chapter 1, page 8.

9. Cf. Engelhardt, *Foundations*, 197: "To see a phenomenon as a disease, deformity, or disability is to see something wrong with it. Diseases, illnesses, and disfigurements are experienced as failures to achieve an expected state, a state held to be proper to the person afflicted. This may be a failure to achieve an expected level of freedom from pain or anxiety. It may involve a failure to achieve an expected realization of human form or grace. Or it may involve a failure to achieve what is an expected span of life. These genres of judgments characterize a circumstance as one of suffering, one of pathology, one of a problem to be solved."

10. Kluge, *Biomedical Ethics,* 341.

11. Let me repeat a point made in chapter 1. Clinical genetics is only partly engaged in the practice of prevention: it also uses genetic information to discover risks, to explain patterns of hereditary disease, to diagnose existing people—including disabled people—so that the quality of their lives can be enhanced. I am not assuming, therefore, that clinical genetics as such is committed to the practice of prevention, even though its tools and techniques can be used for that purpose. I will return to this point in the last section below.

12. See chapter 3.

13. Genetic diseases of the first class are, for example, Tay Sachs syndrome, Lesch Nyhan disease, Duchenne's muscular dystrophy, cystic fibrosis, and Huntington's chorea; genetic diseases of the second class are, for example, Klinefelter's syndrome, retinitis pigmentosa, hemophilia, Down syndrome, and the milder cases of fragile X and spina bifida.

14. Cf. T. S. Spradley and J. P. Spradley, *Deaf Like Me* (Washington: Gallaudet University Press, 1995).

15. Consider the report by Walter E. Nance, a clinical geneticist who, in counseling a couple about the heredity of their deafness, discovered that he saw their condition quite differently from the way this couple did: "I suddenly realized how insensitive I had been and how value laden the words I had used were: words like 'defect', 'abnormality', 'affected', 'malformation', or 'recurrence risk' instead of more neutral terms such as 'trait', or 'deafness', or 'chance' instead of 'risk'." As he discovered that the value the couple attached to their culture developed through signing, Nance realized: "Is it any wonder that they view their deafness as a defining cultural characteristic rather than a handicap? The couple I was counseling came to the clinic not because of any concern they had about having a deaf child but rather because of their interest in learning about the cause of their own deafness" (quoted in Ronald Cole-Turner and Brent Waters, *Pastoral Genetics: Theology and Care at the Beginning of Life* (Cleveland: Pilgrim Press, 1996), 52.

16. This argument is made by Terrence R. Dolan and Alan Buchanan, "Gene Therapy: Promises and Concerns," *Japanese Journal of Developmental Disabilities* 17 (1996): 243–60. According to the authors, the view that the genetics approach entails a devaluation of persons

with disabilities is a "central tenet" of disabilities advocates. They claim that this view requires "the complete unification of the person and the disability into a single entity and fails to recognize the value of the individual independent of the compromising condition associated with the disability."

17. "We can care for the cancer patients by trying to alleviate their cancer without destroying the patient, but you cannot eliminate retardation without destroying the person who is retarded" (Hauerwas, *Dispatches from the Front*, 164).

18. Cf. M. V. Gibbs and J. G. Thorpe, "Personality Stereotype of Noninstitutionalized Down Syndrome Children," *American Journal of Mental Deficiency* 87 (1983): 601–5; J. G. Wishart and F. H. Johnston, "The Effects of Experience on Attribution of a Stereotyped Personality to Children with Down Syndrome: A Comparative Study," *Journal of Mental Deficiency Research* 34 (1990): 409–20.

19. I borrow this phrase from Will Kymlicka, "Liberalism and Communitarianism," *Canadian Journal of Philosophy* 18 (1988): 181–203, 183.

20. Cf. R. M. Hare, *Moral Thinking: Its Levels, Method, and Point* (Oxford: Oxford University Press, 1981), 101–6. Hare distinguishes between 'now-for-now' preferences, 'now-for-then' preferences and 'then-for-then' preferences. The question raised in the present context regards the former two: I judge my life from a first-person point of view with respect to the question of how I value the life I now have and with respect to the question how I will value my life in the future. At a later stage of this inquiry I will move to the third category of 'then-for-then' preferences when we discuss the possibility that if we knew now what (most) parents of disabled children know, i.e., that parenting such a child can be a rewarding experience, we might conclude that at *that* time we might come to think differently about issues regarding the prevention of disabled lives by means of genetic testing (see chapter 11).

21. Symptoms of fragile X syndrome include mental impairment, ranging from learning disabilities to mental retardation; attention deficit and hyperactivity; autistic behaviours; long face, large ears, and hyperextensible joints, especially fingers. See Kenneth L. Jones, *Smith's Recognizable Patterns of Human Malformation*, 4th ed. (Philadelphia: W. B. Sounders, 1988), 126.

22. Quoted from Leon R. Kass, "Implications of Prenatal Diagnosis for the Human Right to Life," in Thomas A. Mappes and Jane S. Zembaty, *Biomedical Ethics*, 3d ed. (New York: McGraw-Hill, 1991), 495–507, 501.

23. I follow here an argument developed by Steven D. Edwards in his essay "The Moral Status of Intellectually Disabled Individuals," *Journal of Medicine and Philosophy* 22 (1997): 29–42, who argues for the view that "disabilities are not detachable from selves" (40).

24. Much later in this inquiry we will explore the possible meaning of this statement; see chapters 10 and 11. The objection that this statement betrays extreme selfishness on the part of parents, suggesting that one can find virtue in 'enduring' a disabled child, will be addressed in chapters 11 and 12. To anticipate the answer, 'meaning' and 'grace' in parenting a disabled child can be received as a free and unsolicited by-product of sharing one's life with a disabled child, but 'enduring' such a child cannot be instrumental to that objective. In other words, although there can be 'nobility' in overcoming adversity (Christopher Lasch, "Engineering the Good Life: The Search for Perfection," *This World* 26 (1989), 9, quoted in Cole-Turner and Waters, *Pastoral Genetics*, 147, note 5), there is certainly no nobility in seek-

ing adversity suffered by others to become virtuous. I owe Henry Jansen for pressing this point.

25. In reflecting on Michael Berube's *Life As We Know It: A Father, a Family, and an Exceptional Child* (New York: Pantheon Books, 1996), Hauerwas notes: "With great candor Berube tells us that he and his wife are as pro-choice after the birth of Jamie [born with Down syndrome] as they were prior to his birth. Indeed, he notes that they intentionally did not use amniocentesis, assuming they would 'just love the baby all the more' if the baby was born with Down's syndrome. Berube confesses such a stance was 'blithe and uninformed' and that if they had known that their child's life 'would be suffering and misery for all concerned' they might have chosen to have an abortion. Berube notes, however, that it is extremely difficult to discuss Jamie in this way. Just as it was hard to talk about him as a medicalized being when he was at the ICU, it is still harder 'to talk about him in terms of our philosophical beliefs about abortion and prenatal testing. That's partly because these issues are so famously divisive and emotionally charged, but it's also because we can no longer frame any such questions about our child now that he is there.'" (Hauerwas, *Sanctify Them*, 143–56, 146).

26. This, it seems to me, is the point of Hauerwas's remark on Michael Berube's confession in the previous note.

27. See A. Lippmann, "Prenatal Genetic Testing and Screening: Constructing Needs and Reinforcing Inequities," *American Journal of Law and Medicine* 17 (1991): 15–50. Also Ted Peters, "Genes, Theology, and Social Ethics: Are We Playing God?," in Peters, *Genetics*, 1–45, 15–20.

28. Robert N. Proctor, "Genomics and Eugenics: How Fair Is the Comparison?" in Annas and Elias, *Gene Mapping*, 57–93, 76; also Evelyne Shuster, "Determinism and Reductionism: A Greater Threat Because of the Human Genome Project?" in Annas and Elias, *Gene Mapping*, 115–27.

29. Cf. the comments by the National Bioethics Advisory Commission in its report "The Science and Application of Cloning": "As social and biological beings we are creatures of our biological, physical, social, political, historical, and psychological environments. Indeed, the great lesson of modern molecular genetics is the profound complexity of both gene-gene interactions and gene-environment interactions in the determination of whether a specific trait or characteristic is expressed. In other words, there never will be another you" quoted in Martha C. Nussbaum and Cass R. Sunstein, eds., *Clones and Clones: Facts and Fantasies about Human Cloning* (New York: W. W. Norton, 1998), 29–40, 39. See also Barbara Katz Rothman on genetics as ideology in her contribution to that volume, "On Order," 280–88.

30. For a detailed account see Elizabeth Thomson, "Genetic Counselling," in John F. Kilner, Rebecca D. Pentz, and Frank E. Young, eds., *Genetic Ethics: Do the Ends Justify the Genes?* (Grand Rapids: Wm. B. Eerdmans, 1997), 146–55.

31. This is even accepted by feminists who claim that free choice implies that society has no business in limiting women's rights to decide for themselves. Their claim is not that women do not need to have good reasons for wanting an abortion, but that the authority to judge what counts as a good reason in this case should left to women themselves. See Maura G. Ryan, "The Argument for Unlimited Procreative Liberty: A Feminist Critique," *Hastings Center Report* 20 (1990): 6–12.

FIVE *Disability, Prevention, and Discrimination*

1. The distinction I will be elaborating in this and the following paragraphs bears resemblance to Derek Parfit's distinction between reasons that depend on self-interest and reasons that depend on value judgments or ideals (see Derek Parfit, *Reasons and Persons* (Oxford, New York: Oxford University Press, 1986), 153 f. Two qualifications explain the distinction in the sense in which I will use it. First, reasons dependent on self-interest are understood to depend on interests *of* the self, which are distinct from interests *in* the self. These reasons I will call reasons regarding quality of life. Second, reasons dependent on value judgments and ideals are understood as depending on *moral* value judgments and ideals. These reasons I will call reasons based on moral standing.

2. Parfit, *Reasons and Persons*, 153.

3. This explains why reasons based on 'moral standing' typically create the problem of 'marginal' cases in a moral taxonomy. In contemporary philosophical literature, the classical example of this kind of problem is presented by the issue of whether the human fetus is a person. See for example Feinberg, *Problem of Abortion*.

4. This example is inspired by a case presented by Thomas Nagel and discussed in Parfit in the context of 'self-interest theory' (Parfit, *Reasons and Persons*, 154).

5. For the distinction and its relation to moral belief, see Hare, *Moral Thinking*, 28–31. See also Bernard Williams, *Ethics and the Limits of Philosophy* (London: Fontana Press/ Collins, 1985), 177 f.

6. It may be objected that the distinction between preferences and beliefs is too strong here. We can think about our moral beliefs in terms of preferences if we think about them as expressing certain ideals, e.g., the ideal to be a particular kind of person. For example, the ideal of the woman with the belief about children as a gift from God is to be the kind of person who acts faithfully according to that belief. It is her preference to be that kind of person. If we think this way we should at least recognize that moral ideals generate preferences of a distinct kind. A preference for acting upon a given belief is not merely a preference for a *state of experience* of the self but for being *a particular kind* of self. In deciding to spend a few days with your friend in the mountains instead of staying at home with your lover, you do not 'fail yourself' in the same way that the woman in our case fails herself when she rejects a child with Down Syndrome. You fail yourself only if you promised your friend that you would join her and then decided to stay home with your lover and break your promise. Given your belief that promises ought to be kept, you surely will incur a self-critical judgment about *yourself* for having failed to keep a promise that *you* made. Overriding a preference for a particular state of experience of yourself is very different from overriding your preference for being a particular self. We may actually go one step further and say that even the possibility of feeling good about being a particular self *as* a state of experience should be distinguished from being that self. The latter is not a state of experience at all. Believing truly that a disabled child is a gift from God does not preclude the possibility of overriding that belief on grounds of the expected quality of life. The consequence of overriding one's moral belief, however, will most likely be the experience of guilt rather than of dissatisfaction. Presumably, the experience of guilt can be outweighed by the prospect of a lasting dissatisfaction with one's disabled child. But even then a judgment balancing the consequences of

abandoning one's moral belief is very different from a judgment that does not have a state of experience but *oneself* as object. This shows that MS reasons cannot be changed into QL reasons without giving up the belief that created the problem in the first place. Even if I forgive myself for my failure to act upon my moral belief, this presupposes that what I did was wrong. In other words, the act of forgiving presupposes that treating my moral belief as just another preference was a mistake in the first place.

7. This claim is defended in Ronald Dworkin's version of liberal theory (see *Rights,* 272–78). See also Ronald Dworkin, "Liberalism," in *Matter of Principle,* 181–204.

8. With regard to disabilities, the United States passed the *Americans with Disabilties Act* (ADA) in 1992.

9. What is true for public policy is also true for scientific journals and organizations in this field. For example, the International Association of the Scientific Study of Mental Retardation (IASSMR) has been rebaptized as the International Association of the Scientific Study of Intellectual Disability (IASSID).

10. Given the details of the case under consideration, the importance of self-esteem betrays a limitation with respect to this example. In particular, profoundly mentally disabled people cannot esteem themselves. This point will be taken into consideration below.

11. Cf. the quote from Isaiah Berlin's essay "Two Concepts," 118–72, 156, preceeding the present chapter. Berlin discusses the importance of status and recognition for our conception of ourselves: "For if I am not so recognized [e.g. as having my own conception of myself], then I may fail to recognize, I may doubt, my own claim to be a fully independent human being. For what I am is, in large part, determined by what I feel and think; and what I feel and think is determined by the feeling and thought prevailing in the society to which I belong, of which . . . I form not an isolable atom, but an ingredient (to use a perilous but indispensable metaphor) in a social pattern" (157). The interesting point here is that, according to Berlin, my claim to be a fully independent human being cannot survive without my being dependent on social recognition. This implies that discrimination is a matter of the social recognition of the equal worth of another person.

12. On this cf. chapter 4, 57 f.

13. Interesting counterexamples to my argument multiply once we consider the fact that the history of public health has developed many policies for no other reason than to prevent disabled lives. From control of the water supply to safety procedures in transportation and traffic, not to mention practices such as childcare and vaccination campaigns, each of these policies has been aimed at diminishing disabling diseases. Does my argument imply that each of them reflected a discriminatory attitude? The correct response, it seems, must be that the answer depends on the type of reason for which these policies were implemented. A particularly relevant example in this connection is the distribution of folic acid to young women to prevent the birth of children with neural tube defects. It has been reported that successful campaigns of this kind have been carried out among poor peasants in Central America using the slogan "For a healthy baby!" This slogan indicates how the above question should be answered.

First, participation in a campaign for using folic acid during pregnancy does not imply the same connection with the prospect of conceiving a disabled child as does participation in prenatal testing. The difference does not reside in the different technologies but in the perspective of those who are involved. In the folic acid case the guiding question is, Do you want a healthy baby? Of course we do! Everybody does. However, the preference for a healthy baby in this case in no way entails an answer to the question faced by those who are involved in genetic testing: Will we accept a disabled child? An explicit judgment on the life of a disabled child is necessarily implied in the latter but not in the former.

Second, one must again consider the point about intention. Presumably, women in Central America who become pregnant can be described as doing a number of different things. They are fulfilling their heart's desire, securing their families' sources of income, satisfying cultural beliefs about marital duties, and contributing to the demographic problem of overpopulation. Which of these act-descriptions are relevant in assessing the morality of what they are doing? In my view, the connection between intention and action serves a moral purpose. As human beings, we have strong reasons for emphasizing the importance of describing our actions in terms of our intentions. If not, we dissolve the connection that makes it possible to regard them as *our own* actions in the first place. Consequently, if a folic acid campaign can be said to have the same effects as genetic testing combined with selective abortion, this does not necessarily mean that they are guided by the same intention. By the same token, it does not mean that this campaign presupposes a negative judgment on disabled lives. Without either the intention or the judgment in question, the issue of discrimination cannot arise as it can in connection with genetic testing. Whether the difference between these cases obtains depends on the perspective from which the intentions guiding them take shape. In this connection, the distinction between disease prevention and positive health promotion is relevant for appreciating the differences between both cases. See Verwey, "Preventive Medicine," 14–18.

14. For a recent discussion along these lines see Kitcher, *Lives to Come.* See also Annas and Elias, *Gene Mapping.*

15. Kitcher, *Lives to Come,* 127–55.

16. Cf. Jane R. Mercer, "The Impact of Changing Paradigms of Disability on Mental Retardation in the Year 2000," in Rowitz, *Mental Retardation,* 15–38.

17. Silver, *Remaking Eden,* 9.

18. Cf. Ted Peters's comments on a scenario of this kind: "This scenario may happen gradually, unevenly, and unnecessarily. Geneticists estimate that each of us carries five to seven lethal recessive genes as well as a larger number of genes that make us susceptible to developing multifactorial diseases. There is probably no one whose genome is disease free. Yet this may not be obvious in the initial years that society wrestles with this problem. Those who are tested in the early years will suffer discrimination because of their apparent singularity. Although it will never be the case that all people will face identical genetic risk, eventually, we are likely to find that differences are minimal. Only later, when we discover again the relative equality of risk distribution, will the pressure for stigma be released. However, this may come only after considerable social damage has been done" ("Genes," 1–45, 5). There is at least one reason to be cautious with this suggestion because the relative equality of risk distribution does not include the equal distribution of risk for genetic disorders that cause *mental* disabilities. The relevance of this consideration is illuminated by Krebs's distinction between disease as an 'exceptional' state and mental disability as a special case with regard to health (see above chapter 3, note 14). We may all—sooner or later in our lives—be in for some exceptional states, but that still does not make us 'special' in the way the mentally disabled are 'special.'

19. For recent assessments of the 'state of the art' from a philosophical (or theological) point of view, see Annas and Elias, *Gene Mapping;* Kitcher, *Lives to Come;* Silver, *Remaking Eden.* See also John Harris, *Wonderwoman and Superman: The Ethics of Human Biotechnology* (Oxford: Oxford University Press, 1992) and Peters, *Playing God?*

20. Cf. Martha Newsome, professor of biology at Tomball College, Houston: "In spite of, perhaps because of, misconceptions about genetics, the demand for such technologies will be great. It is *natural* to seek these devices to forecast or control one's future or the future of the next generation—spurred on by the fear of the unknown and the possibility of fatal illness" (Martha Newsome, "The Educational Challenge," in Kilner, Pentz, and Young, *Genetic Ethics,* 156–67, 158; italics added). This appears to be a perfect example of what McKenny identifies as a commitment to 'the Baconion project' that is incapable of recognizing itself as rooted in a particular contingent discourse (see above chapter 1, notes 24 and 32). If this represents the view of those who are engaged in 'the challenge of education' we can be sure that the demand for gene technology will be massive indeed.

21. Cf. Gregory J. Hayes, "Social Responsibility: Genetics and the Developmentally Disabled," in Linda J. Hayes et al., eds., *Ethical Issues in Developmental Disabilities* (Reno: Context Press, 1994), 183–97: "The new genetics will be seductive. The public will want to believe that perfection can indeed become the norm and they will be susceptible to pronouncements of what is imperfect or undesirable, pronouncements which, while often value judgments at their root, will be cloaked in the objectivity of the genome. The new genetics will ultimately make it possible to eliminate many conditions deemed unacceptable" (191).

22. For example, population effects of genetic testing have already been seen in the incidence of Tay Sachs disease, which has dropped since the 1970s to about one-tenth of previous levels. See Proctor, "Genomics," 57–93, 70. See also Arno G. Motulsky and Jeffrey Murray, "Will Prenatal Diagnosis with Selective Abortion Affect Society's Attitude toward the Handicapped?" *Research Ethics* (1983): 277–91.

23. Cf. McKenny: "The goal of an optimally healthy and reproductive population . . . now operates through stimulation (by means of everything from health information to advertising of the desire of couples to have perfect children, through myriads of forms of prenatal and neonatal monitoring and screening, and through the fear of having an imperfect child in a normalizing society that values persons according to their usefulness and that constantly measures their chances of success according to societal standards of success. Power no longer requires draconian policies but operates through our choices. As expressions of biopower, eugenic goals produce new genetic knowledge as the truth about our bodies which we, well schooled by our society to fear imperfect babies, are eager to seize on" (McKenny, *To Relieve the Human Condition,* 206). In this connection, see also the contemporary version of Huxley's Brave New World in Silver, *Remaking Eden,* 1–11.

24. Proctor notices that in the United States state and federal laws requiring notification of health conditions are expanding, which leads him to suggest that "the stigma against genetic disease may result in an extension of coercive powers of public health" ("Genomics," 71).

25. Kitcher, *Lives to Come,* 135. See also Bartha Knoppers, "Towards Genetic Justice," in Eike H. Kluge, ed., *Readings in Biomedical Ethics: A Canadian Focus* (Scarborough: Prentice Hall Canada, 1993), 478–81: "We may fail to examine our political system, which leaves those with genetic disabilities less insured than those without. We may exert pressure on individuals

to control their reproductive outcome according to our view of normality, and promote the elimination of the handicapped by abortion rather than making the world a better place for them" (479).

26. This is an important point because the inference is concerned with the political consequences of what people may believe to be true regardless of whether or not it is true. Not what is the case, but what the public believes to be the case is the politically relevant fact. The deplorable—but unavoidable—counterpart of this fact is the politician who does not tell her voters what she thinks is the case, but what she thinks her voters want to believe is the case. For public policy in representative democracy to defy misguided perception is a hard task indeed. For a provocative and humorous comment on Dolly the cloned sheep in view of ideology and myth, see Stephen Jay Gould, "Dolly's Fashion and Louis's Passion, " in Nussbaum and Sunstein, *Clones and Clones,* 41–53.

27. Cf. Seymour B. Sarason and John Doris, *Educational Handicap, Public Policy, and Social History: A Broadened Perspective on Mental Retardation* (New York: Free Press, 1979) observe that mental disability is a concept that "both describes and judges interactions of an individual, a social context, and the culturally determined values, traditions and expectations that give shape and substance to that context at a particular time" (17). For historical arguments claiming that classification schemes vary with political, economic, and cultural shifts see Trent, *Inventing the Feeble Mind,* and Ryan and Thomas, *Politics of Mental Handicap.*

28. Here I concur with Wolterstorff's argument against Robert Audi's view that coercive policies limiting citizens of a liberal democratic state in their freedom lack an adequate moral basis if they fail to persuade these citizens provided that they are fully rational and in the possession of the relevant facts. That liberal democracy somehow fails its own standards if it does not generate a *consensus* on coercive laws—which for Audi is not merely majority rule—strikes me as an utterly implausible conception because it makes the concept of liberal democracy an empty one. On Audi's conception there is no single instance of liberal democracy to be found, nor will there ever be one (Wolterstorff, "Audi on Religion," 145–65, 152 ff.).

s i x *Restrictions on Reproductive Choice?*

1. In this connection John Rawls introduced the distinction between 'interests *in* the self' and 'interests *of* the self'. See his *Political Liberalism,* 51 where he writes that rational agents are not solely self-interested, and then continues: "that is, their interests are not always interests in benefits to themselves. Every interest is an interest of a self (agent), but not every interest is in benefits to the self that has it." Cf. also his *Theory of Justice,* 127.

2. This point is well taken in Engelhardt's claim that the moral justification of public policy must respect neutrality between what he calls 'content-full moralities' (*Foundations,* 7 f.). This is a necessary but not a sufficient condition for moral justification in public morality, for there is the further requirement that individuals respect the equal freedom of others. According to Engelhardt his theory of secular morality is different from theories that try to establish a secular ethics based on rational choice theory. For a recent proponent of this approach, see D. Gauthier, *Morals by Agreement* (Oxford: Clarendon Press, 1986). Engelhardt,

Foundations, 55–56, criticizes this approach because he thinks that the problem of coordinating individual choices requires a common ranking of values and a common understanding of moral rationality (56). As was argued in chapter 2, my view is that his own foundational theory that is based on assent and agreement works if and only if it presupposes the same requirement.

3. Robert G. Edwards and David J. Sharpe, "Social Values and Research in Human Embryology," *Nature* 231 (1971): 87–94, 87. The view is not quite generally accepted though, when we take into account recent feminist voices that reject 'pronatalism'. See Jean E. Veevers, *Childless by Choice* (Toronto: Butterworths, 1980); see also Susan Sherwin, *No Longer Patient*. However, both authors accept the pervasiveness of the attitude that they criticize (Veevers, 109 f.; Sherwin, 130 f.).

4. Quoted from Collins's foreword in Peters, *Playing God?*, x–xi. See also Leroy Hood, "Biology and Medicine in the Twenty-First Century," in Daniel J. Kevles and Leroy Hood, eds., *Code of Codes* (Cambridge: Harvard University Press, 1992), 158.

5. Kitcher, *Lives to Come*, 132. The author stresses that in answering this question it is important to distinguish between the various contexts in which genetic information can be applied: the contexts of health insurance, the labor market, and everyday relations. I will focus solely on the analysis of his argument for social justice in the first context.

6. Kitcher, *Lives to Come*, 133.

7. Kitcher, *Lives to Come*, 136 f.

8. Rawls, *Theory of Justice*, 136–42.

9. In his *Theory of Justice* Rawls attempted to provide a twofold justification for his principles of distributive justice as grounded both in equal respect for persons and in rational choice theory (cf. 175–83). Robert Nozick, among others, has criticized the rationality of choosing a redistribution principle to enhance the welfare position of the least advantaged on the grounds of the so-called 'maximin' rule. See Nozick, *Anarchy*, 189–97. The 'later' Rawls has abandoned the element of rational choice in his theory in the sense that he no longer claims the theory of justice to be part of the theory of rational choice. Cf. his *Political Liberalism*, 53, note 7.

10. Cf. Engelhardt, *Foundations*, 51 f. where the author offers a similar criticism of hypothetical choice theory in general.

11. This idea of a fair equality of opportunity continuously returns as the fundamental moral premise of Kitcher's reasoning; cf. his last chapter, "The Unequal Inheritance," *Lives to Come*, 309–26.

12. Daniel Wikler has an interesting suggestion on why people think certain behaviors that endanger one's health, such as smoking cigarettes, are targeted by the charge of irresponsible behavior, while others—such as accepting a very stressful job, sports, moving into a polluted urban area—are not: the targeted behaviors are considered to be vices. In other words, there is a strong moralistic overtone in the charge of irresponsible behavior that has little to do with a careful consideration of the case at hand. See D. Wikler, "Personal Responsbility for Illness," in D. Vandeveer and T. Regan, eds., *Health Care Ethics: An Introduction* (Philadelphia: Temple University Press), 1987, 326–58, 342. If I am right that implied in decisions to prevent birth of a handicapped child is a negative judgment on the lives of handicapped people, then Wikler's suggestion may lead us to expect

that the failure to submit oneself to prenatal testing when pregnant will come to be seen as a vice.

13. On the implications of this prospect, with particular regard to the possibilities of human cloning, see Silver, *Remaking Eden,* 91–132.

14. See Retsinas, "Impact of Prenatal Technology." The author discusses in particular Joseph Fletcher's argument about 'irresponsible reproductive behavior' (92 ff.).

15. In 1991 the American Society of Human Genetics recommended that legislation of abortion should include provisions for allowing the termination of pregnancies where the fetus "is likely to have a serious genetic or congenital disorder" ("American Society of Human Genetics Statement on Clinical Genetics and Freedom of Choice," *American Journal of Human Genetics* 48 (1991): 1011.

16. Cf. Adrienne Asch and Gail Geller, "Feminism, Bioethics, and Genetics," in Wolf, *Feminism and Bioethics,* 318–50, 335 ff.

17. See Overall, *Future of Human Reproduction,* and Holmes and Purdy, *Feminist Perspectives.*

18. The symptoms of the disorder of Lesch Nyhan develop in the first year of infancy. They are progressive mental retardation, uncontrollable muscular spasms, and compulsive self-mutilative behavior. The last symptom in particular renders the qualification 'hostile to human life'—as distinct from 'incompatible with human life'—appropriate. The seriousness of self-mutilative behavior in children with Lesch Nyhan induced Paul Ramsey, an ardent critic of 'selective nontreatment', to accept this condition as a possible exception because of insurmountable pain. P. Ramsey, *Ethics at the Edges of Life* (New Haven: Yale University Press, 1978), 190 ff.

19. Cf. Robinson, "Potential Impact," 215–25: "As long as the premises of *Roe v. Wade* remain intact, however, a woman would have the legal right to terminate a pregnancy on the basis of such genetic information if she so desires. If a woman might abort because the pregnancy is unwanted, an inquiry into her reasons for finding the pregnancy unwanted would be barred" (219).

20. Cf. Kluge, *Biomedical Ethics,* 337 f.: "The overriding logical fact is that our lives and the life of society constantly require decision-making. Decision-making, in turn, if it is done rationally, involves considering and weighing competing options. However, options are not really options if they are not known. We cannot choose what we cannot know." What follows—according to Kluge—is that we should seek to know as much as possible about our genetic dispositions. 'Deliberate ignorance' is apparently beyond the pale of moral possibilities. There is a problem with this claim to rational decision making, however, here as elsewhere in the debate on genetic testing. The option of 'deliberate ignorance' is most emphatically rejected by those who prefer to ignore the social and political context of clinical genetics, and who refrain from asking political questions about whether the widespread proliferation among the population may result in an underclass of people with 'bad genes'. Apparently what is seen as 'rational decision making' depends very much on what the objectives are.

21. See Joseph C. Fletcher, "Ethics and Public Policy: Should Sex Choice Be Discouraged?" in N. G. Bennet, ed., *Sex Selection of Children* (New York: Academic Press, 1983), 213–52; Mary A. Warren, *Gendercide: The Implications of Sex Selection* (Totowa: Rowan &

Allenfield, 1985); and Dorothy Wertz and John C. Fletcher, "Fatal Knowledge? Prenatal Diagnosis and Sex Selection," *Hastings Center Report* 19 (1989): 21–27.

22. I leave aside the further problem of establishing a canonical conception of disease that arises from the discussion about the objective and subjective aspects of our understanding of health and disease. On this problem see Engelhardt, *Foundations*, 197–207. For a defense of a 'middle ground' between 'normativists' and 'non-normativists' on the concept of disease see Caplan, "Gene Therapy," 128–41.

23. The Tay Sachs syndrome develops its symptoms approximately six months after birth. The symptoms are progressing loss of motor reactions, muscular atrophy, blindness, and mental degeneration. Death occurs on average at the age of three or four.

24. Tay Sachs is among the genetic disorders for which a widespread agreement is frequently claimed with regard to their seriousness. See for example Arval A. Morris, "Law, Morality, and Euthanasia for the Severely Defective Child," in Marvin Kohl, ed., *Infanticide and the Value of Life* (Buffalo: Prometheus Books, 1978), 149: "I think there is widespread agreement that the use of the modern arsenal of modern technology in an attempt to prolong the biological existences of defective newborns such as the ones just described [including Tay Sachs] is a misguided or wrongful act that results in cruelty, is contrary to the better interests of the infant, and violates the important maxim of medical ethics, *primum non nocere.*" For a contrasting view see Ramsey, *Ethics*, 178: "There is no reason for saying that six months in the life of a baby born with invariably fatal Tay Sachs disease are a life span of lesser worth to God than living seventy years before the onset of irreversible degeneration."

25. Cf. Jones, *Smith's Recognizable Patterns:* "Generally 'good babies' and happy children, individuals with Down syndrome tend toward mimicry, are friendly, have a good sense of rhythm, and enjoy music. Mischievousness and obstinacy may also be characteristics, and 13 percent have serious emotional problems. Coordination is often poor, and the voice tends to be raucous. Early developmental enrichment programs for Down syndrome children have resulted in improved rates of progress during the first four or five years of life. Whether such training programs will alter their ultimate level of performance remains to be undetermined" (11).

26. Hoedemaekers and his colleagues report that the Duth Health Council, the Nuffic Council on Bioethics, and the Danish Council of Ethics decline to include in their guidelines specifications of the seriousness of genetic disorders in their reports on genetic screening. See Hoedemaekers et al., "Genetic Screening," 135–41, 136.

SEVEN *The Inclusion of the Mentally Disabled*

1. Engelhardt, *Foundations of Bioethics*; Rawls, *Theory of Justice*; Rawls, *Political Liberalism.*

2. Engelhardt, *Foundations*, 239.

3. Engelhardt, *Foundations*, 147.

4. "Persons who are moral agents have rights that are integral to the very character of general secular morality. The rights of persons in a social sense are created by particular communities" (Engelhardt, *Foundations*, 150).

5. "Perhaps, one develops a suggestion from Kant regarding the need to support practices that will, in general, lead to the protection of persons. To find grounds for protecting such individuals [sc nonpersons], one will need to look at the justification for certain social practices in terms of their importance for persons" (Engelhardt, *Foundations*, 147). For a similar argument see Mary Gore Forrester, *Persons, Animals, and Fetuses: An Essay in Practical Ethics* (Dordrecht: Kluwer Academic Press, 1996). Forrester calls nonrational beings 'extended persons' and argues that we treat those not only with beneficence but also with fairness: "Since we all look with horror on the possibility that we will, when old and senile, be sent to a nursing home where we will be ridiculed and physically neglected, we have a strong interest in insuring that the senile are given equal consideration. The same remarks apply to all forms of mental disability" (79).

6. Engelhardt, *Foundations*, 148.

7. Engelhardt discusses the example where animals are used in drug experiments. In that case it would be rational, according to the author, to outweigh the harm done to animals: "The greater good of persons will likely be seen as having a higher position in the hierarchy of goods than the good of experimental animals who will need to be sacrificed in the course of medical experimentation and research" (*Foundations*, 141). The suggestion that a similar argument holds for the comparison between 'real' persons and the (profoundly) mentally disabled is certainly not outrageous from the point of view of 'general secular morality' as Engelhardt understands it. As matter of fact, it is his view that much of the bioethical literature is far from being candid about the shallowness of public morality in liberal society.

8. Engelhardt, *Foundations*, 109.

9. Engelhardt, *Foundations*, 105: "The principle of beneficence is not required for the coherence of the moral world."

10. Engelhardt, *Foundations*, 107; italics added.

11. Engelhardt, *Foundations*, 72, 75, 78, 84, 102.

12. Engelhardt, *Foundations*, 150.

13. "One only derives from a hypothetical-choice theory those choices which one has ordained or predestined by an antecedent choice of a particular thin theory of the good, moral sense, cluster of moral intuitions, or notion of moral rationality" (Engelhardt, *Foundations*, 51).

14. Rawls, *Theory of Justice*, 142 f.

15. Rawls, *Theory of Justice*, 178.

16. See Loretta M. Kopelman and J. C. Moskop, eds., *Ethics and Mental Retardation* (Dordrecht/Boston: Reidel Publishing Company, 1984). Cf. particularly the contributions by Jeffery G. Murphy, "Rights and Borderline Cases," 3–17; Joseph Margolis, "Applying Moral Theory to the Retarded," 19–35; Engelhardt, "Joseph Margolis, John Rawls, and the Mentally Retarded," 37–43. See also, Daniel Wikler, "Paternalism and the Mildly Retarded," *Philosophy and Public Affairs* 8 (1979): 377–92.

17. It may be objected at this point that I have not taken into account the 'original position', which is Rawls's device for excluding partiality in the choice for the principles of justice, and that the inclusion of the disabled is secured by that device. Since the parties do not know anything about their own identity, they cannot choose a conception of justice to their own advantage. Given this informational constraint, the objection runs, the position of disabled people will not be disregarded since anybody might find her- or himself in that posi-

tion. This argument fails, however, because the construction of the original position already presupposes Rawls's concept of the moral person, which means that the disabled are excluded from the very beginning. They do not qualify as 'parties' to the hypothetical agreement because they are incapable of reciprocating the requirements of justice.

18. Rawls, *Theory of Justice*, 504.

19. Rawls, *Theory of Justice*, 490–504.

20. Murphy argues for a defense of Rawls's hypothetical choice theory on this point that is entirely based on the mutual advantage claim. Given that people in the original position are unaware of their own assets, they have to consider the possibility of being the parent of a disabled child. This consideration is sufficient, according to Murphy, for guaranteeing the rights of the mentally disabled (cf. Murphy, "Rights," 11 ff). The argument here also works by means of substitution, as did Engelhardt's argument: the rights eventually assigned to the disabled depend on the rights assigned to their parents.

21. Rawls, *Theory of Justice*, 497.

22. Rawls, *Theory of Justice*, 512.

23. In this connection Rawls refers us to the task of metaphysics. "One of the tasks of metaphysics is to work out a view of the world which is suited for this purpose; it should identify and systematize the truths decisive for these questions. How far justice as fairness will have to be revised to fit into this larger theory it is impossible to say" (Rawls, *Theory of Justice*, 512).

24. Rawls, *Political Liberalism*, xv–xvi.

25. Rawls, *Political Liberalism*, 50–51.

26. Rawls points out that the idea of society as a fair system of social cooperation is grounded in reciprocity rather than mutual advantage (*Political Liberalism*, 17). In other words, there is no longer the claim that justice as fairness can be justified from the point of individual interest. The 'rational' is no longer the more basic source of justification.

27. Rawls now speaks of creatures who do not fit the description of "a political conception of the person" (*Political Liberalism*, 29).

28. Rawls, *Political Liberalism*, 21.

29. Rawls, *Political Liberalism*, 214.

30. Rawls, *Political Liberalism*, 215.

31. Rawls, *Political Liberalism*, 217 f.

32. It may be asked whether Rawls's theory of natural duties can provide any help to solve the problem under consideration. There are several reasons for thinking that this is not the case. First, Rawls confines the operation of natural duties to the realm of interpersonal relations. They are not necessarily attached to institutions or social arrangements (*Theory of Justice*, 114 f.). Thus we have a natural duty to another person not to be cruel, or to help her, regardless of who that person is and irrespective of the institutional settings in which we interact. Since the problem of including the disabled occurs in connection with institutions and social arrangements, the theory of natural duties does not seem to offer much help. Second, and more importantly, Rawls deals with the justification of natural duties within the context of his justice as fairness. Thus he answers the question of which principles of natural duties the parties in the original position would have chosen (*Theory of Justice*, 333 f.). Since the construction of this contractual device creates the problem for Rawls in the first

place, it is difficult to see how the appeal to natural duties, i.e., the duty to mutual aid, could solve that problem. Third, one could consider the duty to mutual aid as a 'sub-class' of the duty of benevolence and then ask whether the inclusion of severely disabled persons cannot be justified as a matter of benevolence rather than justice. This solution is forfeited by Rawls's argument that his justice as fairness does not need to rely on benevolence because combined with the original position the condition of mutual disinterestedness will secure the effects of good will. The theoretical advantage of this construction, he says, is that we do not need so 'strong a condition' as to assume that people have benevolent desires towards others (*Theory of Justice*, 148 f.). The aim of my criticisms in this chapter is precisely to show that this theoretical advantage is obtained at the cost of an irresolvable problem for liberal theory. We have already seen that Engelhardt's resort to the principle of beneficence did not fare any better. In the end, both theorists do need to assume this 'stronger condition' of people having benevolent desires towards others.

33. In the case of my example—e.g., the belief that nonpersons are owed equal respect because their lives have been woven into the relationships that constitute our society as a moral community—it is clear that its notion of society as a moral community per se exceeds the limits of liberal thinking because it regards social relationships rather than individuals *qua* individuals as constitutive of the moral community.

34. There is a communitarian defense of liberalism that probably escapes this critique in that it regards liberal morality as a particular content-full morality—to borrow Engelhardt's phrase. This defense necessarily fails in the eyes of liberal theorists such as Rawls and Engelhardt because it reflects a particular conception of the good. For an example see Galston, *Liberal Purposes*. Galston presents a version of liberalism as the 'content-full' morality of a particular society, namely that of the United States of America.

35. It can be argued that apart from the two claims mentioned above, a claim to equality is a third feature that is characteristic of liberal theory. If this is accepted, a theory of public morality such as Engelhardt's probably would have to be classified as libertarian rather than as liberal because it distances itself from egalitarian interpretations of public morality. The distinction between both types of theory is not important for my purposes, however, because I intend to show that equality cannot solve the problem of moral standing of defective persons.

36. I have already considered the implication of the belief that being affected by a genetic disorder will become more and more a matter of individual responsibility. As was argued in chapter 6, this belief will undermine the force of the principle of equality of opportunity because it fosters the perception that irresponsible reproductive behavior causes society to pay the price for special needs that could have been prevented.

37. Let me illustrate this claim by reference to Ronald Dworkin's version of egalitarian liberalism, which would seem to support the kind of objection under consideration here. Dworkin has consistently argued for a particular conception of equality as 'the nerve of liberalism' (cf. his widely published essay "Liberalism," in *Matter of Principle*, 181–204, the quote is on 183). The conception of equality defended by Dworkin is based on a distinction between two different principles. The first principle requires that the government "treat all those in its charge *as equals*, that is, as entitled to its equal concern and respect." The second demands that it treat "all those in its charge *equally* in the distribution of some resource of

opportunity" (190). According to Dworkin the first principle, which he calls 'the principle of equal concern and respect,' is constitutive while the second is only derivative.

This constitutive principle can be taken in two different but incompatible interpretations, the first of which supposes "that government must be neutral on what might be called the question of the good life" while the second supposes that such neutrality is impossible because the government "cannot treat its citizens as equal human beings without a theory of what human beings ought to be" (191). Dworkin defends the first alternative as the proper liberal position.

Two questions are relevant to see whether his conception of equality can solve the problem that the theories of Rawls and Engelhardt fail to solve. The first question is What makes certain individuals eligible for being treated as equals? The answer appears to be simply that they hold the legal status of citizenship. Although Dworkin does not provide a *moral* reason for why people should be treated as equals (cf. Rosenberg, "Political Philosophy," 1–31, 18), he does seem to presuppose a particular moral reason, which will be seen when we raise the second question: What is the point of government treating its citizens as equals in such a way as to abstain from any judgment about their conception of the good life? This question he does answer, namely in explaining why liberals reject that they are governed by other people's preferences for the good life: "the domination of one set of *external* preferences, that is, preferences people have about what others shall do or have . . . invades rather than enforces the right of citizens to be treated as equals," (196). Apparently, the principle of equal concern and respect is a principle that applies to persons who can choose their own conception of the good and act accordingly (which is confirmed by the fact that, according to Dworkin, the question of what it means for the government to treat its citizens as equals is the same as the question of what it means "to treat all citizens as free, or as independent, or with equal dignity" (191).

I conclude, therefore, that (1) the principle of equal opportunity as provided by Dworkin's theory of liberalism does only manage to include disabled people because it does not answer the question of why we owe other people what liberal morality demands, and (2) should we try to infer an answer to that question from his theory, it would fail for exactly the same reason as Rawls's and Engelhardt's theories fail: everything it says presupposes a conception of human beings as independent agents in the possession of reason and free will. See in this connection also Alan H. Goldman's justification of equal opportunity that appeals to the requirement of equal concern and respect as a fundamental moral principle ("The Justification of Equal Opportunity," in Paul et al., *Equal Opportunity*, 88–103): "At the highest level of abstraction, the appeal here may be simply to the property of being human, and to the claim that all persons deserve equal respect and concern simply in virtue of their common humanity. Or, more concretely, it can be pointed out that all persons have desires, form plans and goals, enjoy satisfactions and suffer frustrations in relation to these goals, and share basic needs. Equally relevant is the fact that all normally rational agents share certain second order desires: all desire to have their needs satisfied, to be able to do what they want, and to obtain the means for satisfying their first order desires" (89 f.). It occurs to me that this is the kind of justification that one would expect from liberals, including egalitarian liberals like Ronald Dworkin, and that, therefore, the objection that liberal theory is capable of including the disabled on the basis of equality necessarily fails.

38. I should qualify this explanation with regard to Rawls. He himself does not go beyond the claim that he thinks my question regarding the standing of non-persons can be answered by his political liberalism. However, he has no room to show how (*Political Liberalism*, 21 f., 245).

39. I should qualify this verdict, again, with respect to Rawls. In *Political Liberalism* he more than once mentions the importance of what he calls a background culture which is formative of the beliefs that people have, including moral beliefs, but it remains entirely unclear how the beliefs of this background culture are relevant to Rawls's theory. See *Political Liberalism*, 14, 215, 220. The background culture is the social realm where nonpublic reasons are exchanged: "Nonpublic reasons comprise the many reasons of civil society and belong to what I have called the 'background culture', in contrast with the public political culture." (220). Rawls's concern is precisely to provide a justification of political liberalism *independently* from this background culture.

EIGHT *Imperatives of the Self*

1. See Richard B. Brandt, *A Theory of the Good and the Right* (Oxford: Oxford University Press, 1979); Hare, *Moral Thinking.*

2. Singer and Kuhse, *Should the Baby Live?;* Harris, *Value of Life;* Kuhse, *Sanctity of Life;* P. Singer, *Rethinking Life and Death: The Collapse of Our Traditional Ethics* (Oxford: Oxford University Press), 1995.

3. See Singer's essay "Unsanctifying Human Life," in John Ladd, *Ethical Issues Relating to Life and Death* (Oxford: Oxford University Press, 1979), 41–61 where he presents anthropological and historical material to show that other cultures hold different views from those reflected by the sanctity of life doctrine. The presentation of this material is preceded by the following remark: "To refute a doctrine it is necessary to produce sound arguments against it. Unfortunately, when a doctrine is very deeply embedded in people's moral intuitions, it is sometimes necessary to do more than refute the doctrine in order to convince people that it is false (55–56). A similar strategy is found in *Should the Baby Live?* where Singer and Kuhse claim "to show by rigorous argument that the sanctity of life principle is unsound. Perhaps what we have said in earlier chapters [presenting case studies and other material] will have already persuaded some of our readers of this conclusion; but we have a more ambitious aim than the persuasion of those already sympathetic to our views on these questions. The argument we shall present is so clear-cut that henceforth the onus will be on those who invoke the sanctity of life principle to show where our refutation goes wrong" (118). Apparently people's 'deeply embedded moral intuitions' have to be demolished by critical thinking regardless of what this does to their moral character and integrity.

4. Zygmunt Bauman presents a poignant description of this feature of modern moral philosophy when he writes: "Properly ethical statements are such as do not depend for their truthfulness on what people are actually doing or even on what they believe they ought to be doing. If what ethical statements say and what people do or believe are at odds with each other, this is assumed to mean, without need of further proof, that it is the people who are in the wrong. Only ethics can say what *really* ought to be done so that the good be served."

According to Bauman, this derogatory view of the ethical competence of nonexperts is closely connected to the project of providing philosophically ascertained foundations for morality. Within this project "true foundations must be stronger and less volatile than ordinary people's erratic habits and their notoriously unsound and mercurial opinions. What is more, those foundations must be placed at a distance from the hurly-burly of daily life, so that ordinary people will not see them from the places in which they conduct their ordinary business, and will not be able to pretend that they know them unless told, taught or trained by the experts" (*Life in Fragments: Essays in Postmodern Morality* [Oxford: Blackwell Publishers, 1995], 11).

5. Cheryl N. Noble, "Normative Ethical Theories," in Stanley G. Clarke and E. Simpson, eds., *Anti-Theory in Ethics and Moral Conservatism* (Albany: State University of New York Press, 1989), 49–64, 61.

6. Kenzaburo Oë, *A Personal Matter,* trans. John Nathan (New York: Grove Weidenfeld, 1969). See also Nancy Dew Taylor and Ryuki Kassai, "The Healer and the Healed: Works and Life of Kenzaburo Oë," *The Lancet* 352 (1998): 642–44.

7. I am most indebted to professor MacIntyre for permission to use his unpublished paper "Human Identity, Accountability and Disablement" (April 1994) and to quote from it extensively, even if that means that the reader—other than the author himself—cannot check my use of his analysis against the original text.

8. Here are Oë's own comments in an interview in 1995 in which he told that despite a successful literary career he had in his mid-twenties "lost all sense of identity" and he explained: "In 1963, my son was born. This little baby was a kind of personification of my unhappiness. He looked like a baby with two heads. There was a huge growth on his head that made him look like that. This was the most important crisis in my life. The doctors made us decide whether or not to operate. Without an operation, Hikari would have died very quickly. With the operation, he might live, but with terrible, terrible difficulties. My son was born on the thirteenth of June, and I went to Hiroshima on August 1st. . . . I was escaping from my baby. These were shameful days for me to remember. I wanted to escape to some other horizon. I'd been asked to do some reportage in Hiroshima, and so I went there, fled there" (quoted in Taylor and Kassai, "Healer and the Healed," 643).

9. Thus the point that lends overriding moral importance to the existence of his disabled son is not that he is a member of the human species. From the perspective of Singer and Kuhse's impartialist utilitarianism, the capacity of having valuable experiences as a moral criterion would probably give less moral weight to the life of a profoundly mentally disabled child than it would give to the life of a healthy chimpanzee (for explorations of this claim see Paola Cavalieri and Peter Singer, *The Great Ape Project: Equality beyond Humanity* [New York: St. Martin's Press, 1994]). From the perspective of Oë's novel, however, the important point is that the chimp, for all that its life is worth, could not be the father's son. The moral importance of the child's existence is embedded in this relationship rather than in its inherent characteristics.

10. Cf. Taylor and Kassai, "Healer and Healed," 643.

11. See also Michiko N. Wilson, *The Marginal World of Kenzaburo Oë: A Study in Themes and Techniques* (New York: M. E. Sharpe, 1986).

12. Alasdair MacIntyre, "Human Identity" 4. In this section I will focus only on the connection between identity and accountability as MacIntyre sees it. I will ignore here what

he has to say on the connection between both these concepts and the condition of disability and leave that for another occasion.

13. MacIntyre, "Human Identity," 10.

14. I cannot resist giving one more superb example of Oë's imaginative powers to illustrate the point. Waiting for the desired deterioration in the son's condition, Bird visits the clinic once more. He is disappointed to see that the baby does not look like a creature on the point of death and that it is even somewhat bigger than before. Bird notices how its little fingers are furiously rubbing behind its ears as if to get rid of the lump on its head. Reassured by the doctor that the 'crisis' is soon to be expected, he leaves the hospital. Then Oë depicts the power that the child has over Bird in this way: "The minute the door closed Bird regretted not having made clear his desire to the doctor once again. He put his hand behind his ears as he walked along the corridor and began to rub his head just below the hairline with the fleshy pads of his thumbs. Gradually he arched backward, as if a heavy weight were attached to his head. He stopped short a minute later when he realized he was imitating the baby's gestures, and glanced around him nervously" (*A Personal Matter,* 123).

15. The extent to which we can choose who we want to be is one of the issues to be discussed in chapter 12.

16. I borrow this phrase from Brandt, *Theory of the Good,* 11 f.

N I N E *Responsibility for Dependent Others*

1. The argument here is confined to a claim about a sufficient condition for accepting responsibility for the disabled, leaving aside whether this claim also amounts to a stronger claim about a necessary condition. As has been explained, the argument is intended to defeat moral views grounded in a conception of disengaged reason as failing to provide a sufficient reason for accepting responsibility. To make the stronger claim I would have to show that the position defended in this chapter is superior to other positions that oppose moral views grounded in disengaged reason along similar lines, which is more than I intend to do.

2. Knut E. Løgstrup, *The Ethical Demand,* trans. T. L. Jensen (Philadelphia: Fortress Press, 1971). A newer edition is introduced by Hans Fink and Alasdair MacIntyre (Notre Dame, Ind.: University of Notre Dame Press, 1997).

3. For Bauman's interpretation of modern moral philosophy (i.e., 'ethics') and the importance of Løgstrup's work for attacking it, I will draw on *Postmodern Ethics* (Oxford: Blackwell Publishers, 1993) and *Life in Fragments.*

4. It is a failure according to Rawls's own standard of justice as fairness as a theory of political morality. Since the mentally disabled are accepted as citizens, such a theory should at least explain this fact. Because it does not succeed in giving an independent account of the moral standing of these people in terms of public reason, the contractualist method on which the theory is grounded apparently does not yield the kind of convictions it needs in order to succeed.

5. That is to say, these intuitions are going to be decisive *also* from the perspective of indirect utilitarianism. The result from both strands in modern ethical theory, Kantianism and utilitarianism, is therefore the same: it appears to be impossible for these theories to answer

the question in dispute independently from particular moral convictions and beliefs that exceed their respective conceptions of disengaged reason.

6. Løgstrup, *Ethical Demand,* 9. For a general account of Løgstrup's work see Kees van Kooten Niekerk, "Knud E. Løgstrups 'Norm und Spontaneität': eine Einführung," *Zeitschrift für Evangelische Ethik* 35 (1991): 51–59, 51. The author, to whom I owe many improvements of my account in the present chapter, provides a richly documented analysis of Løgstrup's background in existentialist thought as well in the Danish tradition of *Lebensphilosophie.* For our present purposes I will limit my account to Løgstrup's moral phenomenology.

7. It is interesting to ask whether Løgstrup's account covers *all* types of engagement between human beings. Is it true of all social interactions that the agent places herself somehow in the power of the other? In a sense it is true, as can be seen from the analysis of games presented by rational choice theory, such as, for example, the 'prisoner's dilemma'. The fact that *A* does not know how *B* will respond to his decision makes him keenly aware of his dependency on *B.* To the extent that he cannot really be sure about *B*'s response, their exchange is frustrated by a lack of trust, which is precisely what causes the 'suboptimal' result. This suggests that even strictly self-interested agents, who simply want to use others as a resource, are aware of the fact that they *do* place themselves in one another's hands in cooperative enterprises. Since this awareness is what hinders them in their engagement, it appears that also for self-interested agents trust is indispensable. See Mackie's discussion of this point in his *Ethics,* 115–20.

8. Løgstrup, *Ethical Demand,* 20 f.

9. Løgstrup, *Ethical Demand,* 23. Because of this qualification some of his commentators have read him as a 'situationist'. See Van Kooten Niekerk, "Knud Løgstrup," 55. Even though this interpretation is not surprising—given Løgstrup's existentialist background—it seems to be mistaken, as will be explained below.

10. Løgstrup, *Ethical Demand,* 22; 59–63.

11. Note how accurately this observation describes the strategy adopted by modern moral philosophy both of the utilitarian and Kantian variety.

12. Løgstrup, *Ethical Demand,* 26. Even the reciprocation of enlightened self-interest must depend on trust, however. Apparently, the author himself did not see how his description of what is involved in social interaction does include interactions motivated by self-interest, as I tried to show by referring to rational choice theory.

13. Løgstrup, *Ethical Demand,* 46.

14. Van Kooten Niekerk, "Knud Løgstrup," 53.

15. The text of this chapter in the first English edition of Løgstrup's book, chapter 2, is unnecessarily muddled by rendering the translation of Danish terms like *formidlede, mediet, formidlingen, mediumløse* by derivations from the English term 'motive,' whereas the correct translation appears to be 'mediation' (cf. the German equivalent *Vermittlung*). The correction is found in the revised edition: Knut Eljert Løgstrup, *The Ethical Demand,* 2d ed., intro. by Hans Fink and Alasdair MacIntyre (Notre Dame: University of Notre Dame Press, 1997). My references are to the first edition.

16. Løgstrup, *Ethical Demand,* 58: "The social norms give comparatively precise directives about what we shall do and what we shall refrain from doing. We are usually able to conform to these directives without even having to consider the other person, much less take

244 Notes to Pages 145–146

care of his life. We may very well live in harmony with at least many of the social norms even though we may have entirely different purposes in doing so."

17. It is important to notice that Løgstrup—at least at this stage of his thought—does not believe in the practical possibility of immediate spontaneity as a guide to moral action. Human beings do not interact morally in an unmediated, spontaneous way without threatening other persons in their otherness. On this aspect of Løgstrup's thought, see Van Kooten Niekerk, "Knud Løgstrup," 53 f. Although in his early work—including *The Ethical Demand*—Løgstrup shared the ideal of a spontaneous 'unmediated' moral life, he did not believe that it would ever be realized because of the condition of human sinfulness. In his later work, Løgstrup developed the theory of the spontaneous expressions of life in which he argued that these expressions are irresistable. We do not choose to fulfill them: they are more like inclinations than possibilities. But they can also be blocked by turning away from the other, which is why the ethical demand is not redundant. See on the connection between the demand and Christian themes of sinfulness and forgiveness, Joseph L. Allen's review article, "The Significance of a Christian Outlook on Ethics," *Journal of Religion* 53 (1973): 239–46.

18. Løgstrup, *Ethical Demand*, 44, 60–66, 111 f. See also Van Kooten Niekerk, "Knud Løgstrup," 55.

19. Løgstrup, *Ethical Demand*, 20 f., 41–45, 55–59.

20. Here Løgstrup uses the illuminating example of the difference between the parental duty to take care of a child's education, which can be done simply by sending it to school at the prescribed age, even if this is motivated by the wish to get rid of the child for at least a couple of hours each day, on the one hand, and, on the other, the duty to help the child become independent. The latter cannot be discharged by the same selfish motive but requires parental love if the child is not to become pathologically dependent on others for fear of being abandoned (*Ethical Demand*, 65).

21. Løgstrup, *Ethical Demand*, 123–25, 154 f., 165. I understand the phrase 'outlook on life' as referring to the convictions and beliefs that guide us in how we conduct our lives. In the terms of our earlier analysis, it refers to a wide conception of morality that is grounded in a substantial vision of the good life for human beings.

22. At this point we may consider the philosophical debate on the so-called golden rule. Against the interpretation that reads the golden rule as a principle of rational consistency, which is found in the writings of philosophers like Alan Gewirth and R. M. Hare, Paul Ricoeur has suggested to read it in the context of what he calls an 'economy of gift'. Thus interpreted, the rule prescribes: Since you have received, give in return. As Ricoeur explains, the fact of being cared for comes to be understood as a source of obligation to do the same for others. See Paul Ricoeur, *Amour et Justice: Mit einer deutschen Parallelübersetzung von Matthias Raden* Oswald Baier, ed. (Tübingen: J. C. B. Mohr, 1990), 48; see also by the same author, "The Golden Rule: Exegetical and Theological Perplexities," *New Testament Studies* 36 (1990): 392–97, 395; "Entre Philosophie et Théologie: La Règle d'Or en Question," *Revue d'Histoire et de Philosophie Religieuse 69* (1989): 3–9. For a discussion of the philosophical debate that follows Ricoeur's suggestion, see my essay, "The Golden Rule between Philosophy and Theology," in Alberto Bondolfi, Stefan Grotefeld, and Rudi Neuberth, eds., *Ethics, Reason and Rationality* (Münster: LIT Verlag, 1996), 145–68. The central idea of this essay is

to view moral responsibility for dependent others as motivated by gratitude rather than en-ligthened self-interest.

23. Van Kooten Niekerk made me see this point.

24. In this connection the ambiguity attached to the idea of the ethical demand as a human possibility continuously gives Løgstrup pause to reflect upon the extent of human sinfulness (see above, n. 17). His account is typically Lutheran in the sense of understanding the human condition as caught in contradiction from which only faith can save us—*simul justus ac peccator*—without paying much attention to the question of how faith may actually alter our lives (*Ethical Demand*, 126 f., 146–49, 154 f., 173–83). He writes: "From the stand-point of our very existence [e.g., the fact that we live in company with one another] . . . the demand is indeed fulfillable. Along with the blessing in which the demand is incorporated, life has provided us with all that is necessary for its fulfillment" (175). On the other hand, however, Løgstrup maintains that the failure to fulfill the demand in actual practice is a sign of human sinfulness. As indicated, this apparent tension in his view changes in his later work with the development of his theory of spontaneous expressions of life. See Van Kooten Niekerk, to whom I owe this point, "Knud Løgstrup," 54.

25. Løgstrup, *Ethical Demand*, 124. According to the author the reverse is also the case: "a person may well dispute theoretically that he has received his life as a gift while in fact he does accept it as such."

26. Bauman, *Postmodern Ethics*, 1–15; *Life in Fragments*, 10–43.

27. Bauman, *Life in Fragments*, 23.

28. Bauman, *Life in Fragments*, 11 f.

29. Bauman, *Life in Fragments*, 36 f., 42 f.; *Postmodern Ethics*, 12–5.

30. Bauman, *Postmodern Ethics*, 78 f. Having quoted Løgstrup's observation that "social convention has the effect of reducing both the trust that we show and the demand that we care for the other person's life, Bauman adds, "Conventions make life comfortable: they safe-guard life lived in the pursuit of self-interest. It only seems, on the surface, that following conventional courtesy is the intrument of togetherness. In fact, separation is the effect." See also, *Life in Fragments*, 55 f.

31. Bauman, *Life in Fragments*, 61 f.

32. In Bauman's view, the state of emotionality caused by the encounter is decisive. The moral content of the emotion itself—sympathy, fellow-feeling—is only secondary. The ex-planation is that Bauman wants to pitch the state of emotionality against the world of con-ventionality where the other is 'stereotyped'. For Bauman, responsibility is necessarily char-acterized by uncertainty and ambiguity ("Pointing my finger at the rules, re-presenting my nod with the Other as an item in the set of similar bonds, a specimen of a category, a case of a general rule—I avoid all responsibility except a procedural one" [*Life in Fragments*, 63]). Thus the state of emotionality is itself understood as "neutral in relation to good and evil" (62). The problem with this view is that negative emotions—repulsion, envy, con-tempt, disgust—cannot trigger a sense of responsibility in the agent. Bauman apparently conflates the emotional state of responding sympathetically with the state of knowing how to act following upon that response. But sympathy does not imply that the agent knows what to do. It only implies that she feels responsible for doing something *for or with* the other rather than remaining indifferent. The kind of emotion that signals the response cannot

be secondary but forces itself upon the agent. At least, that is what I take Løgstrup's view to be. One cannot be a moral agent without having the emotion of sympathy, or, more accurately, being a moral agent manifests itself in the fact that one experiences this emotional state as being present in oneself.

33. See Van Kooten Niekerk, "Knud Løgstrup," 58.

34. These remarks draw on Løgstrup's later book *Norm und Spontaneität* (Tübingen: J. C. B. Mohr, 1989), where he explains obedience—as distinct from acceptance—as *Ersatzmotiv*, a second-rate motive, which renders the agent's response to the demand as being a matter of her duty (see Van Kooten Niekerk, "Knud Løgstrup," 54).

35. The issue of how activity and passivity interact in the process of shaping our lives will be the subject of extensive discussion in the last chapter, but a brief comment is appropriate here. The issue at stake is that of the relation between freedom and fulfillment. When human beings abrogate the traditional lives they are living, they aspire to change some aspects of their own identity. This may be because they have discovered a new self, so that to change their lives is, in a way, to make it fit with what they have come to see as their true selves. However, self-deception is always a possibility. That is to say, in criticizing and rejecting (certain aspects of) what has been handed down to us by previous generations, we may believe ourselves to have arrived at the stage of true freedom. But it may also be the case that we have fallen prey to the latest cultural and intellectual fashion. Løgstrup addresses this issue when he considers the modern view that individuals should be sovereign over their own lives with regard to their cultural heritage and background. He believes this to be a mistake: "The changes we are able to accomplish in this respect are extremely limited. We are in the power of the psychic content of our various particular relationships and institutions, a content which they had prior to our growing up in them or even getting into them. . . . Our disposition, our individuality, our personality, and whatever other part of our make-up we might want to mention have simply been constituted and shaped by this content" (Logstrup, *Ethical Demand,* 107).

36. Again, this is not to deny the wounded selves of those among us that have been, or still are, the victim of habitual oppression, abuse, or neglect. But it is to deny that an account of the moral life should take the perversion of moral relationships that manifests itself in oppression, abuse, and neglect as paradigmatic. It is also to deny, therefore, that this account must proceed from the notion of the moral life being dominated by the dynamics of power and inequality. To proceed in that way, it seems to me, is to conflate the ethical and the political, which is largely what modern moral philosophy appears to have been engaged in doing.

37. Bauman thinks that no modern ethical theory has been more thorough in destroying the primordial moral impulse in facing the other than utilitarianism. The reason is that it turned the original intention of caring for the other into a universal law: "The utilitarian recipe for universal happiness differs from loving care the way the latest tariff of welfare handouts differs from sharing a meal" (*Postmodern Ethics,* 103).

38. According to Van Kooten Niekerk, the suggestion that the task of articulating the ethical demand with the appropriate motive should be linked to the need for developing the moral character required for that capability, would probably have offended Løgstrup's Lu-

theran sensibilities. Mainstream Protestantism in general never had much use for the notion of developing moral character as a way to attain personal growth, given its all-consuming preoccupation with human sinfulness.

39. Recognition of the gift of life in the sense explained is never free from the danger of being subverted or ignored because, and insofar as, createdness is never present in our lives without being disrupted by the condition of fallenness—hence the possibility that people receive less than they should because others fail to give what they themselves have received.

TEN *The Presumption of Suffering*

1. Kathryn Ida Scorgie, "From Devastation to Transformation: Managing Life when a Child is Disabled" (Diss., University of Alberta, 1996). The author reviews the professional literature on counseling parents with disabled children (1–3, 22–72, 73–79). She found that the main focus is on the negative effects of parenting a child with disabilities (22).

2. "The desire to have children must be among the most basic of human instincts" (Edwards and Sharpe, "Social Values," 87–94, 87). See also chapter 6, note 4 for references to feminist discussions of 'pronatalism'. For a general discussion see Kenneth D. Alpern, "Genetic Puzzles and Stork Stories: On the Meaning and Significance of Having Children," in Alpern, *Ethics,* 147–69, 149 f.

3. Engelhardt, *Foundations,* 239.

4. As an example, cf. this assertion by Wertz and Fletcher: "The writings of parents of children with disabilities present a mixed message. Although generally intended to inspire by presenting triumphs over adversity, many of these biographies describe the immense effort and sacrifice on the part of the parents. There is no clear outcome that might be labeled 'joy'. Instead, many parents write as if the grieving process that began at the child's birth continues throughout the child's life, as a never ending sense of loss" ("A Critique of Some Feminist Challenges," 385–403, 389). For a similar account see Singer and Kuhse, *Should the Baby Live?,* 152.

5. See Robert Wuthnow, *Learning to Care: Elementary Kindness in an Age of Indifference* (New York: Oxford University Press, 1995), 6–11, 76–81. The author criticizes the tendency in contemporary culture to reduce moral language to language about feelings. He argues that inquiring into the reasons that motivate people to care for others is important in order to understand how self-understanding enters into their behavior.

6. There is, of course, the literature on attitudes towards the disabled both in society and in the realm of politics. There is also literature where experiences of parents are narrated autobiographically (see below, note 17). But there is not much in the *ethical* literature that evaluates these reports. Among the few exceptions is Hauerwas, *Suffering Presence;* also by the same author *Naming the Silences: God, Medicine and the Problem of Suffering* (Grand Rapids: Wm. B. Eerdmans, 1990). For a brief discussion of rational inquiry into the reasons governing human reproduction, see Alpern, *Ethics,* 149 ff. For a typical example of dealing with reproduction and disabilities within a liberal framework see Kluge, "The Right to Have Children," *Bioethics in a Canadian Context* (Scarborough: Prentice Hall, 1992), 302–29.

7. In this chapter I will therefore ignore questions about whether one should abstain from procreation in order to prevent the suffering of a future child. This means that the responsibilities that parents have toward their children will not be discussed here as an independent problem. It does not mean that there is no problem. For parental responsibilities toward their unborn children see the literature on 'wrongful' life. For example: M. D. Bayles, "Harm to the Unconceived," *Philosophy and Public Affairs* 5 (1976): 292–304; George Annas, "Righting the Wrong of Wrongful Life," *Hastings Center Report* 11 (February 1981); P. G. Peters, "Protecting the Unconceived: Nonexistence, Avoidability, and Reproductive Technology," *Arizona Law Review* 31 (1989): 487–548; Kluge, *Biomedical Ethics,* 341–44.

8. Robert F. Weir, *Selective Nontreatment of Handicapped Newborns: Moral Dilemmas in Neonatal Medicine* (New York: Oxford University Press, 1984), 59–90 is still one of the best discussions in this area.

9. A famous court case in the Netherlands involved a decision to withhold surgery from a newborn infant with Down syndrome for a duodenal atresia, which is a blockage of the intestines that prevents food from being absorbed by the body. Expert testimonies regarding the quality of life of children with Down syndrome were radically opposed. See R. W. M. Croughs, "Recht op leven van ernstig gehandicapte kinderen" (The right to life of severely handicapped children), *Medisch Contact* 44 (1989): 647–51 and J. Molenaar et al., "Geneeskunde, dienares der barmhartigheid" (Medicine, the servant of mercy), *Nederlands Tijdschrift voor Geneeskunde* 132 (1988): 1913–17.

10. See the references to the debate between 'normativism' and 'non-normativism' with regard to the concept of disease in chapter 3, 44–46.

11. In assessing expectations of suffering attached to reproductive decisions one factor should not be left unnoticed, namely the suffering that results from the decision to terminate a pregnancy. Given the fact that in most cases the pregnancy was very much wanted, parents often do mourn intensely, sometimes even for years, after the termination of a pregnancy for reasons of fetal abnormality. See D. M. Zuskar, "The Psychological Impact of Prenatal Diagnosis of Fetal Abnormality: Strategies for Investigation and Intervention," *Women and Health* 12 (1987): 91–103; Margaretha C. A. White-Van Mourik et al., "The Psychological Sequela of a Second Trimester Termination of Pregnancy for Fetal Abnormality over a Two Year Period," in Gerry Evers-Kieboom et al., eds., *Psychosocial Aspects of Genetic Counseling* (New York: John Wiley & Sons, 1992), 61–74; Margaretha C. A. White-Van Mourik, "Looking from the Outside—Reactions to a Termination of Pregnancy for Fetal Abnormality From the Point of View of Those Who Care," in L. Abramsky and J. Chapple, eds., *Prenatal Diagnosis: The Human Side* (London: Chapman & Hall, 1994), 181–201.

12. For a discussion that touches upon similar points covered in this chapter, but with respect to issues of death and dying, see Daniel Callahan, *The Troubled Dream of Life: Living with Mortality* (New York: Simon & Schuster, 1993), chs. 4–7.

13. Hauerwas, *Suffering Presence,* 165–68. Let me quote McKenny's account of 'Hauerwas' geography of suffering,' as he calls it: "First is the suffering that has a point because it either (1) fits into or at least does not disrupt our moral projects (which may mean that it is not suffering in the strict sense), or (2) occurs as a result of our moral convictions. Second is suffering that is pointless and which either (3) cannot be cured without violating one or more moral convictions, (4) cannot be cured at all (whether in general or for a specific indi-

vidual) due to the limitations or the tragic nature of medicine, or (5) can be cured and does not fit into our moral projects" (McKenny, *To Relieve the Human Condition,* 180–81). McKenny's point is that modern technological medicine is based on the Baconian view that reduces all forms of suffering to (5). My account of Hauerwas's distinctions focuses on a different point, which is the question of whether (1) can be explained as a mediation between (2) and (4).

14. This by no means necessarily expresses a shortsighted—let alone selfish—point of view, because it is very likely that people fear the suffering of a life *with* a disabled child because they fear witnessing the suffering *of* their child. Again, this possibility is ignored in the present chapter because we are considering judgments about lives affected by genetic disorders that cause impairments without illness. The disabled individuals in question have problems, but ordinarily those problems do not stem from ill health. Disabled children within this category may suffer indeed, but, if they do, it is suffering caused by the limitations imposed on them by society and social attitudes.

15. Hauerwas, *Suffering Presence,* 166.

16. See A. P. O'Connor et al., "Understanding the Cancer Patient's Search for Meaning," *Cancer Nursing* 13 (1990): 167–75.

17. For parental testimonies see A. Fraiberg and L. Fraiberg, *Insights from the Blind: Comparative Studies of Blind and Sighted Infants* (New York: New American Library, 1979); Alex F. DeFord, *The Life of a Child* (New York: The American Library, 1984); M. Forecki, *Speak to Me* (Washington, D.C.: Gallaudet University Press, 1985); Spradley and Spradley *Deaf Like Me;* M. Dorris *The Broken Cord* (New York: Harper & Row, 1989); D. Meyer, ed., *Uncommon Fathers: Reflections on Raising a Child with a Disability* (Bethesda: Woodbine House, 1995); and Frances M. Young, *Face to Face: A Narrative Essay in the Theology of Suffering* (Edinburgh: T. & T. Clark, 1990).

18. John Stuart Mill, *Utilitarianism, On Liberty, and Considerations on Representative Government,* ed. H. B. Acton (London: Dent, 1992), 10.

19. See Isaiah Berlin, "John Stuart Mill and the End of Life," in *Four Essays,* 173–206. According to Berlin, Mill opposed the doctrine of utilitarianism as taught by Bentham and his own father, James Mill, precisely because they argued for the maximization of happiness as pleasurableness by whatever means were the most effective: "Bentham and [James] Mill believed in education and legislation as the roads to happiness. But if a shorter way had been discovered, in the form of pills to swallow, techniques of subliminal suggestion, or other means of conditioning human beings . . . they might well have accepted this as a better, because more effective and perhaps less costly, alternative than the means that they had advocated. John Stuart Mill, as he made plain both by his life and by his writings, would have rejected with both hands any such solution. He would have condemned it as degrading the nature of man. For him man differs from animals primarily neither as the possessor of reason, nor as the inventor of tools and methods, but as a being capable of choice. . . . The seeker of ends, and not merely of means, ends that he pursues, each in his own fashion" (177 f.).

20. The experiment was first presented in *Anarchy,* 42–45. Here I follow Nozick's discussion of the same idea in his *The Examined Life* (New York: Simon and Schuster, 1986), 104–8.

21. Nozick, *The Examined Life,* 106. For an argument that neither our desires nor our reflective responses to our desires should be taken at face value because of the possibility of self-deception see Alpern, "Genetic Puzzles," 152–57.

22. As Nozick puts it: "We care about more than just how things feel to us from the inside; there is more to life than feeling happy. We are about what actually is the case. We want certain situations we value, prize, and think important to actually hold and be so. . . . We want to be importantly connected to reality, not to live in a delusion" (*The Examined Life*, 106).

23. On Berlin's interpretation, this is what made John Stuart Mill critical of Benthamite utilitarianism. The idea that the satisfaction of desire—'feeling good'—constituted the comprehensive good deprived individuals of the necessity to try new 'experiments' in living their lives, to create diversity, to transform themselves so as to find out what they are capable of achieving (see "John Stuart Mill," 180 ff.). Mill believed, according to Berlin: "that man is spontaneous, that he has freedom of choice, that he moulds his own character, that as a result of the interplay of men with nature and with other men something novel continuously arises, and that this novelty is precisely what is most characteristic and most human in men" (189).

24. For this notion of by-product, see Jon Elster, *Sour Grapes: Studies in the Subversion of Rationality* (Cambridge: Cambridge University Press, 1983). The theme of fulfillment as 'unsolicited gift' will be extensively discussed in the last chapter when we look into modern conceptions of the meaning of life.

25. Scorgie, "From Devastation to Transformation," 74.

26. See C. J. Palus, "Transformative Experiences of Adulthood: A New Look at the Seasons of Life," in J. Demick et. al., eds., *Parental Development* (Hillsdale: Erlbaum, 1993), 39–58. The author defines a transformative experience as "a life event and its outcome, such that the event is given a central role within a self-narrative in causing, catalyzing, or symbolizing substantial, lasting psychological change" (40). For studies that report positive change in terms of personal growth as a by-product of crisis experiences see A. M. Aldwin, *Stress, Coping, and Development: An Integrative Perspective* (New York: Guilford Press, 1994); R. Janoff-Bulman, *Shattered Assumptions: Towards a New Psychology of Trauma* (New York: Macmillan, 1992); R. Moos, ed., *Coping with Life Crises: An Integrated Approach* (New York: Plenum Press, 1986). The exploration of the notion of parenting a disabled child as the cause of personal transformation will be continued in the next chapter.

27. The danger here is in the suggestion that facing the difficulties that a life with hardships can bring is an option that can be *chosen* as a *means* to attaining the good life, which turns the argument into something like a secular 'theodicy': there is a way to make sense of human suffering which consists in the fact that it enables us to become better people. Contrary to his intentions, McKenny comes close to falling into this trap when he talks about accepting the finitude and mortality of the body as a 'self-regarding concern' (*To Relieve the Human Condition*, 222). Crucial in this connection is that we avoid an instrumentalist account of suffering, which is the reason why I press the characterization of personal growth and fulfillment as a by-product (see above, note 24). We cannot say that facing the task of parenting a disabled child is a way to develop moral character because it takes moral character to do so. The enrichment claim is explained in retrospect, not prospectively. People explain what facing this task did with them in their lives, but they do not explain this as if it were a rational plan of life. What distinguishes these parents is that they have managed to face their own pain and disappointment, that they have integrated it into the story of their life, and that in doing so, they have been shown capable of attending the hardships of

their disabled children. The convictions and beliefs that enabled them to face this task were not attuned to a self-regarding concern about their own character, but to an other-regarding concern, namely the task of accepting responsibility for their child as the other that is delivered into their hands (to use Løgstrup's phrase). If this is correct, it implies that people who in facing reproductive decisions resolve to accept this task, will more likely be guided by reasons from moral standing rather than by reason from quality of life. If the future of one's own life is the object of reflection, one probably will not find reasons to accept it, which is likely to be the best result. If the question is what to think of a disabled child is the object, however, things may be different. This explains why people who are guided by MS reasons can find fulfillment as an unsolicited by-product, and why people guided by QL reasons are prone to block themselves from receiving such a gift.

28. See Callahan, *The Troubled Dream,* 94–100.

29. Cf. Hauerwas: "In a way, modern medicine exemplifies the predicament of the Enlightenment project, which hopes to make society a collection of individuals free from the bonds of necessity other than those we choose. In many ways that project has been accomplished, only now we have discovered that the very freedom we sought has, ironically, become a kind of bondage. Put in the language of theodicy, we now suffer from the means we tried to use to eliminate suffering" (*Naming the Silences,* 108).

30. See above, p. 165.

31. The meaning of learning this task probably explains to some extent why very recently some AIDS patients who have reconciled themselves with the fact of impending death experience difficulty in accepting the possibility of prolonged life after the development of new drugs. I owe this information to personal communication with Marli Huijer.

32. Cf. McKenny's claim that the effort to render ourselves immune to suffering "restricts our freedom and power to make what happens to us our own and deprives us of the skills and practices of caring that are the only appropriate response to suffering that cannot be cured. It is also destructive to others. It subordinates persons to diseases, subjects patients to further (avoidable) suffering by its unwillingness to accept the inevitability of some pointless suffering, and is willing in the interest of eliminating suffering to eliminate those who suffer. In short, far from resolving the problem of alienation, the Baconian project, by replacing the traditional moral commitments of medicine with its utopian and illusory dream of eliminating suffering, merely perpetuates it, since the inevitable limits of medicine as a tragic profession guarantee that there will always be pointless suffering and some sufferers who will remind us of our subjection to contingency and fortune" (*To Relieve the Human Condition,* 174). How the modern preoccupation with control over our lives may affect practices of caring for the disabled will be the subject of our discussion in chapter 12.

33. Callahan, *The Troubled Dream,* 153: "We none of us like to imagine ourselves utterly deprived of a right and an ability to make choices about our lives, to make our lives our own. We cannot, in any case, live with modern medicine without making choices. Mere passivity and sheer resignation will not do: we can too easily be used and abused. But we can become our own person in our choices, and that person can be someone who sees the subtle but real traps in an overwhelming urge to achieve full and perfect control. My target has been the mistaken belief that a *necessary* condition of our self-worth is our control of our lives" (see also 220–23).

34. Here we return to the paradox of health that was noticed already in chapter 1: the more people pay attention to their health status the lesser the confidence they have in the solidity of their health. See Verwey, "Preventive Medicine," 83–86.

35. In commenting on the view of happiness as the ultimate value, Nozick observes with regard to the Freudian 'reality principle' that it requires that we refrain from seeking satisfaction, given certain facts about the world, because it is more expedient for the goal of satisfaction to accept detour or delay. According to Nozick, the Freudian reality principle demands a kind of prudential behavior (*The Examined Life*, 102). In contradistinction to this principle Nozick presents a second reality principle, which tells us to seek true beliefs about ourselves that enable us to be in touch with reality as a means of responding adequately to it (*The Examined Life*, 106).

36. Callahan, *The Troubled Dream*, 154 f.: "It is an enormous error to act as if the possession of choice could obviate the need for the kind of individual character necessary either to make good choices when we have to make them, or to live well and without despair in the absence of choice. We can only live without choice if we have become the kind of person who can be a person while lacking choice. To make our sense of well-being and dignity dependent upon a capacity to control and manipulate our circumstances is already to have set ourselves up for a fall. We will have become the kind of person who has lost sight of reality, who has found and wallowed in the ultimate evasion of hard truth, thinking our death cannot be meaningful unless a self-creation, or [cannot be] tolerable unless devoid of suffering and self-determination."

ELEVEN *The Transformation Experience*

1. Scorgie, "From Devastation to Transformation." Later in this chapter I will draw extensively on the insights provided by this study.

2. David M. Biebel, "The Riddle of Suffering," in Kilner, Pentz, and Young, *Genetic Ethics*, 3–6, 4.

3. See H. Lane et al., *A Journey into the Deaf-World* (San Diego: Dawn Sign Press, 1996); Spradley and Spradley, *Deaf Like Me*.

4. See above chapter 4, notes 14 and 15.

5. See D. Wasserman, "Some Moral Issues in the Correction of Impairments," *Journal of Social Philosophy* 27 (1996): 128–45, 138.

6. It is important to note that people who adopt this position are not saying that they *now* think that they should have chosen to prevent the life of their child had there been a choice, but that they believe that *at that time* they might have made this choice.

7. T. Nagel, *The View from Nowhere* (Oxford: Oxford University Press, 1986), 210. In this section I will use Nagel's account as an explanatory device. I will later raise some critical questions, particularly with regard to the suggested inevitability of the tension between our 'objective' and 'subjective' selves, eventually mounting to absurdity.

8. Here I have in mind predominantly children with profound mental disabilities. Within this category there are no people who would be capable of living lives of their own, not even under the most favorable social conditions.

9. It should be noted that this claim is hypothetical: if people are ambivalent about the lives of disabled children, this does not necessarily mean that they are incoherent or confused. This ambivalence can be explained by an inner division between the 'objective' and 'subjective' selves.

10. Nagel, *View from Nowhere*, 214.

11. A parent of a child with a rare metabolic condition says: "If I look at the big picture with L——, it's a very difficult picture. And I don't like to look at it. I don't choose to look at it" (Scorgie, "From Devastation to Transformation," 129).

12. Nagel locates this possibility in the realm of aesthetics: "The experience of great beauty tends to unify the self: the object engages us immediately and totally in a way that makes distinctions among points of view irrelevant" (*View from Nowhere*, 223).

13. Scorgie, "From Devastation to Transformation," 1–3. See also W. Wolfensberger, "Counseling Parents of the Retarded," in A. Baumeister, ed., *Mental Retardation: Appraisal, Education and Rehabilitation* (Chicago: Aldine Press, 1967), 329–400.

14. Scorgie's main theoretical source is Aldwin, *Stress, Coping, and Development*. This author suggests that when how people deal with crises in their lives is researched only in terms of reducing the negative psychological effects of the 'stress factor,' possible positive outcomes of such crises will be overlooked (Scorgie, "From Devastation to Transformation," 73).

15. Scorgie's study is based on a series of semi-structured interviews with parents from fourteen families resulting in the formation of nine themes on the basis of which a 'Life Management Survey' was constructed. The survey was used to assess the extent to which a larger sampling of parents with disabled children corroborated the earlier findings. I will ignore methodological aspects of the study and its results. Nor am I concerned with the extent to which her conclusions are representative for other groups of parents. For our purposes we can be content that they hold for some and ask what makes it possible that some people find a blessing where others can experience only a curse. However, it is important to understand that Scorgie's study aims at explaining why families with disabled children manage to do well. This implies that she has neither been investigating families that fail nor why they fail.

16. Scorgie, "From Devastation to Transformation," 5.

17. Scorgie, "From Devastation to Transformation," 146–54.

18. The transformation experiences may therefore not only be viewed as a result but also as a condition. Scorgie suggests something similar when she says that transformations may be foundational to positive outcomes ("From Devastation to Transformation," 197). She quotes Aldwin: "Rather than simply a homeostatic function, the more important role of coping may be transformation" (Aldwin, *Stress, Coping, and Development*, 270). The suggestion is not that in due course the journey of life may turn out to be a rewarding one because one finds oneself to be positively transformed. It is rather that being transformed is part of what makes the journey possible.

19. Scorgie, "From Devastation to Transformation," 105.

20. Scorgie, "From Devastation to Transformation," 113 ff., 194.

21. Scorgie, "From Devastation to Transformation," 194.

22. Scorgie, "From Devastation to Transformation," 30–33.

23. In a paper commenting and elaborating on Scorgie's study, Dick Sobsey refers to some of the older literature that discusses the experience of disintegration, that is, the collapse

of one's expectations and hopes with regard to one's future. The major crisis of the birth of a disabled child affects one's self-esteem and self-confidence, and renders the meaning of life incoherent. Many researchers tend to regard this experience of disintegration the normal parental response. Any claim to positive aspects of parenting is interpreted as 'denial'. In view of this literature, Scorgie's—and Sobsey's—interpretation works just the other way around. Ignoring transforming experiences is a denial of the hope that parents have: not the hope that the disability will be miraculously cured but the hope that energizes creative responses (Scorgie, "From Devastation to Transformation," 195 f.). Disintegration is thus not taken as a permanent state with which people must learn to cope—"something we grow *in spite of*," as Sobsey puts it—but as the first step toward transformation that allows the reintegration of the self. To the extent that parents try to continue their 'formative' lives by incorporating the care for their disabled child in their daily routine they are most likely to experience negative coping. Only if they allow themselves and their lives to be changed the possibility of transformation appears. See D. Sobsey, "Family Transformation: From Dale Evans to Neil Young," in R. Friedlander and Sobsey, eds., *Conference Proceedings: Through the Lifespan* (Kingston: National Association for Persons with Developmental Disabilities and Mental Health Needs, 1996), 13–16.

24. R. Haughton, *The Transformation of Man: A Study of Conversion and Community* (New York: Paulist Press, 1967), 12. I am indebted to Prof. Stanley Hauerwas for drawing my attention to Haughton's rich book.

25. Haughton, *Transformation of Man*, 107.

26. Haughton has an antagonistic conception of the relation between formation and transformation. They have nothing in common, she says, but "Without the long process of formation there could be no transformation, yet no amount of careful formation can transform. Transformation is a timeless point of decision, yet it can only operate in the personality formed throught time-conditioned stages of development, and its effects can be only worked out in terms of that formation" (*Transformation of Man*, 32). Transformation thus conceived indicates a crisis of the 'old' self that is overcome by means of reintegrating the devastating experience into a 'new' self.

27. Cf. Sobsey: "Failure to be adequately shattered by the experience of parenting an atypical child is frequently viewed as denial and considered grounds for a dose of 'reality' to eliminate 'false hope'. Professionals rarely consider the possibility that parental hope might be justified or beneficial. They rarely consider the possibility that the so-called 'reality therapy' that they are pushing might be 'false despair' and that false despair may be a thousand times more destructive than false hope" ("Family Transformation," 14). See also C. Goodey, "Fools and Heretics: Parents' Views of Professionals," in T. Booth, ed., *Learning for All* (London: Routledge, 1991), 165–76.

28. This is one of the leading concerns in Robert Wuthnow's study (*Learning to Care*) on the motivational structure of volunteering in contemporary America. Similar concerns are expressed by Robert Bellah and his colleagues in *Habits of the Heart: Individualism and Commitment in American Life* (New York: Harper & Row, 1985).

29. Haughton, *Transformation of Man*, 111.

30. H. J. Karp, "If Not Always the Victor, Always the Hero," in Meyer, *Uncommon Fathers*, 102–12.

31. A recent Dutch study collected a number of historical testimonies of parents who received their disabled child 'for the second time', for example in cases where the child was supposed to die but survived, upon which they decided to accept it, not unlike what happens in Kenzaburo Oë's novel *A Personal Matter*. See Inge Mans, *Zin der zotheid: Vijf eeuwen cultuurgeschiedenis van zotten, onnozelen en zwakzinnigen* (The sense of folly: Five centuries of the cultural history of fools, innocents and the mentally retarded) (Amsterdam: Bert Bakker, 1998), 88 ff. Mans describes the phenomenon in connection with the ancient rituals regarding the so-called changeling, where by means of some mysterious event parents received their disabled children back from evil spirits. See C. Haffter, "The Changeling: History and Psychodynamics of Attitudes to Handicapped Children in European Folklore," *Journal of the History of Behavioral Sciences* 4 (1968): 55–62 and C. Goodey, "John Locke's Idiots in the Natural History of the Mind," *History of Psychiatry* 4 (1994): 215–50.

32. Sobsey, "Family Transformation," 15.

TWELVE *The Meaning of Life in Liberal Society*

1. This is the central theme in W. Stoker, *Is The Quest for Meaning the Quest for God? The Religious Ascription of Meaning in Relation to the Secular Ascription of Meaning: A Theological Study,* trans. Lucy Jansen and Henry Jansen (Amsterdam/Atlanta: Rodopi, 1996). See particularly 170–79 where Stoker opposes the philosophical positions that take both notions as representing alternative conceptions of meaning, respectively the 'objectivist' (finding) and 'subjectivist' (giving). He considers both positions to be false, because the subjective and objective aspects of meaning cannot be separated (171).

2. Vincent Brümmer, *Theology and Philosophical Inquiry: An Introduction* (London: Macmillan, 1981), 121.

3. See R. Nozick, *Philosophical Explanations* (Oxford: Oxford University Press, 1981), 594.

4. This is, again, Thomas Nagel's point about the perspective on our lives from the outside that we discussed in the previous chapter. In Nagel's view, it will be recalled, the threat of alienation is irradicably attached to this perspective, which accounts for the experience of the absurd in human existence.

5. Stoker, *Quest*, 6–7.

6. An interesting question is how one should conceive of the connections between various levels and structures. Traditonally, theologians are the ones who think that religion—and therefore ultimately God—is the most encompassing 'entity' for conferring meaning upon our lives. That is to say, in their view God is equivalent to 'ultimate reality' (to borrow Paul Tillich's term) or to 'the whole of reality' (as Wolfgang Pannenberg has it). Stoker's book is a theological attempt to take seriously the rejection of this particular claim by secular thinkers. The opposite position regards the outstanding feature of modern existence to be the fact that people construct their own images and hierarchies of heaven and earth. Consequently, in this view, being a fan of Amsterdam's famous soccer club *Ajax* is just as capable of conferring meaning upon one's daily experience as any religion may do.

7. The belief in ontological freedom—i.e., the belief that objects are not just instances of an essence that determines what they 'really' are, with the result that their particular properties are merely 'accidental'—does not stand on its own, but is on a par with other beliefs such as the belief that any statement about the essence of things cannot be separated from our conceptual schemes. I owe this point to Jan Bransen.

8. Claude Lévi-Strauss, *The Savage Mind* (Chicago: University of Chicago Press, 1966), 17.

9. See Jeffrey Stout, *Ethics after Babel: The Languages of Morals and Their Discontents* (Cambridge: James Clarke & Co., 1988), 74 f. It will be recalled that Lévi-Strauss uses the metaphor of *bricolage* in order to characterize the premodern mind that operates in a non-constructionist way.

10. Cf. R. Braidotti, *Nomadic Subjects: Embodiment and Sexual Difference in Contemporary Feminist Theory* (New York: Columbia University Press, 1995).

11. R. Rorty, *Contingency, Irony and Solidarity* (Cambridge: Cambridge University Press, 1989), 3–22; 23–43.

12. See Rorty, *Contingency,* 39 f. where he explains the shift towards radical contingency in authors such as Nietzsche and Proust as the appreciation of the power of redescription, which is "the power of language to make new and different things possible and important—an appreciation which becomes possible only when one's aim becomes an expanding repertoire of alternative descriptions rather than The One Right Description. Such a shift in aim is possible only to the extent that both the world and the self have been de-divinized."

13. Rawls, *Theory of Justice,* 563 f.

14. Kymlicka, *Liberalism,* 50 f.

15. Kymlicka, *Liberalism,* 165.

16. This account of Kymlicka's views may make him look unduly 'decisionistic', however, since in his later work he stresses the fact that revising our commitments and convictions is a very hard and difficult process which may take us a lifetime to achieve (see Kymlicka, *Multicultural Citizenship,* 84–93). Furthermore, it should be noted that Kymlicka's argument addresses issues concerning the political philosophy of liberalism, which makes his interest primarily to be individual freedom. Ultimately, the meaning of life is for Kymlicka a matter of private judgment according to which experiences are meaningful *because* we have chosen to be engaged in them.

17. See G. M. van Asperen, "Eén temidden van velen: zingeving en ethiek" (One among many: The quest for meaning and ethics), in G. A. Van der Wal and F. L. C. M. Jacobs, red., *Vragen naar zin* (The quest for meaning) (Baarn: Ambo, 1992), 86–103. The author argues that freedom of choice in liberal society creates a peculiar paradox with regard to the quest for meaning: "This freedom is not so much the freedom to forge social ties *ex nihilo,* but to leave the ties in which we no longer feel at home. That freedom summons a demand for reflexivity: one does not do things just of the sake of doing them, but one needs to be justified in doing them, if only before oneself. The demand for reflexivity in modern societies is incomparably more intense than in a traditional society, where there is an undisputed consensus about meaning and purpose. Whenever the (legitimate) demand for reflexivity is translated as a demand for total transparency, as the demand to give a rational foundation for that by which one is motivated, then this has asked too much" (97, trans. by the present author).

18. There is an analogy between how liberal theorists such as Kymlicka construct 'meaning' as the object of deliberate evaluation and choice on the one hand and how Harry Frankfurt, on the other, does the same with desire (see H. Frankfurt, "Freedom of the Will and the Concept of a Person," in John Christman, ed., *The Inner Citadel* (Oxford: Oxford University Press, 1989), 63–76). Frankfurt distinguishes between two levels on which I can have desires. On the first level what traditionally were called the natural inclinations are operative, being the kind of things that human beings ordinary feel an urge to do or possess: to eat, drink, have sex, play, talk, and so on. On the second level the person develops self-critical desires with regard to her first-level desires. Herein lies the possibility of her free will and autonomy. Natural inclinations are given to us but in the sense of presenting themselves as the object of deliberate evaluation and choice. A problem for Frankfurt is to explain the source of our self-critical second-level desires. His theory is threatened by an infinite regress that he can stop only by claiming that at some point the agent "makes up her mind" and identifies herself with her most prominent desires concerning herself (see H. Frankfurt, "Identification and Wholeheartedness," in H. Frankfurt, *The Importance of What We Care About* (Cambridge: Cambridge University Press, 1988), 159–76). However, this solution does not work because the question then is, What causes the agent to make up her mind in this particular way? The infinite regress will not go away, which suggests that the transparency of the self that is presupposed in Frankfurt's notion of free will is illusory. The reason for this is not hard to find, because the will only finds itself 'willing'. That is to say, we confront our will only in a state of desiring something, as Augustine already recognized. An analoguous problem haunts all attempts to construe the self as the source of meaning. We succeed in finding meaning in things because and insofar as we are already attached to them. (On the problem of infinite regress that threatens Frankfurt's solution see Jan Bransen, "Identification and the Idea of an Alternative of Oneself," *European Journal of Philosophy* 4 (1996): 1–16.)

19. Stoker, *Quest*, 203.

20. A. MacIntyre, *After Virtue: A Study in Moral Theory* (Notre Dame: University of Notre Dame Press, 1981), 175 f.

21. We should recall the point about the nature of choice and control that parents of disabled children who manage to live rewarding lives underlined in connection with the notion of living with uncertainty (see above, chapter 11). In their account, the values attached to reflective activity—self-confidence, being in control, the will to succeed—are qualities of knowing how to respond. These qualities were achieved only *after* having surrendered and given in to the fact that their lives were going to be very different from what they previously expected them to be.

22. See Van Asperen, "Eén temidden van velen", 97, where she argues that "the experiental dimension of meaning precedes the fact of its being consciously and explicitly ascertained."

23. Kymlicka, *Liberalism*, 52.

24. This notion is found in Elster, *Sour Grapes*, 43–108.

25. Scorgie, "From Devastation to Transformation," 151 ff.

Bibliography

Aldwin, A. M. *Stress, Coping, and Development: An Integrative Perspective.* New York: Guilford Press, 1994.

Allen, Joseph L. "The Significance of a Christian Outlook on Ethics." *Journal of Religion* 53 (1973): 239–46.

Alpern, Kenneth D. "Genetic Puzzles and Stork Stories: On the Meaning and Significance of Having Children." In Kenneth D. Alpern, ed., *The Ethics of Reproductive Technology,* pp. 147–69. New York, Oxford: Oxford University Press, 1992.

Alpern, Kenneth D., ed. *The Ethics of Reproductive Technology.* New York, Oxford: Oxford University Press, 1992.

American Psychiatric Association. *Diagnostic and Statistical Manual of Mental Disorders.* DSM-4. 4th ed. Washington, D.C.: APA, 1994.

"American Society of Human Genetics Statement on Clinical Genetics and Freedom of Choice." *American Journal of Human Genetics* 48 (1991): 1011.

Annas, George. "Righting the Wrong of Wrongful Life." *Hastings Center Report* 11 (February 1981).

Asch, Adrienne. "Reproductive Technology and Disability." In S. Cohen and N. Taub, eds., *Reproductive Laws for the 1990s,* pp. 69–127. Clifton: Humana Press, 1989.

Asch, Adrienne, and Gail Geller. "Feminism, Bioethics, and Genetics." In Susan Wolf, ed., *Feminism and Bioethics,* pp. 318–50. New York: Oxford University Press, 1996.

Bauman, Zygmunt. *Life in Fragments: Essays in Postmodern Morality.* Oxford: Blackwell, 1995.

———. *Postmodern Ethics.* Oxford: Blackwell, 1993.

Bayles, Michael D. "Harm to the Unconceived." *Philosophy & Public Affairs* 5 (1976): 292–304.

Beauchamp, Tom L. "The Four Principles Approach." In Raanan Gillon, ed., *Principles of Health Care Ethics,* pp. 3–12. Chichester: John Wiley, 1994.

Beauchamp, Tom L., and James F. Childress. *Principles of Biomedical Ethics.* 4th ed. New York/Oxford: Oxford University Press, 1994.

Beauchamp, Tom L., and LeRoy Walters, eds., *Contemporary Issues in Bioethics.* 4th ed. Belmont, Calif.: Wadsworth, 1994.

Beiner, Ronald. "Liberalism in the Cross-Hairs of Theory." In Ronald Beiner, ed., *Philosophy in a Time of Lost Spirit,* pp. 3–17. Toronto: University of Toronto Press, 1997.

Bellah, Robert et al. *Habits of the Heart: Individualism and Commitment in American Life.* New York: Harper & Row, 1985.

Berlin, Isaiah. "John Stuart Mill and the End of Life." In I. Berlin, *Four Essays on Liberty,* pp. 173–206. Oxford: Oxford University Press, 1969.

———. "Two Concepts of Liberty." In *Four Essays on Liberty,* pp. 118–72. Oxford: Oxford University Press, 1969.

Billings, Paul R., et al. "Discrimination as a Consequence of Genetic Testing." In Tom L. Beauchamp and LeRoy Walters, eds., *Contemporary Issues in Bioethics,* 4th ed, pp. 637–43. Belmont, Calif.: Wadsworth, 1994.

Boorse, Christopher. "On the Distinction between Disease and Illness." In Arthur L. Caplan et al., eds., *Concepts of Health and Disease: Interdisciplinaty Perspectives,* pp. 545–60. London: Addison-Wesley, 1981.

Braidotti, Rosi. *Nomadic Subjects: Embodiment and Sexual Difference in Contemporary Feminist Theory.* New York: Columbia University Press, 1995.

Brandt, Richard B. *A Theory of the Good and the Right.* Oxford: Oxford University Press, 1979.

Bransen, Jan. "Identification and the Idea of an Alternative of Oneself." *European Journal of Philosophy* 4 (1996): 1–16.

Brincat, Cynthia A. "The Foundations of the *Foundations of Bioethics:* Engelhardt's Kantian Underpinnings." In Brendan P. Minogue et al., eds., *Reading Engelhardt,* pp. 189–203. Dordrecht: Kluwer Academic Publishers, 1997.

Brock, Dan W. "The Non-Identity Problem and Genetic Harms—the Case of Wrongful Handicaps." *Bioethics* 9 (1995): 269–75.

Brown, H., and H. Smith, eds. *Normalization—A Reader for the Nineties.* London: Tavistock and Routledge, 1989.

Brümmer, Vincent. *Theology and Philosophical Inquiry: An Introduction.* London: Macmillan, 1981.

Callahan, Daniel. *Abortion: Law, Choice and Morality.* London: Collier Macmillan, 1971.

———. *The Troubled Dream of Life: Living with Mortality.* New York: Simon & Schuster, 1993.

Caplan, Arthur L. "If Gene Therapy Is the Cure, What Is the Disease?" In George J. Annas, and S. Elias, eds., *Gene Mapping: Using Law and Ethics as Guides,* pp. 128–41. Oxford: Oxford University Press, 1992.

Cavalieri, Paola, and Peter Singer. *The Great Ape Project: Equality Beyond Humanity.* New York: St. Martin's Press, 1994.

Charlesworth, Max. *Bioethics in a Liberal Society.* Cambridge: Cambridge University Press, 1993.

Cole-Turner, R., and B. Waters. *Pastoral Genetics: Theology and Care at the Beginning of Life.* Cleveland: Pilgrim Press, 1996.

Croughs, R. W. M. "Recht op leven van ernstig gehandicapte kinderen." (The right to life of severely handicapped children.) *Medisch Contact* 44 (1989): 647–51.

DeFord, Alex F. *The Life of a Child.* New York: American Library, 1984.

Dokecki, Paul R. "Ethics and Mental Retardation: Steps towards the Ethics of Community." In Louis Rowitz, ed., *Mental Retardation in the Year 2000,* pp. 39–51. New York: Springer Verlag, 1992.

Dolan, Terrence R., and Alan Buchanan. "Gene Therapy: Promises and Concerns." *Japanese Journal of Developmental Disabilities* 17 (1996): 243–60.

Dorris, M. *The Broken Cord.* New York: Harper & Row, 1989.

Dosen, Antal, and F. J. Menolascino, eds., *Depression in Mentally Retarded Children and Adults.* Leiden: Logon Publications, 1990.

Dworkin, Ronald. "Liberalism." In R. Dworkin, *A Matter of Principle,* pp. 181–204. Cambridge: Harvard University Press, 1985.

———. *Life's Dominion: An Argument about Abortion and Euthanasia.* London: Harper/Collins, 1993.

———. *Taking Rights Seriously.* London: Duckworth, 1977.

Edwards, Robert G., and David J. Sharpe. "Social Values and Research in Human Embryology." *Nature* 231 (1971): 87–94.

Edwards, Steven D. "The Moral Status of Intellectually Disabled Individuals." *Journal of Medicine and Philosophy* 22 (1997): 29–42.

———. "Nordenfelt's Theory of Disability." *Theoretical Medicine and Bioethics* 19 (1998): 89–100.

Engelhardt, H. Tristam, Jr. "The Concepts of health and Disease." In Arthur L. Caplan, et al., eds., *Concepts of Health and Disease: Interdisciplinary Perspectives,* pp. 31–45. Reading, Mass.: Addison-Wesley, 1981.

———. "Joseph Margolis, John Rawls, and the Mentally Retarded." In Loretta M. Kopelman, and John C. Moskop, eds., *Ethics and Mental Retardation,* pp. 37–43. Dordrecht, Boston: Reidel, 1984.

———. *The Foundations of Bioethics.* 2d ed. New York, Oxford: Oxford University Press, 1996.

———. "The Foundations of Bioethics and Secular Humanism: Why Is There No Canonical Moral Content?" In Brendan P. Minogue et al., eds., *Reading Engelhardt Jr.,* pp. 259–85. Dordrecht: Kluwer Academic Publishers, 1997.

Elster, Jon. *Sour Grapes: Studies in the Subversion of Rationality.* Cambridge: Cambridge University Press, 1983.

Feinberg, Joel, ed., *The Problem of Abortion.* Belmont, Calif.: Wadsworth, 1984.

Fletcher, Joseph C. "Ethics and Public Policy: Should Sex Choice Be Discouraged?" In N. G. Bennet, ed., *Sex Selection of Children,* pp. 213–52. New York: Academic Press, 1983.

———. *The Ethics of Genetic Control.* New York: Doubleday, 1974.

———. *Morals and Medicine.* Princeton: Princeton University Press, 1954.

Forecki, M. *Speak to me.* Washington, D.C.: Gallaudet University Press, 1985.

Forrester, Mary Gore. *Persons, Animals, and Fetuses: An Essay in Practical Ethics.* Dordrecht: Kluwer Academic Press, 1996.

Fraiberg, A., and L. Fraiberg. *Insights from the Blind: Comparative Studies of Blind and Sighted Infants.* New York: New American Library, 1979.

Frankfurt, Harry. "Freedom of the Will and the Concept of a Person." In John Christman, ed., *The Inner Citadel,* pp. 63–76. Oxford: Oxford Univerity Press, 1989.

———. "Identification and Wholeheartedness." In H. Frankfurt, *The Importance of What We Care About,* pp. 159–76. Cambridge: Cambridge University Press, 1988.

Galston, William. *Liberal Purposes.* Cambridge: Cambridge University Press, 1992.

Gauthier, David. *Morals by Agreement.* Oxford: Clarendon Press, 1986.

Gibbs, M. V., and J. G. Thorpe, "Personality Stereotype of Noninstitutionalized Down Syndrome Children." *American Journal of Mental Deficiency* 87 (1983): 601–5.

Gillon, Raanan. "On Sterilizing Severely Mentally Handicapped People." *Journal of Medical Ethics* 13 (1987): 59–61.

Goldman, Alan H. "The Justification of Equal Opportunity." In Ellen F. Paul et al., eds., *Equality of Opportunity,* pp. 88–103. Oxford: Basil Blackwell, 1987.

Goodey, C. "Fools and Heretics: Parent's Views of Professionals." In T. Booth, ed., *Learning for All,* pp. 165–76. London: Routledge, 1991.

————. "John Locke's Idiots in the Natural History of the Mind." *History of Psychiatry* 5 (1994): 215–50.

Gorovitz, Samuel, et al., eds., *Moral Problems in Medicine.* 2d ed. Englewood Cliffs, N.J.: Prentice Hall, 1983.

Gray, John N. "On the Contestability of Social and Political Concepts." *Political Theory* 7 (1977): 331–48.

————. "Political Power, Social Theory and Essential Contestability." *British Journal of Political Science* 1978: 385–402.

Green, Ronald M. "Parental Autonomy and the Obligation Not to Harm One's Child Genetically." *Journal of Law, Medicine & Ethics* 25 (1997): 5–15.

Grubb, Andrew, and David Pearl. "Sterilization and the Courts." *Cambridge Law Journal* 46 (1987): 439–64.

Haffter, C. "The Changeling: History and Psychodynamics of Attitudes to Handicapped Children in European Folklore." *Journal of the History of Behavioral Sciences* 4 (1968): 55–62.

Hare, R. M. *Moral Thinking: Its Method, Levels and Point.* Oxford: Oxford University Press, 1981.

Harris, John. *The Value of Life: An Introduction to Medical Ethics.* London: Routledge & Kegan Paul, 1985.

————. *Wonderwoman and Superman: The Ethics of Human Biotechnology.* Oxford: Oxford University Press, 1992.

Hauerwas, Stanley M. *Dispatches from the Front: Theological Engagements with the Secular.* Durham, N.C.: Duke University Press, 1994.

————. *Naming the Silences: God, Medicine and the Problem of Suffering.* Grand Rapids, Mich.: Wm. B. Eerdmans, 1990.

————. "Not All Peace Is Peace: Why Christians Cannot Make Peace with Engelhardt's Peace." In Brendan P. Minogue et al., eds., *Reading Engelhardt,* pp. 31–44. Dordrecht: Kluwer Academic Publishers, 1997.

————. *Sanctify Them in the Truth: Holyness Exemplified.* Nashville: Abington Press, 1998.

————. "Suffering the Retarded: Should We Prevent Retardation?" In *Suffering Presence: Theological Reflections on Medicine, the Mentally Retarded, and the Church,* pp. 159–81. Notre Dame: University of Notre Dame Press, 1986.

Haughton, Rosemary. *The Transformation of Man: A Study of Conversion and Community.* New York: Paulist Press, 1967.

Hayes, Gregory J. "Social Responsibility: Genetics and the Developmentally Disabled." In Linda J. Hayes et al., eds., *Ethical Issues in Developmental Disabilities,* pp. 183–97. Reno: Context Press, 1994.

Hoedemaekers, Roger, et al. "Genetic Screening: A Comparative Analysis of three Recent reports." *Journal of Medical Ethics* 23 (1997): 135–41.

Holland, Barry, and Charalambos Kyriacou, eds., *Genetics and Society.* Wokingham: Addison-Wesley, 1993.

Holmes, Helen B., and Laura M. Purdy, eds., *Feminist Perspectives in Medical Ethics.* Bloomington, Ind.: Indiana University Press, 1992.

Holtzman, Neil A. "Genetic Screening: For Better or for Worse?" In Samuel Gorovitz, et al., eds., *Moral Problems in Medicine,* 2d ed., pp. 375–77. Englewood Cliffs, N.J.: Prentice Hall, 1983.

Hood, Leroy. "Biology and Medicine in the Twenty-First Century." In Daniel J. Kevles and Leroy Hood, eds., *Code of Codes.* Cambridge, Mass.: Harvard University Press, 1992.

Hume, David. *A Treatise of Human Nature.* Trans. and ed. P. H. Nidditch. 2d ed. Oxford: Clarendon Press, 1978.

International League of Societes for Persons with Mental Handicaps (ILSPMH). *Just Technology? From Principles to Practice in Bioethical Issues.* North York, Ontario: L'Institut Roeher, 1994.

Irwin, Terence. *Plato's Ethics.* New York: Oxford University Press, 1995.

Janoff-Bulman, R. *Shattered Assumptions: Towards a New Psychology of Trauma.* New York: Macmillan, 1992.

Jones, Kenneth L. *Smith's Recognizable Patterns of Human Malformation.* 4th ed. Philadelphia: W. B. Sounders, 1988.

Jonsen, Albert R. *The New Medicine and the Old Ethics.* Cambridge, Mass.: Harvard University Press, 1990.

Kaplan, Deborah. "Prenatal Screening and Its Impact on Persons with Disabilities." *Clinical Obstetrics and Gynaecology* 36 (1993): 605–12.

Karp, H. J. "If Not Always the Victor, Always the Hero." In D. Meyer, ed., *Uncommon Fathers: Reflections on Raising a Child with a Disability,* pp. 102–12. Bethesda, Md.: Woodbine House, 1995.

Kass, Leon. "Implications of Prenatal Diagnosis for the Human Right to Life." In Thomas A. Mappes and Jane S. Zembaty, eds., *Biomedical Ethics,* 3rd ed., pp. 495–507. New York: McGraw-Hill, 1991.

Kitcher, Philip. *Lives to Come: The Genetic Revolution and Human Possibilities.* London: Penguin Books, 1996.

Kluge, Eike Henner W. *Biomedical Ethics in a Canadian Context.* Scarborough: Prentice Hall, 1992.

Knoppers, Bartha. "Towards Genetic Justice." In Eike H. Kluge, ed., *Readings in Biomedical Ethics: A Canadian Focus,* pp. 478–81. Scarborough: Prentice Hall Canada, 1993.

Kopelman, Loretta M., and John C. Moskop, eds., *Ethics and Mental Retardation.* Dordrecht, Boston: Reidel, 1984.

Kovesi, Julius. *Moral Notions.* London: Routledge and Kegan Paul, 1967.

Krebs, Heinz. "Social Medicine and Social Ethics on Health and Disease of Persons with a Mental Handicap." In Bishop Beckers Foundation, *Workshop Bioethics and Mental Handicap: Report on The European Workshop 6–8 November 1989,* pp. 28–37. Utrecht: Bishop Beckers Foundation, 1990.

Krishef, C. H. "State Laws on Marriage and Sterilization." *Mental Retardation* 10 (1972): 36–38.

Kuhse, Helga. *The Sanctity of Life Doctrine: A Critique.* London: Clarendon Press, 1987.

Kymlicka, Will. "Liberalism and Communitarianism." *Canadian Journal of Philosophy* 18 (1988): 181–203.

———. *Liberalism, Community, and Culture.* Oxford: Clarendon Press, 1991.

———. *Multicultural Citizenship: A Liberal Theory of Minority Rights.* Oxford: Clarendon Press, 1995.

Lane, H. et al. *A Journey into the Deaf-World.* San Diego: Dawn Sign Press, 1996.

Lévi-Strauss, Claude. *The Savage Mind.* Chicago: University of Chicago Press, 1966.

Lippmann, A. "Prenatal Genetic Testing and Screening: Constructing Needs and Reinforcing Inequities." *American Journal of Law and Medicine* 17 (1991): 15–50.

Løgstrup, Knut E. *The Ethical Demand.* Trans. T. L. Jensen. Philadelphia: Fortress Press, 1971.

———. *Norm und Spontaneität.* Tübingen: J. C. B. Mohr, 1989.

Luckasson, R., D. A. Coulter, E. A. Polloway et al. *Mental Retardation: Definition, Classification and Systems of Supports.* Washington, D.C.: AAMR, 1992.

MacIntyre, Alasdair. *After Virtue: A Study in Moral Theory.* Notre Dame: University of Notre Dame Press, 1981.

———. "Human Identity, Accountability and Disablement." Unpublished paper, April 1994.

———. "The Privatization of the Good: An Inaugural Lecture." *Review of Politics* 52, 3 (1990): 344–61.

———. *Whose Justice, Which Rationality?* Notre Dame: University of Notre Dame Press; London: Duckworth, 1988.

Mackie, John L. *Ethics: Inventing Right and Wrong.* Harmondsworth: Penguin Books, 1977.

Macklin, Ruth. "Moral Issues in Human Genetics: Counseling or Control?" In Samuel Gorovitz, et al., eds., *Moral Problems in Medicine,* 2d ed., pp. 364–75. Englewood Cliffs, N.J.: Prentice Hall, 1983.

Mans, Inge. *Zin der zotheid: Vijf eeuwen cultruugeschiedenis van zotten, onnozelen en zwakzinnigen.* (The Sense of Folly: Five Centuries of the Cultural History of Fools, Innocents and the Mentally Retarded.) Amsterdam: Bert Bakker, 1998.

Mansell, J., and K. Eriksson, eds., *Deinstitutionalization and Community Living.* London: Chapman & Hall, 1996.

Margolis, Joseph. "Applying Moral Theory to the Retarded." In Loretta M. Kopelman, and John C. Moskop, eds., *Ethics and Mental Retardation,* pp. 19–35. Dordrecht, Boston: Reidel, 1984.

McKenny, Gerald P. *To Relieve the Human Condition. Bioethics, Technology, and the Body.* Albany: State University of New York Press, 1997.

McKusick, Victor A. "The Human Genome Project: Plans, Status and Applications in Biology and Medicine." In Tom L. Beauchamp, and LeRoy Walters, eds., *Contemporary Issues in Bioethics,* 4th ed., pp. 622–29. Belmont, Calif.: Wadsworth, 1994.

Mensch, Elizabeth, and Alan Freeman. *The Politics of Virtue: Is Abortion Debatable?* Durham, N.C.: Duke University Press, 1993.

Mercer, Jane R. "The Impact of Changing Paradigms of Disability on Mental Retardation in the Year 2000." In Louis Rowitz, ed., *Mental Retardation in the Year 2000*, pp. 15–38. New York: Springer Verlag, 1992.

Meyer, D., ed., *Uncommon Fathers: Reflections on Raising a Child with a Disability.* Bethesda, Md.: Woodbine House, 1995.

Mill, John Stuart. *Utilitarianism, On Liberty and Considerations on Representative Government.* Ed. H. B. Acton. Everyman's Library. London: Dent, 1992.

Minogue, Brendan P. "Engelhardt, Historicism and the Minimalist Paradox." In Brendan P. Minogue et al., eds., *Reading Engelhardt*, pp. 205–219. Dordrecht: Kluwer Academic Publishers, 1997.

Minogue, Brendan P., et al., eds., *Reading Engelhardt: Essays on the Thought of H. Tristam Engelhardt, Jr.* Dordrecht: Kluwer Academic Publishers, 1997.

Molenaar, Jan, et al. "Geneeskunde, dienares der barmhartigheid." (Medicine, the Servant of Mercy.) *Nederlands Tijdschrift voor Geneeskunde* 132 (1988): 1913–17.

Moos, R., ed. *Coping with Life Crises: An Integrated Approach.* New York: Plenum Press, 1986.

Morris, Arval A. "Law, Morality, and Euthanasia for the Severely Defective Child." In Marvin Kohl, ed., *Infanticide and the Value of Life.* Buffalo: Prometheus Books, 1978.

Moser, Hugo W. "Prevention of Mental Retardation (Genetics)." In Louis Rowitz, ed., *Mental Retardation in the Year 2000*, pp. 140–48. New York: Springer Verlag, 1992.

Motulsky, Arno G., and Jeffrey Murray. "Will Prenatal Diagnosis with Selective Abortion Affect Society's Attitude toward the Handicapped." *Research Ethics* (1983): 277–91.

Murphy, Jeffry G. "Rights and Borderline Cases." In Loretta M. Kopelman, and John C. Moskop, eds., *Ethics and Mental Retardation*, pp. 3–17. Dordrecht, Boston: Reidel, 1984.

Nagel, Thomas. "Moral Conflict and Political Legitimacy." *Philosophy and Public Affairs* 16, 3 (1987): 215–40.

———. *The View from Nowhere.* Oxford: Oxford University Press, 1986.

Nelson, James L. "Everything Includes Itself in Power: Power and Coherence in Engelhardt's *Foundations of Bioethics.*" In Brendan P. Minogue, et al., eds., *Reading Engelhardt*, pp. 15–29. Dordrecht: Kluwer Academic Publishers, 1997.

Newsome, Martha. "The Educational Challenge." In John F. Kilner, Rebecca D. Pentz, and Frank E. Young, eds., *Genetic Ethics: Do the Ends Justify the Genes?* pp. 156–67. Grand Rapids: Wm. B. Eerdmans, 1997.

Nirje, B. "The Principle of Normalization and its Human Management Implications." In R. Kugel and W. Wolfensberger, *Changing Patterns in Residential Services for the Mentally Retarded.* Washington, D.C.: The President's Committee on Mental Retardation, 1969.

Noble, Cheryl N. "Normative Ethical Theories." In Stanley G. Clarke and E. Simpson, eds., *Anti-Theory in Ethics and Moral Conservatism*, pp. 49–64. Albany: State University of New York Press, 1989.

Nordenfelt, L. *On the Nature of Health.* Dordrecht: Kluwer, 1995.

Nozick, Robert. *Anarchy, State, and Utopia.* New York, Basic Books, 1974.

———. *The Examined Life.* New York, Simon and Schuster, 1986.

———. *Philosophical Explanations.* Oxford: Oxford University Press, 1981.

Nuffic Council on Bioethics. *Genetic Screening: Ethical Issues.* London: Nuffic Council on Bioethics, 1993.

O'Connor, A. P., et al. "Understanding the Cancer Patient's Search for Meaning." *Cancer Nursing* 13 (1990): 167–75.

Nussbaum, Martha C., and Cass R. Sunstein, eds. *Clones and Clones: Facts and Fantasies About Human Cloning,* pp. 29–40. New York: W. W. Norton, 1998.

Oë, Kenzaburo. *A Personal Matter.* Trans. John Nathan. New York: Grove Weidenfeld, 1969.

Overall, Christine, ed. *The Future of Human Reproduction.* Toronto: The Women's Press, 1989.

Palus, C. J. "Transformative Experiences of Adulthood: A New Look at the Seasons of Life." In J. Demick et al., eds., *Parental Development,* pp. 39–58. Hillsdale, N.J.: Erlbaum, 1993.

Parfit, Derek. *Reasons and Persons.* Oxford / New York: Oxford University Press, 1986.

Perrin, B. *Beyond Normalization: Its Continuing Relevance for the 1990s–and Beyond.* Helsinki: IASSID 10th World Congress, 1996.

Petchesky, R. P. "Reproduction, Ethics and Public Policy: the Federal Sterilization Regulation." *The Hastings Center Report* 9 (1979): 29–41.

Peters, P. G. "Protecting the Unconceived: Nonexistence, Avoidability, and Reproductive Technology." *Arizona Law Review* 31 (1989): 487–548.

Peters, Ted. "Genes, Theology, and Social Ethics: Are We Playing God?" In Ted Peters, ed., *Genetics: Issues of Social Justice,* pp. 1–45. Cleveland: Pilgrim Press, 1998.

———. *Playing God? Genetic Determinism and Human Freedom.* New York: Routledge, 1997.

Peters, Ted, ed. *Genetics: Issues of Social Justice.* Cleveland: Pilgrim Press, 1998.

Plato. *Protagoras.* Trans. C. C. W. Taylor. Oxford: Clarendon Press, 1976.

Proctor, Robert N. "Genomics and Eugenics: How Fair is the Comparison?" In George A. Annas, and S. Elias, eds., *Gene Mapping: Using Law and Ethics as Guides,* pp. 57–93. Oxford: Oxford University Press, 1992.

Purdy, Laura M. "Can Having Children Be Immoral?" In Samuel Gorovitz, et al., eds., *Moral Problems in Medicine,* 2d ed., pp. 377–84. Englewood Cliffs, N.J.: Prentice Hall, 1983.

Ramsey, Paul. *Ethics at the Edges of Life.* New Haven: Yale University Press, 1978.

Rawls, John. *Political Liberalism.* New York: Columbia University Press, 1993.

———. *A Theory of Justice.* Oxford: Oxford University Press, 1971.

Raz, Joseph. *The Morality of Freedom.* Oxford: Clarendon Press, 1986.

Reilly, Philip J. *The Surgical Solution: A History of Involuntary Sterilization in the United States.* Baltimore: John Hopkins University Press, 1991.

Reinders, Hans S. "The Golden Rule between Philosophy and Theology." In Alberto Bondolfi, Stefan Grotefeld, and Rudi Neuberth, eds., *Ethics, Reason and Rationality,* pp. 145–68. Münster: LIT Verlag, 1996.

Rescher, Nicholas. *Pluralism: Against the Demand of Consensus.* Oxford: Clarendon Press, 1993.

Retsinas, Joan. "The Impact of Prenatal Technology upon Attitudes toward Disabled Infants." *Research in the Sociology of Health Care* 9 (1991): 75–102.

Ricoeur, Paul. *Amour et Justice: Mit einer deutschen Parallelübersetzung von Matthias Raden*. Oswald Baier, ed. Tübingen: J. C. B. Mohr, 1990.

———. "Entre Philosophie et Théologie: La Règle d'Or en Question." *Revue d'Histoire et de Philosophie Religieuse* 69 (1989): 3–9.

———. "The Golden Rule: Exegetical and Theological Perpexleties." *New Testament Studies* 36 (1990): 392–97.

Robinson, John A. "The Potential Impact of the Human Genome Project on Procreative Liberty." In George J. Annas and Sherman Elias, eds., *Gene Mapping: Using Law and Ethics as Guides*, 215–25. New York: Oxford University Press, 1992.

Rorty, Richard. *Contingency, Irony and Solidarity.* Cambridge: Cambridge University Press, 1989.

Rosenberg, Alexander. "The Political Philosophy of Biological Endowments: Some Considerations." In Ellen F. Paul et al., eds., *Equality of Opportunity*, pp. 1–31. Oxford: Basil Blackwell, 1987.

Ryan, Joanna, and Frank Thomas. *The Politics of Mental Handicap*. Harmondsworth: Penguin Books, 1980.

Ryan, Maura. "The Argument for Unlimited Procreative Liberty: A Feminist Critique." *Hastings Center Report* 20 (1990): 6–12.

Sarason, Seymour B., and John Doris. *Educational Handicap, Public Policy, and Social History: A Broadened Perspective on Mental Retardation.* New York: Free Press, 1979.

Scheerenberger, R. C. *A History of Mental Retardation*. Baltimore: Brookes, 1983.

Scorgie, Kathryn I. "From Devastation to Transformation: Managing Life When a Child is Disabled." Dissertation, University of Alberta, 1996.

Sherwin, Susan. "Feminist and Medical Ethics: Two Different Approaches to Contextual Ethics." In Helen B. Holmes, and Laura M. Purdy, eds., *Feminist Perspectives in Medical Ethics*, pp. 17–31. Bloomington: Indiana University Press, 1992.

Sherwin, Susan. *No Longer Patient: Feminist Ethics and Health Care*. Philadelphia: Temple University Press, 1992.

Shuster, Evelyne. "Determinism and Reductioniswm: A Greater Threat Because of the Human Genome Project?" In George A. Annas, and S. Elias, eds., *Gene Mapping: Using Law and Ethics as Guides*, pp. 115–27. Oxford: Oxford University Press, 1992.

Sidgwick, Henry. *The Method of Ethics*. 6th ed. London: Macmillan, 1901.

Silver, Lee. *Remaking Eden: Cloning and Beyond in a Brave New World*. New York: Avon Books, 1997.

Silvers, Anita. "(In)equality, (Ab)normality, and the Americans with Disabilities Act." *Journal of Medicine and Philosophy* 21 (1996): 209–24.

Singer, Peter. *Rethinking Life and Death: The Collapse of Our Traditional Ethics*. Oxford: Oxford University Press, 1995.

———. "Unsanctifying Life." In John Ladd, ed., *Ethical Issues Relating to Life and Death*, pp. 41–61. Oxford: Oxford University Press, 1979.

Singer, Peter, and Helga Kuhse. *Should the Baby Live?: The Problem of Handicapped Infants.* Oxford: Oxford University Press, 1985.

Smith, J., et al. "Institutionalization, Involuntary Sterilization, and Mental Retardation: Profiles from the History of the Practice." *Mental Retardation* 31 (1993): 208–14

Sobsey, Dick. "Family Transformation: From Dale Evans to Neil Young." In R. Fried-
lander and D. Sobsey, eds., *Conference Proceedings: Through the Lifespan*, pp. 13–16.
Kingston: National Association for Persons with Developmental Disabilities and
Mental Health Needs, 1996.

Sorensen, K. *Klinefelter's Syndrome in Childhood, Adolescence and Youth: A Genital,
Clinical, Developmental, Psychiatric and Psychological Study.* Chippenham: Parthenon
Publishing, 1987.

Spradley, T. S., and J. P. Spradley. *Deaf Like Me.* Washington, D.C.: Gallaudet University
Press, 1998.

Steinbock, Bonnie. *Life Before Birth: The Moral and Legal Status of Embryos and Fetuses.*
Oxford: Oxford University Press, 1992.

Stoker, Wessel. *Is the Quest for Meaning the Quest for God? The Religious Ascription of
Meaning in Relation to the Secular Ascription of Meaning. A Theological Study.* Trans. Lucy
Jansen and Henry Jansen. Currents of Encounter, vol. 11. Amsterdam, Atlanta: Rodopi,
1996.

Stout, Jeffrey. *Ethics after Babel: The Languages of Morals and Their Discontents.*
Cambridge: James Clarke, 1988.

Strawson, Peter F. "Social Morality and Individual Ideal." In G. Wallace, and A. D. M.
Walker, eds., *The Definition of Morality*, pp. 98–118. London: Methuen, 1970.

Sumner, Lewis W. *Abortion and Moral Theory.* Princeton: Princeton University Press, 1981.

Taylor, Nancy D., and Ryuki Kassai. "The Healer and the Healed: Works and Life of
Kenzaburo Oë." *The Lancet* 352 (August 22 1998): 642–44.

Thomson, Elizabeth. "Genetic Counselling." In John F. Kilner, Rebecca D. Pentz, and
Frank E. Young, eds., *Genetic Ethics: Do the Ends Justify the Genes?* pp. 146–155. Grand
Rapids: Wm. B. Eerdmans, 1997.

Tooley, Michael. *Abortion and Infanticide.* London: Clarendon Press, 1983.

Trent, James. *Inventing the Feeble Mind: A History of Mental Retardation in the United
States.* Berkeley: University of California Press, 1994.

United Nations. "Decade of Disabled Persons 1983–1992." *World Programme of Action
Concerning Disabled Persons.* New York, United Nations, 1983.

Van Asperen, Gertrude M. "Eén temidden van velen: zingeving en ethiek." ("One Among
Many: The Quest for Meaning and Ethics.") In G. A. Van der Wal and F. L. C. M.
Jacobs, eds., *Vragen naar zin* (The Quest for Meaning), pp. 86–103. Baarn: Ambo, 1992.

Van Kooten Niekerk, Kees. "Knud E. Løgstrups 'Norm und Spontaneität': eine Einführung." *Zeitschrift für Evangelische Ethik* 35 (1991): 51–59.

Veatch, Robert M. "Models for Ethical Medicine in a Revolutionary Age." In Daniel
Callahan, ed., *Ethical Issues in Professional Life.* New York, Oxford: Oxford University
Press, 1988.

Veevers, Jean E. *Childless by Choice.* Toronto: Butterworths, 1980.

Verwey, Marcel. *Preventive Medicine—Between Obligation and Aspiration.* Dissertation,
Utrecht University, 1998.

Vries, L. B. A. de. "The Fragile X syndrome: Clinical, Genetic and Large Scale Diagnostic
Studies among Mentally Retarded Individuals." Dissertation, Erasmus Universiteit
Rotterdam, 1997.

Waldschmidt, Anne. "Against Selection of Human Life—People with Disabilities Oppose Genetic Counseling." *Issues in Reproductive and Genetic Engineering* 5 (1992): 155–67.

Walters, Leroy. "Religion and the Renaissance of Medical Ethics in the United States: 1965–1975." In Earl A. Shelp, ed., *Theology and Bioethics: Exploring the Foundations and Frontiers*, pp. 3–16. Dordrecht/Boston: Reidel, 1985.

Walzer, Michael. *Spheres of Justice: A Defense of Pluralism and Equality.* Oxford: Blackwell, 1983.

Warnock, Baroness Mary. "The Problem of Knowledge." In Barry Holland and Charalambos Kyriacou, eds. *Genetics and Society,* pp. 103–117. Wokingham: Addison-Wesley, 1993.

Warnock, Geoffrey J. *The Object of Morality.* London: Methuen, 1971.

Warren, Mary A. *Gendercide: The Implications of Sex Selection.* Totowa, N.J.: Rowan & Allenfield, 1985.

Wasserman, David. "Some Moral Issues in the Correction of Impairments." *Journal of Social Philosophy* 27 (1996): 128–45.

Watson, James. "The Human Genome Initiative." In Barry Holland and Charalambos Kyriacou, eds., *Genetics and Society,* pp. 13–26. Wokingham: Addison-Wesley, 1993.

Weir, Robert F. *Selective Nontreatment of Handicapped Newborns: Moral Dilemmas in Neonatal Medicine.* New York: Oxford University Press, 1984.

Wendell, Susan. "Toward a Feminist Theory of Disability." In Helen B. Holmes, and Laura M. Purdy, eds., *Feminist Perspectives in Medical Ethics*, pp. 63–81. Bloomington, Ind.: Indiana University Press, 1992.

Wertz, Dorothy, and John C. Fletcher. "Fatal Knowledge? Prenatal Diagnosis and Sex Selection." *Hastings Center Report* 19 (1989): 21–27.

Wertz, Dorothy C., and John C. Fletcher. "A Critique of Some Feminist Challenges to Prenatal Diagnosis." In Françoise Baylis et al., eds., *Health Care Ethics in Canada,* pp. 385–403. Toronto, Montreal: Harcourt Brace, 1995.

West, Richard. "Ethical Aspects of Generic Disease and Genetic Counseling." *Journal of Medical Ethics* 14 (1988): 194–97.

White-Van Mourik, M. "Looking from the Outside—Reactions to a Termination of Pregnancy for Fetal Abnormality from the Point of View of Those Who Care." In L. Abramsky and J. Chapple, eds., *Prenatal Diagnosis: The Human Side,* pp. 181–201. London: Chapman & Hall, 1994.

White-Van Mourik, Margaretha C.A., et al. "The Psychological Sequela of a Second Trimester Termination of Pregnancy for Fetal Abnormality over a Two Year Period," in Gerry Evers-Kiebooms et al., eds., *Psychosocial Aspects of Genetic Counseling,* pp. 61–74. New York: John Wiley, 1992.

Wikler, Daniel. "Paternalism and the Mildly Retarded." *Philosophy and Public Affairs* 8 (1979): 377–92.

———. "Personal Responsibility for Illness." In D. Vandeveer, and T. Regan, eds., *Health Care Ethics: An Introduction,* pp. 326–58. Philadelphia: Temple University Press, 1987.

Williams, Bernard. *Ethics and the Limits of Philosophy.* London: Fontana Press/Collins, 1985.

Wilson, Michiko N. *The Marginal World of Kenzaburo Oë: A Study in Themes and Techniques.* New York: M. E. Sharpe, 1986.

Wishart, J. G., and F. H. Johnston. "The Effects of Experience on Attribution of a Stereotyped Personality to Children with Down Syndrome: A Comparative Study." *Journal of Mental Deficiency Research* 34 (1990): 409–20.

Wolf, Susan, ed. *Feminism and Bioethics*. New York: Oxford University Press, 1996.

Wolfensberger, Wolf. "Counseling Parents of the Retarded." In A. Baumeister, ed., *Mental Retardation: Appraisal, Education and Rehabilitation*, pp. 329–400. Chicago: Aldine Press, 1967.

———. *The Principle of Normalization in Human Services*. Toronto: National Institute on Mental Retardation, 1972.

———. "Social Role Valorisation: A Proposed New Term for the Principle of Normalization." *Mental Retardation* 21 (1983): 234–39.

Wolterstorff, Nicholas. "Audi on Religion, Politics, and Liberal Democracy." In Robert Audi, and Nicholas Wolterstorff, *Religion in the Public Square: The Place of Religious Convictions in Political Debate*, pp. 145–65. Lanham, Md.: Rowman & Littlefield, 1997.

World Health Organization. *International Classification of Impairments, Disabilities and Handicaps*. Geneva, WHO, 1980.

Wuthnow, Robert. *Learning to Care: Elementary Kindness in an Age of Indifference*. New York: Oxford University Press, 1995.

Young, Frances M. *Face to Face: An Essay in the Theology of Suffering*. Edinburgh: T.&T. Clark, 1990.

Zuskar, D. M. "The Psychological Impact of Prenatal Diagnosis of Fetal Abnormality: Strategies for Investigation and Intervention." *Women and Health* 12 (1987): 91–103.

Index

abortion, 23, 131, 227n.25, 248n.11
    on demand, 37, 49, 95–96, 234n.19
    and gene therapy, 58–59
    restrictions on, 47, 50, 64, 101, 221n.3,
        227n.31
    Roe v. Wade, 221n.8, 234n.19
    as selective, 4, 8, 15, 38, 39, 40–42, 51, 55,
        56, 78, 91–92, 93, 94–96, 221n.6,
        230n.13, 231n.25, 234n.15
    See also prevention of disabilities
Aldwin, A. M., 253nn.14, 18
alienation, 180–82, 187, 190–91, 251n.32,
    255n.4
American Association of Mental Retardation
    (AAMR), 221n.12
American Psychiatric Association (APA),
    221n.12
American Society of Human Genetics, 234n.15
Audi, Robert, 214n.36, 232n.28
autonomy, 35, 71, 122, 153, 213nn.25, 29,
    216n.6, 257n.18
    vs. dependence, 44, 142–43, 210n.10,
        229n.11
    as modern value, 171–73, 193, 196–97,
        205–6, 210n.10, 214n.33, 251n.32
    See also control; freedom, individual

Bauman, Zygmunt, 139
    on commitment/conventionality, 149–51,
        245n.30
    on Løgstrup, 149–50
    on moral philosophy, 140, 148–49,
        240n.4, 246n.37

on moral responsibility, 140, 141–42,
    245n.32
Beauchamp, Thomas L., 215n.2
Beiner, Ronald, 21
Benhabib, Seyla, 21
Bentham, Jeremy, 167, 249n.19, 250n.23
Berlin, Sir Isaiah, 22, 66–67, 229n.11,
    249n.19, 250n.23
Berube, Michael, 227n.25
bioethics, 217n.22, 218n.31, 247n.6
    critical method in, 123
    McKenny on, 212n.25, 214n.33
    medical paradigm in, 1–5, 7–8, 10, 12, 25,
        52, 64–65, 74–75, 76, 77, 98, 161,
        210n.8, 212n.21
    normalization paradigm in, 2–4, 8, 17–18,
        35–36, 72, 75, 210n.9
    See also Engelhardt, H. Tristam, Jr.; moral
        philosophy
biological determinism, 61–63
Boorse, Christopher, 223n.18
Brandt, Richard, 123
Brave New World, 76
Brincat, Cynthia, 218nn.25, 31
Brümmer, Vincent, 195
Buchanan, Alan, 225n.16

Callahan, Daniel, 159, 251n.33, 252n.36
cancer, 44, 165, 172–73
    vs. genetic disorders, 55, 56, 226n.17
Caplan, Arthur L., 211n.17, 223n.20
Charlesworth, Max, 222n.16
Childress, James F., 215n.2

choice, free. *See* freedom, individual
Christianity, 34, 150–52, 245n.24, 246n.38
clinical genetics. *See* genetic testing/screening
Collins, Francis S., 1, 87
conscience, moral, 122, 123
control
  over nature, 173–74, 213n.25, 251n.32,
    252n.36
  over one's life, 143, 153, 171–72, 185–87,
    190–91, 196–203, 204, 251nn.32, 33,
    257n.21
  See also autonomy; freedom, individual
Crick, Francis, 212n.19
cystic fibrosis, 45, 54, 161, 225n.13

deafness, 3, 54, 97, 177–78, 207, 225n.15
denial, 188–89, 254n.23
dependence, 16–17, 26
  vs. autonomy, 44, 142–43, 210n.10, 229n.11
  See also control
disabilities
  as biological, 3, 210n.7
  as defects, 2, 3, 4–5, 39, 52, 74–75, 161
  vs. genetic disorders, 43, 44–46, 53,
    222n.14, 230n.18
  vs. handicaps, 42–43
  vs. illnesses, 97, 222n.17
  as impairments, 97, 161
  mental vs. physical, 3, 38, 43–44, 207,
    214n.34
  non-genetic sources of, 81–83
  and personal identity, 54, 59–61, 62–63,
    225n.16
  as socio-culturally determined, 3, 42–43,
    45–46, 53–54, 81–82, 100, 210n.7,
    221n.12, 225n.15, 232n.27
  See also disabled people; genetic disorders;
    prevention of disabilities
disabled people
  care for, 4, 5, 14–15, 16–18, 25–26, 34–35,
    36, 76, 79, 81, 86, 94, 105–21, 122–38,
    139–42, 146, 153–55, 207–8, 231n.25,
    250n.27
  equality of, 2, 34–35, 65, 71–73, 101–2, 105,
    118–20, 206, 238nn.36, 37
  vs. genetic disorders, 52–65

as gifts, 70, 152, 186, 190, 192, 206, 207–8,
    228n.6, 250nn.24, 27
  meaning in lives of, 15, 57–58, 193–94,
    203, 205–6, 207
  moral standing of, 15–16, 68–70, 71–73,
    92–93, 97, 105–7, 108–10, 112–21, 153,
    162, 228nn.1, 6, 236n.7, 237nn.20, 32,
    238n.37, 242n.4, 250n.27
  negative evaluations of lives of, 3, 4, 50,
    52–53, 54, 55–65, 67, 74–75, 85, 91–92
  personal identity of, 51, 54, 59–61, 62–63,
    225n.16
  personhood of, 23, 139–40
  as reasonably happy, 99–100, 161–62,
    173–74, 235n.25
  respect for, 1, 68, 72–74, 93, 101–2
  self-esteem of, 66–67, 74, 229n.10
  social relationships involving, 124–38,
    139–40, 153–55, 241n.9
  welfare programs for, 5, 14–15, 76, 79, 81,
    86, 94, 119, 146, 231n.25
  See also disabilities; genetic disorders; par-
    ents of disabled people; prevention of
    disabilities; public policy; quality of
    life; suffering
discrimination, 70–76, 229n.11
  in actions, 68, 70–71
  in attitudes, 68, 71–75, 91–93
  based on normality, 71–73
  and exclusion, 70–73
  as genetically based, 7, 14–15, 18, 50, 52,
    55, 67–68, 86–91, 92–93, 94, 97, 101–2,
    106, 162, 206
  and intentions, 74, 93, 229n.13
  public policies against, 23–24, 35, 72, 76,
    106, 216n.8
  See also equality
diseases, genetic. *See* genetic disorders
Distinction between Person and Condition
    (DPC) argument, 52–53, 55–63
Dolan, Terrence R., 225n.16
Doris, John, 232n.27
Down syndrome, 56–57, 70, 93
  quality of life with, 45, 54, 99–100, 161,
    162, 210n.7, 225n.13, 227n.25, 235n.25,
    248n.9

Duchenne's muscular dystrophy, 45, 46, 161, 225n.13
Dworkin, Ronald, 87, 215n.37, 238n.37

Edwards, Robert G., 85, 233n.3
Edwards, Steven, 222n.17
employment, 68, 71, 75, 87, 101, 233n.9
Engelhardt, H. Tristam, Jr., 87, 107–13, 160, 213n.29, 222n.16, 225n.9
    on content-full morality, 22, 27, 29, 32, 34–35, 101, 108, 111, 217nn.20, 21, 218n.30, 223n.22, 232n.2
    on human good, 21–22, 26–27, 34, 118, 238n.34
    and Kant, 30, 31, 32, 33, 109, 111–12, 123–24, 218n.31, 219nn.36, 37, 236n.5
    on moral diversity, 26, 27–28, 30, 217n.20
    on moral friends, 27, 32–33, 111–12, 217nn.17, 20, 218n.30
    on moral strangers, 27, 31, 32–34, 108, 112, 217nn.17, 22, 218n.30, 219nn.34, 38
    on personhood, 32–34, 108–10, 111–13, 115, 120, 141, 219n.37, 235n.4, 236n.7, 238n.37
    on principle of beneficence, 110–12, 216n.15, 237n.32
    on principle of permission, 27–34, 108, 111–12, 216n.15, 218n.30, 219nn.34, 37, 38
    on procedural morality, 22, 27, 29, 32, 34–35, 111, 219n.34
    on public morality, 26–36, 108–9, 112, 121, 123, 141, 218n.30, 220n.42, 223n.22, 232n.2, 238n.35
    vs. Rawls, 107, 113–14, 115, 118–21, 123, 141, 240n.39
    on the social sense of persons, 108–9, 121, 235n.4
equality, 86–91, 233n.9
    of disabled people, 2, 34–35, 65, 71–73, 101–2, 105, 118–20, 206, 238nn.36, 37
    and justice, 106, 114
    in liberalism, 13–14, 15, 18, 23–24, 32–36, 65, 71–73, 77, 79–80, 85, 87, 101–2, 106–7, 206, 238nn.35, 37

restrictions on, 71–72
    See also discrimination
Ethical Demand, The, 140, 142–48
ethics. See moral philosophy
euthanasia, 5

feminism, 51, 212n.21, 213nn.27, 28, 225n.7, 227n.31, 233n.3
fetuses, human, 23, 41, 62, 94–95, 221n.8, 228n.3
Fletcher, John C., 225n.7, 247n.4
folic acid, 221n.6, 229n.13
Forrester, Mary Gore, 236n.5
Foundations of Bioethics, The, 21–22, 26–36, 107–13. See also Engelhardt, H. Tristam, Jr.
fragile X syndrome, 45, 58, 60–61, 63, 99, 161, 163, 209n.2, 225n.13, 226n.21
Frankfurt, Harry, 257n.18
freedom, individual, 212nn.21, 25, 218n.31, 251n.32, 256nn.7, 16
    in liberalism, 7, 8–9, 13, 15–16, 22–23, 34–35, 76–78, 79–80, 84–102, 161, 198–99, 206, 256n.17, 257n.18
    and public morality, 46–50, 65, 84–85, 92
    and public policy, 7, 8, 13–15, 46–50, 65, 77, 84
    restrictions on, 15, 39–40, 41, 47–50, 64–65, 67–68, 77, 84–102, 221n.3, 227n.31, 246n.35, 251n.33
    See also autonomy; control; reproductive choice; responsibility, individual
Freeman, Alan, 221n.8
Freudian reality principle, 175, 252n.35
fulfillment, 177, 187, 203–4, 207–8, 250nn.24, 27
    vs. happiness, 166–71, 249n.19

Galston, William, 215n.37
gene technology. See genetic research; genetic testing/screening
gene therapy, 58–59, 61, 62–63, 176–77
genetic counseling. See genetic testing/screening
genetic disorders, 39
    vs. cancer, 55, 56, 226n.17

genetic disorders (*cont.*)
    cystic fibrosis, 45, 54, 161, 225n.13
    vs. disabilities, 3, 43, 44–46, 53, 222n.14,
        230n.18
    vs. disabled people, 52–65
    as diseases, 1–2, 43, 44–46, 53–54
    Down syndrome, 45, 54, 56–57, 70, 93,
        99–100, 161, 162, 210n.7, 225n.13,
        227n.25, 235n.25, 248n.9
    Duchenne's muscular dystrophy, 45, 46,
        161, 225n.13
    fragile X syndrome, 45, 58, 60–61, 63, 99,
        161, 163, 209n.2, 225n.13, 226n.21
    hemophilia, 40, 225n.13
    Huntington's chorea, 45, 161, 225n.13
    vs. illnesses, 44–46, 53–54, 161, 223n.18
    as impairments, 44–45
    Klinefelter's syndrome, 45, 99, 223n.19,
        225n.13
    Lesch Nyhan disease, 95, 225n.13,
        234n.18
    retinitis pigmentosa, 225n.13
    spina bifida, 73–74, 99, 163, 225n.13
    Tay Sachs syndrome, 99, 225n.13, 231n.22,
        235nn.23, 24
    See also disabilities; disabled people;
        prevention of disabilities
geneticization, fallacy of, 61–63
genetic research, 1–7, 211n.17, 212n.19
    assumptions of, 9–10, 92
    funding for, 4–5
    gene therapy, 58–59, 62–63
    public control of, 6–7, 8
    public policy influenced by, 4–5, 8, 14–15,
        37–39
    reproductive choice enhanced / influenced
        by, 2, 52, 64, 68, 74–75, 77–79, 94,
        206, 224n.5, 231n.21
    See also genetic testing / screening
genetic screening. *See* genetic testing / screening
Genetics and Society, 6–8
genetic testing / screening, 1–2, 8, 21, 25, 62,
    209n.2, 224nn.1, 5, 225n.11
    and negative evaluations of lives of dis-
        abled, 50, 52–53, 54, 55–65, 74–75, 85,
        229n.13

    public policies related to, 37–39, 47–49,
        83, 84–102
    restrictions on, 96–102, 234n.20
    side effects from, 5–6, 7, 8, 12–13, 14–15,
        18, 36, 49–50, 51–52, 55, 66, 77–78,
        79–80, 83, 85–86, 91–102, 106–7, 206,
        225n.7, 238n.36
    See also genetic research; prevention of
        disabilities
Gewirth, Alan, 244n.22
God, 24, 27–28, 228n.6, 255n.6
Goldman, Alan H., 239n.37
guilt / remorse, 70, 128, 130, 228n.6

handicaps, 42–43, 222n.14. *See also* disabilities
happiness, 252n.35
    vs. fulfillment, 166–71, 249n.19
Hare, Richard M., 123, 226n.20, 244n.22
Harris, John, 123
Hauerwas, Stanley M., 218n.25, 220n.42
    on the disabled, 66, 210n.10, 226n.17,
        227n.25
    on liberalism, 215n.39
    on suffering, 164–66, 172–73, 248n.13,
        251n.29
Haughton, Rosemary, 187–89, 190, 191,
    254n.26
Hayes, Gregory J., 231
health
    as conventional, 97–100, 213n.29
    vs. disease, 97–99
    See also health care, costs of; health
        insurance
health care, costs of, 77, 81, 86, 90–91, 92,
    102, 119
health insurance, 70–71, 75, 80, 87–91, 94,
    96, 102, 231n.25, 233n.5
hemophilia, 40, 225n.13
Heschel, Abraham, 122
Hippocrates, 223n.18
Hobbes, Thomas, 29, 30
human fetuses, 23, 41, 62, 94–95, 221n.8,
    228n.3
Human Genome Project, 87, 211n.17
human good, 11–12, 13, 184, 218n.31,
    244n.21

assumptions concerning, 9–10, 16–17, 160
  Engelhardt on, 21–22, 26–27, 34, 118,
    238n.34
  happiness vs. fulfillment as, 166–71,
    249n.19
  and liberalism, 24, 93, 101, 118
  Mill, John Stuart, on, 249n.19, 250n.23
  privatization of, 21, 25–26
  See also morality
"Human Identity, Accountability and
  Disablement," 241nn.7, 12
Hume, David, 29, 30, 215n.3
Huntington's chorea, 45, 161, 225n.13
Huxley, Aldous, 76

identity, moral, 122, 123, 124, 132–33, 134–38,
    153, 172, 240n.3
  and personal identity, 125, 135–38
identity, personal, 54, 59–63, 66–67, 135–38,
    225n.16, 229n.11
  activity/passivity in construction of, 153,
    196–203, 246n.35
  as constructed, 196–98
  of disabled people, 51, 54, 59–61, 62–63,
    225n.16
  MacIntyre on, 125, 135–38, 241n.12
  and moral identity, 125, 135–38
  and suffering, 165, 172–73
  transformations in, 169–70, 175–92,
    182–92, 204, 254n.26
illnesses
  activity/passivity in response to, 165,
    172–73
  vs. disabilities, 97, 222n.17
  vs. genetic disorders, 44–46, 53–54, 161,
    223n.18
  vs. impairments, 44–45, 53–54, 97, 161,
    225n.13, 249n.14
impairments, 42, 81–82
  vs. illnesses, 44–45, 53–54, 97, 161, 225n.13,
    249n.14
Inclusion International, 51
infanticide, 4
insurance, health, 70–71, 75, 80, 87–91, 94,
    96, 102, 231n.25, 233n.5. See also health
    care, costs of

International Association of the Scientific
    Study of Intellectual Disability
    (IASSID), 229n.9
International Classification of Impairments,
    Disabilities and Handicaps (ICIDH),
    42–43
International League of Societies for Persons
    with Mental Handicaps (ILSPMH),
    4–5, 9, 55, 62
IQ tests, 42
Irwin, Terence, 218n.28

job market. See employment
Jonsen, Albert, 223n.18
justice, social, 75, 86–91, 105, 109–18, 233n.9
  and equality, 106, 114
  as fairness, 114–18, 236n.17, 237nn.23, 26,
    32, 242n.4
  See also Rawls, John

Kant, Immanuel
  and Engelhardt, 30, 31, 32, 33, 109, 111–12,
    123–24, 218n.31, 219nn.36, 37, 236n.5
  and moral philosophy, 123–24, 141, 153,
    154, 242n.5, 243n.11
  on personhood, 30, 32, 33, 111, 219n.37
Karp, Henry J., 189–90
Kitcher, Philip, 79–80, 87–91, 233n.5
Klinefelter's syndrome, 45, 99, 223n.19,
    225n.13
Kluge, Eike H., 53, 234n.20
Knoppers, Bartha, 231n.25
Krebs, Heinz, 222n.14, 230n.18
Kuhse, Helga, 123, 240n.3, 241n.9
Kymlicka, Will, 215n.37, 216n.6, 226n.19
  on choice, 198–99, 201–3, 256n.16, 257n.18

labor market. See employment
late onset diseases, 38, 45
Lesch Nyhan disease, 95, 225n.13, 234n.18
Levinas, Emmanuel, 139, 150
Lévi-Strauss, Claude, 197, 256nn.8, 9
liberalism
  equality in, 13–14, 15, 18, 23–24, 32–36, 65,
    71–73, 77, 79–80, 85, 87, 101–2, 106–7,
    206, 238nn.35, 37

liberalism (*cont.*)
  features of, 22–26, 38, 46–50, 65, 214n.36,
    215nn.37, 39, 216nn.6, 8, 222n.16,
    238n.35
  and human good, 24, 93, 101, 118
  individual freedom in, 7, 8–9, 13, 15–16,
    22–23, 34–35, 76–78, 79–80, 84–102,
    161, 198–99, 206, 256n.17, 257n.18
  meaning of life in, 198–99, 201–5, 206–7,
    256n.16
  moral agents in, 15–16, 23, 71–72, 105–7,
    112–13, 114–18, 153, 154, 205–6, 235n.4,
    238n.37
  personhood in, 16–17, 23, 44, 118, 122–24,
    153, 222n.16, 238n.37
  public morality in, 10–12, 13–18, 22, 24–26,
    101–2, 105–21, 153, 214n.33, 236n.7
  See also Engelhardt, H. Tristam, Jr.; public
    morality; Rawls, John
life
  as a gift, 24, 124, 146–48, 150–52, 154–55,
    206–7, 245n.25, 247n.39
  the important things in, 182, 184, 204
  as uncertain, 184, 186, 257n.21
  value of, 10, 23, 24, 50, 52–53, 54, 55–65,
    92, 98, 123, 153, 191, 216n.6, 240n.3
  See also meaning of life; quality of life
Locke, John, 135
Løgstrup, Knud E., 243n.6, 245n.32,
    246n.38
  Bauman on, 149–50
  on ethical demands, 141–48, 149, 150–51,
    154–55, 245n.24, 246n.35, 250n.27
  on life as a gift, 146–48, 150–52
  and religion, 150–52
  on social norms, 144–46, 149–50, 243n.16
  on trust, 142–43, 243nn.7, 12, 245n.30
Lutheranism, 245n.24, 246n.38

MacIntyre, Alasdair, 241n.7
  on accountability, 125, 135–37, 241n.12
  on identity, 125, 135–38, 241n.12
  on internal goods, 201
  on privatization of the good, 25
Mans, Inge, 255n.31
McKenny, Gerald P., 171–72, 231nn.20, 23
  on bioethics, 212n.25, 214n.33

on suffering, 159, 248n.13, 250n.27,
    251n.32
meaning of life, 12, 193–208, 255n.1
  as constructed, 196–205, 207, 255n.1,
    255n.6, 256nn.16, 17
  for disabled people, 15, 57–58, 193–94,
    203, 205, 207
  as discovered, 200–205, 206–8, 250n.24,
    255n.1, 257n.18
medical paradigm, 1–5, 7–8, 76, 210n.8
  disabilities as defects in, 2, 3, 4–5, 52,
    74–75, 161
  doctor-patient relations in, 1–2, 10, 12, 25,
    64–65, 77, 98–99, 100, 212n.21
  See also genetic research; genetic
    testing / screening; normalization
    paradigm
medicine, 171–72, 173–74, 248n.13, 251nn.29,
    32, 33
Mensch, Elizabeth, 221n.8
Mill, James, 249n.19
Mill, John Stuart, 167, 249n.19, 250n.23
Minogue, Brendan P., 218nn.25, 31
moral diversity, 10–12, 22, 24, 113, 116,
    214n.33
  Engelhardt on, 26, 27–28, 30, 217n.20
  See also moral strangers
moral friends, 111–13
  vs. moral strangers, 27, 32–34, 112,
    217n.17, 218n.30
morality
  conventionalist justifications for, 31, 34,
    215n.3
  formalist justifications for, 30, 31–32, 34,
    218n.31, 219n.38
  instrumentalist justifications for, 28–29,
    30–31, 32–33, 34
  narrow vs. wide conceptions of, 11–12, 16,
    22, 27, 29, 32, 34–35, 111, 214n.33,
    219n.34
  and trust, 142–43, 144, 243n.7
  See also human good; moral diversity;
    moral friends; morality, content-full;
    moral philosophy; public morality
morality, content-full, 101, 108, 123, 217nn.20,
    21, 218n.30, 223n.22, 232n.2
  liberal morality as, 238n.34

vs. procedural morality, 22, 27, 29, 32, 34–35, 111, 219n.34
morality, procedural, vs. content-full morality, 22, 27, 29, 32, 34–35, 111, 219n.34
moral philosophy, 11–12, 122, 139, 150, 151, 240n.4, 246n.36
    Bauman on, 140, 148–49, 240n.4, 246n.37
    critical method in, 123–24, 137–38, 140–42, 240n.3
    Kantianism in, 123–24, 141, 153, 154, 242n.5, 243n.11
    reason in, 137–38, 140, 148–49, 154, 242nn.1, 5
    utilitarianism in, 109–10, 123–24, 141, 153, 154, 167, 241n.9, 242n.5, 243n.11, 246n.37, 249n.19, 250n.23
    See also bioethics; Engelhardt, H. Tristam, Jr.; morality; public morality; Rawls, John; responsibility, moral
moral strangers, 219n.34
    vs. moral friends, 27, 32–34, 112, 217n.17, 218n.30
    See also moral diversity
Morris, Alval A., 235n.24
Murphy, Jeffry G., 237n.20

Nagel, Thomas, 177, 179–82, 187, 190–91, 216, 252n.7, 253n.12, 255n.4
Nance, Walter E., 225n.15
National Bioethics Advisory Commission, 227n.29
National Center for Human Genome Research, 1, 87
National Institutes of Health, 59
Nelson, James L., 218n.25, 219n.38
Newsome, Martha, 231n.20
Noble, Cheryl N., 122, 124
non-treatment decisions, 5
Nordenfelt, L., 222n.17
normality, 12, 42–43, 82, 92, 161, 223n.20
    discrimination based on, 71–73
    as issue in prevention of disabilities, 45–46, 54–55, 97, 100, 231n.25
normalization paradigm, 17–18, 72, 210n.9
    and prevention of disabilities, 2–4, 8, 35–36, 75
    See also medical paradigm

Nozick, Robert, 168–69, 171, 215n.37, 233n.9, 250n.22, 252n.35
Nuffield Council on Bioethics, 210n.9

Oë, Kenzaburo, 124–38, 153, 180, 191, 241nn.8, 9, 242n.14, 255n.31

Palus, C. J., 250n.26
parents of disabled people
    ambivalence among, 176–77, 178–81, 191–92, 253nn.9, 11
    convictions/beliefs of, 12, 36, 59–61, 62–63, 110, 124–38, 142–48, 152, 154–55, 160–61, 166–71, 173–74, 176, 184–86, 204, 226n.24, 227n.25, 228n.6, 229n.13, 237n.20, 241n.8, 247n.6, 252n.6
    as coping, 182, 183, 184, 204–5, 253n.23
    as in denial, 188–89, 253n.23, 254n.27
    quality of life for, 9, 39, 51, 67, 68–70, 73–75, 159–74, 226n.20, 249n.14, 257n.21
    transformation experiences among, 169–70, 175–92, 182–92, 194, 204, 250nn.26, 27, 253n.18, 23, 254n.26, 257n.21
    See also reproductive choice
Parfit, Derek, 69, 228n.1
patient rights, 10
peaceableness, 27–34, 218n.30, 219nn.34, 38
Personal Matter, A, 124–38, 153, 180, 191, 241nn.8, 9, 242n.14, 255n.31
personhood, 41, 143, 221n.8
    of disabled people, 23, 139–40
    Engelhardt on, 32–34, 108–10, 111–12, 115, 120, 141, 219n.37, 235n.4, 236n.7, 238n.37
    Kant on, 30, 32, 33, 111, 219n.37
    in liberalism, 16–17, 23, 44, 118, 122–24, 153, 222n.16, 238n.37
    Rawls on, 113–18, 120, 139, 141, 236n.17, 238n.37, 240n.38
Peters, Ted, 230n.18
Plato, 29, 218n.28
pleasure, 167–71, 250n.23
pneumonia, 44

Political Liberalism, 107, 113–14, 116–18,
    240n.39. *See also* Rawls, John
postmodernity, 148–49, 197–98
prevention of disabilities, 11–12, 210n.9,
    221nn.5, 6, 224n.1, 225n.11, 226n.20,
    231n.21
  before conception, 38, 40, 177–78
  illness as issue in, 46, 154
  as issue of reproductive choice, 8–9, 21,
    25, 38
  as morally permissible, 37–38, 39–40
  as morally required, 37–38, 39–40
  moral standing (MS) reasons for, 68–70,
    71–73, 92–93, 97, 162, 228nn.1, 3, 6,
    250n.27
  and negative evaluations of disabled lives,
    50, 52, 53–54, 55–65, 74–75, 85, 91–92,
    93, 162–64, 229n.13, 233n.12
  normality as issue in, 45–46, 54–55, 97,
    100, 231n.25
  and normalization paradigm, 2–4, 8,
    35–36, 75
  as preventing defects, 2, 3, 4–5
  quality of life (QL) reasons for, 68–70,
    73–75, 92–93, 159–64, 170–71, 228nn.1,
    6, 250n.27
  side effects from, 5–6, 7, 8, 12–13, 14–15,
    18, 36, 49–50, 51–52, 55, 66, 77–78,
    79–80, 83, 85–86, 91–102, 106–7, 206,
    225n.7, 238n.36
  See also abortion; disabilities; disabled
    people; discrimination; reproductive
    choice; responsibility, individual
principle of beneficence, 110–12, 216n.15,
    237n.32
principle of permission, 27–34, 108, 111–12,
    216n.15, 218n.30, 219nn.34, 37, 38
Principles of Medical Ethics, 215n.2
Pritchard, Robert, 6–7, 12, 212n.21
privacy
  of genetic information, 75–76
  in reproductive decisions, 35–36, 39–40,
    47, 52, 75–78, 85, 227n.31
privatization of the good, 21, 25
Proctor, Robert, 62, 231n.24
Protagoras, 29, 31, 218n.27

public morality, 37–38
  Engelhardt on, 26–36, 108–9, 112, 121, 123,
    141, 218n.30, 220n.42, 223n.22, 232n.2,
    238n.35
  and individual freedom, 46–50, 65, 84–85,
    92
  in liberalism, 10–12, 13–18, 22, 24–26,
    101–2, 105–21, 153, 214n.33, 236n.7
  Rawls on, 113–18, 121, 123, 141
  social sense of persons in, 108–9, 121,
    122–23, 235n.4
  See also liberalism; morality; moral
    philosophy; public policy
public policy
  debate on, 12, 22, 24–36
  toward the disabled, 5, 14–15, 17–18, 38,
    67–68, 72–73, 76, 77, 79, 84–102, 119,
    146, 231n.25, 232n.26
  against discrimination, 23–24, 35, 72, 76,
    106, 216n.8
  genetic research as influence on, 4–5, 8,
    14–15, 37–39
  related to genetic testing, 37–39, 47–49,
    83, 84–102
  and individual freedom, 7, 8, 13–15,
    46–50, 65, 77, 84
  See also public morality; state, democratic

quality of life, 10, 54, 98, 159–74
  for disabled people, 2, 3, 5, 7–9, 15, 39,
    44–46, 51, 52, 53–55, 67, 68–70, 73–75,
    92, 99–100, 127, 159–64, 173–74, 205,
    228n.6, 234n.18, 249n.14
  with Down syndrome, 45, 54, 99–100,
    161, 162, 210n.7, 225n.13, 227n.25,
    235n.25, 248n.9
  for parents of disabled people, 9, 39, 51,
    67, 68–70, 73–75, 159–74, 226n.20,
    249n.14, 257n.21

Ramsey, Paul, 234
rational choice theory, 116, 232n.2, 233n.9,
    243nn.7, 12
Rawls, John, 88, 89, 107, 198–99, 215n.37,
    222n.16, 232n.1, 233n.9, 238n.34,
    240n.39

vs. Engelhardt, 107, 113–14, 115, 118–21, 123, 141, 238n.37
on justice as fairness, 114–18, 236n.17, 237n.26, 32, 242n.4
and Kant, 123–24
on natural duties, 237n.32
on personhood, 113–18, 120, 139, 141, 236n.17, 238n.37, 240n.38
on public morality, 113–18, 121, 123, 141
on public reason, 117, 141, 242n.4
on reasonable agents vs. rational agents, 116–17
Theory of Justice vs. *Political Liberalism*, 113–14, 116–17
Raz, Joseph, 215n.37
Reading Engelhardt, 218nn.25, 31
religion, 24, 34, 150–52, 245n.24, 246n.38, 255n.6
Remaking Eden, 6, 76
reproductive choice, 170–71, 250n.27
  as enhanced/influenced by genetic research, 2, 52, 64, 68, 74–75, 77–79, 94, 206, 224n.5, 231n.21
  prevention of disabilities as issue of, 8–9, 21, 25, 38
  as private, 35–36, 39–40, 47, 52, 75–78, 85, 227n.31
  responsibility for, 14, 77–81, 85–86, 90–91, 92, 94, 106, 206, 233n.12, 238n.36, 248n.7
  restrictions on, 15, 41, 47–50, 64–65, 84–102, 221n.3, 224n.25, 225n.7, 231n.25
  See also freedom, individual; prevention of disabilities; responsibility, individual
responsibility, individual, 7, 151
  vs. institutional responsibility, 140–42, 146, 153–55
  for reproductive choice, 14, 77–81, 85–86, 90–91, 92, 94, 106, 206, 233n.12, 238n.36, 248n.7
  for responses to disabilities, 185–87
  See also freedom, individual; prevention of disabilities; responsibility, moral
responsibility, institutional, 123, 140–42, 146, 153–55

responsibility, moral, 139–50, 245n.32
  Bauman on, 140, 141–42, 245n.32
  to care for disabled people, 16–18, 121, 123–38, 139–42, 153–55
  Løgstrup on, 141–48, 149, 150–51, 154–55, 245n.24, 246n.35, 250n.27
  See also responsibility, individual
retinitis pigmentosa, 225n.13
Ricoeur, Paul, 244n.22
Robinson, J. A., 224n.25, 234n.19
Roe v. Wade, 221n.8, 234n.19
Rorty, Richard, 198, 256n.12
Rosenberg, Alexander, 210n.7
rubella, 44

Santurri, Edmund N., 105
Sarason, Seymour B., 232n.27
schizophrenia, 54
Scorgie, Kathryn I., 183–89, 190–91, 204, 247n.1, 253nn.14, 15, 18, 23
self-determination. *See* autonomy
self-esteem, 66–67, 74, 93, 136, 229n.10
Sharpe, David J., 233n.3
Sherwin, Susan, 213n.27
Should the Baby Live?, 240n.3
Shuster, Evelyn, 37
Sigerest, Henry, 223n.18
Silver, Lee M., 6, 76–77, 84
Silvers, Anita, 210n.7
Singer, Peter, 123, 240n.3, 241n.9
smoking, 67, 101
Sobsey, Dick, 51, 175, 190, 253n.23, 254n.27
spina bifida, 73–74, 99, 163, 225n.13
state, democratic, 238n.37
  and abortion laws, 41
  interventions of, 15, 22, 23–24, 47–50, 65, 72, 76, 79, 82–83, 84–102, 91, 106, 216n.10, 224n.25, 231n.24, 232n.28
  See also public morality; public policy
Stoker, W., 255nn.1, 6
suffering, 1, 12, 110, 152, 201, 212n.25, 248n.11, 251n.29
  of disabled children, 7–9, 44–46, 51, 52–55, 75, 92, 100, 126, 127, 160,

suffering (*cont.*)
   161–62, 173–74, 176–77, 205, 234n.18,
   249n.14
  Hauerwas on, 164–66, 172–73, 248n.13,
   251n.29
  McKenny on, 159, 248n.13, 250n.27,
   251n.32
  of parents of disabled children, 159–60,
   166, 169–70, 249n.14
  and personal identity, 165–66,
   172–73
  types of, 164–66, 172–73, 248n.13
Sydenham, Thomas, 223n.18

Tay Sachs syndrome, 99, 225n.13, 231n.22,
   235nn.23, 24
Theory of Justice, A, 107, 113–18. *See also*
  Rawls, John
tobacco companies, 67–68
treatment decisions, 5
trust, 142–43, 144, 243nn.7, 12

Uncommon Fathers, 189–90
"Unsanctifying Human Life," 240n.3

utilitarianism, 109–10, 123–24, 141, 153, 154,
   167, 241n.9, 242n.5, 243n.11, 246n.37,
   249n.19, 250n.23

Van Asperen, Gertrude M., 256n.17
Van Kooten Niekerk, Kees, 243n.6, 244n.17,
   246n.38
Veatch, Robert M., 213n.29
Verwey, Marcel, 221nn.5, 6

Walzer, Michael, 215n.37
Warnock, Mary, 7–8, 12
Watson, James, 212n.19
welfare programs, 5, 76, 79, 81, 86, 94, 119,
   146, 231n.25
Wertz, Dorothy C., 225n.7, 247n.4
West, Richard, 224n.1
White, Stephen, 105
Wikler, Daniel, 1, 233n.12
Wolf, Susan, 193
Wolterstorff, Nicholas, 214n.36, 232n.28
World Health Organization, 3, 42
Wuthnow, Robert, 247n.5

Young, Neil, 175